AF817008

RESEARCH FOR THE RADIATION THERAPIST

From Question to Culture

RESEARCH FOR THE RADIATION THERAPIST

From Question to Culture

Edited by

Caitlin Gillan MRT(T) BSc MEd FCAMRT

Radiation Therapist, Radiation Medicine Program,
Princess Margaret Cancer Centre, Toronto, Canada
Assistant Professor, Department of Radiation Oncology,
University of Toronto, Toronto, Canada

Lisa Di Prospero MRT(T) BSc MSc

Manager, Research and Education, Radiation Therapy,
Odette Cancer Centre, Sunnybrook Health Sciences Centre,
Toronto, Canada
Assistant Professor, Department of Radiation Oncology,
University of Toronto, Toronto, Canada

Nicole Harnett MRT(T) ACT BSc MEd

Director, Graduate Programs, Medical Radiation Sciences Program
and Assistant Professor, Department of Radiation Oncology,
University of Toronto, Toronto, Canada

Lori Holden MRT(T) BSc CCRP

Clinical Specialist Radiation Therapist and Vice Chair,
Rapid Response Radiotherapy Program and Bone Metastases Clinic,
Odette Cancer Centre, Sunnybrook Health Sciences Centre, Toronto, Canada
Assistant Professor, Department of Radiation Oncology,
University of Toronto, Toronto, Canada

Apple Academic Press

TORONTO NEW JERSEY

Apple Academic Press Inc.
3333 Mistwell Crescent
Oakville, ON L6L 0A2
Canada

Apple Academic Press Inc.
9 Spinnaker Way
Waretown, NJ 08758
USA

©2014 by Apple Academic Press, Inc.
Exclusive worldwide distribution by CRC Press, a member of Taylor & Francis Group

Cover photos provided by Dawn Danko, Michelle Lau, and Brian Liszewski.

No claim to original U.S. Government works

International Standard Book Number-13: 978-1-926895-98-7 (Hardcover)

This book contains information obtained from authentic and highly regarded sources. Reprinted material is quoted with permission and sources are indicated. Copyright for individual articles remains with the authors as indicated. A wide variety of references are listed. Reasonable efforts have been made to publish reliable data and information, but the authors, editors, and the publisher cannot assume responsibility for the validity of all materials or the consequences of their use. The authors, editors, and the publisher have attempted to trace the copyright holders of all material reproduced in this publication and apologize to copyright holders if permission to publish in this form has not been obtained. If any copyright material has not been acknowledged, please write and let us know so we may rectify in any future reprint.

Trademark Notice: Registered trademark of products or corporate names are used only for explanation and identification without intent to infringe.

Library of Congress Control Number: 2013956385

Library and Archives Canada Cataloguing in Publication

Research for the radiation therapist: from question to culture/edited by Caitlin Gillan MRT(T) BSc MEd FCAMRT, Radiation Therapist, Radiation Medicine Program, Princess Margaret Cancer Centre, Toronto, Canada, Assistant Professor, Department of Radiation Oncology, University of Toronto, Toronto, Canada, Lisa Di Prospero MRT(T) BSc MSc, Manager, Research and Education, Radiation Therapy, Odette Cancer Centre, Toronto, Canada, Assistant Professor, Department of Radiation Oncology, University of Toronto, Toronto, Canada, Nicole Harnett MRT(T) ACT BSc MEd, Director, Graduate Programs, Medical Radiation Sciences Program, and Assistant Professor, Department of Radiation Oncology, University of Toronto, Toronto, Canada, Lori Holden MRT(T) BSc CCRP, Clinical Specialist Radiation Therapist and Vice Chair, Rapid Response Radiotherapy Program and Bone Metastases Clinic, Odette Cancer Centre, Sunnybrook Health Sciences Centre, Toronto, Canada, Assistant Professor, Department of Radiation Oncology, University of Toronto, Toronto, Canada.

Includes bibliographical references and index.
ISBN 978-1-926895-98-7 (bound)

1. Radiotherapy--Research--Canada. 2. Radiotherapy--Canada--Methodology. I. Gillan, Caitlin, author, editor of compilation II. Di Prospero, Lisa, author, editor of compilation III. Harnett, Nicole, author, editor of compilation IV. Holden, Lori (Radiation therapist). author, editor of compilation

RM849.R48 2014 615.8'42072 C2013-908083-X

Apple Academic Press also publishes its books in a variety of electronic formats. Some content that appears in print may not be available in electronic format. For information about Apple Academic Press products, visit our website at **www.appleacademicpress.com** and the CRC Press website at **www.crcpress.com**

ABOUT THE EDITORS

Caitlin Gillan

Caitlin has been a radiation therapist at the Princess Margaret Cancer Centre since 2008, and she is an assistant professor in the Department of Radiation Oncology at the University of Toronto. She graduated from the joint degree and diploma program in Medical Radiation Sciences offered by the Michener Institute for Applied Health Sciences and the University of Toronto in 2007, and completed her Master of Education in 2009. She served on the Canadian Association of Medical Radiation Technologists (CAMRT) Board of Directors from 2009 to 2011, representing those early in their careers. She was also the Student Lead for the ISRRT World Congress and CAMRT Annual General Conference in Toronto in 2012. In June 2013, Caitlin was awarded her Fellowship of the CAMRT (FCAMRT) in St. John's, Newfoundland.

Currently, while practicing as a clinical radiation therapist, Caitlin is the Project Manager for the Accelerated Education Program at the Princess Margaret Cancer Centre. She is also the Associate Director of Curriculum for the Masters in Health Science in Medical Radiation Sciences (MHSc-MRS) program for radiation therapists at the University of Toronto. Her research interests include interprofessional education and practice in light of changing technologies.

Lisa Di Prospero

Lisa is currently the Manager of Education and Research for Radiation Therapy at the Odette Cancer Centre at Sunnybrook Health Sciences Centre and an assistant professor in the Department of Radiation Oncology at the University of Toronto. She received her undergraduate and graduate degree in biology at McMaster University under the supervision of Dr. Andrew Rainbow and graduated from the Toronto-Sunnybrook School of Radiation Therapy in 1996. Throughout her professional career, Lisa has held several appointments in both research and education. Previous to her current appointment, she was a professor in the undergraduate Medical Radiation Sciences program at the Michener Institute for Applied Health Sciences and The University of Toronto. She continues to teach at both the undergraduate and graduate levels. Lisa has authored and coauthored numerous articles and continues to mentor and coach both intra- and inter-professional colleagues. Lisa has been named the Editor-in-Chief of the *Journal of Medical Imaging and Radiation Sciences* (JMIRS), an international, peer-reviewed journal. Her leadership style is transformative, and she leads by the question of "why not?" Her academic, clinical and research interests include interprofessional education and curriculum development, clinical teaching models and creating a research culture for radiation therapists. Lisa currently serves on committees for both the College of Medical Radiation Technologists of Ontario (CMRTO) and the Canadian Association of Medical Radiation Technologists (CAMRT).

Nicole Harnett

Nicole is currently the Director of the Radiation Skills Lab at the Princess Margaret Cancer Centre, the Director of the Medical Radiation Sciences Graduate Program and assistant professor in the Department of Radiation Oncology at the University of Toronto. Nicole became a certified radiation therapist in 1984 and completed her advanced certification in 1990. After completing her Bachelor of Science degree in 1994, she went on to complete a master's degree in Health Professional Education at the University of Toronto in 2003.

She has been involved in education for many years beginning as a radiation therapy clinical instructor and coordinator in Thunder Bay. Over the years, she has participated heavily in the evolution of radiation therapy education including the development of the joint BSc and diploma program offered by the University of Toronto and the Michener Institute for Applied Health Sciences. Nicole coordinated the program upon implementation and eventually served as Dean of Diagnostic Imaging and Therapy at the Michener Institute. Nicole co-led the development of a professional master's program for radiation therapists, which began in 2009, at the University of Toronto—the first of its kind in North America. Nicole also leads the continuing medical educational initiatives within the Accelerated Education Program, including the Image-Guided Radiation Therapy and the Quality and Safety in Radiation Therapy Education Courses, at the Princess Margaret Cancer Centre.

Nicole has been the Principal Investigator for the Clinical Specialist Radiation Therapist Project in Ontario since 2004, a project funded by the provincial Ministry of Health and Long-Term Care, investigating the potential impact of advanced radiotherapy practice on the radiation medicine enterprise.

Lori Holden

Currently, Lori is the Clinical Specialist Radiation Therapist in the Palliative Site at the Odette Cancer Centre at Sunnybrook Health Sciences Centre, and an assistant professor in the Department of Radiation Oncology, at the University of Toronto. In 1998, she graduated from the Hamilton Regional Cancer Centre (Juravinski Cancer Centre), and in 1999, she transferred and began her employment at the Odette Cancer Centre (OCC) at Sunnybrook Health Sciences Centre, in Toronto. During her time at OCC, Lori has been responsible for the development and integration of a variety of new roles within the department such as the Palliative Radiation Therapist and the designated Research Radiation Therapist roles. In 2005, Lori was one of the initial select investigators for the Clinical Specialist Radiation Therapist project. Lori is an Associate Faculty Member, Institute of Medical Sciences, at the University of Toronto, and holds a certification as a Certified Clinical Research Professional (CCRP) from the Society of Clinical Research Associates. In 2010, Lori was the recipient of the prestigious Schulich Award for Nursing and Clinical Excellence—one of only ten awarded annually. Currently, she is the Vice Chair of the Rapid Response Radiotherapy Program/Bone Metastases Site Group at OCC.

CONTENTS

LIST OF CONTRIBUTORS

Kate Bak MSc
Policy Research Analyst, Radiation Treatment Program, Cancer Care Ontario, Toronto, Canada

Ruth Barker MRT(T) BSc MEd
Instructor, Department of Radiation Oncology, University of Toronto, Toronto, Canada

Amanda Bolderston RTT MSc FCAMRT
Provincial Professional Practice and Academic Leader, British Columbia Cancer Agency, Fraser Valley Cancer Centre, Surrey, Canada

Bonnie Bristow MRT(T) BSc
Research Radiation Therapist, Odette Cancer Centre, Sunnybrook Health Sciences Centre, Toronto, Canada

Laura D'Alimonte MRT(T) BSc MHSc
Clinical Specialist Radiation Therapist, Odette Cancer Centre, Sunnybrook Health Sciences Centre, Toronto, Canada
Lecturer, Department of Radiation Oncology, University of Toronto, Toronto, Canada

Carol-Anne Davis RTT ACT MSc
Clinical Educator, Radiation Therapy Services, Nova Scotia Cancer Centre, Queen Elizabeth II Health Sciences Centre, Halifax, Canada

Colleen Dickie MRT(T) MRT(MR) MSc
Radiation Therapist, Radiation Medicine Program, Princess Margaret Cancer Centre, Toronto, Canada
Assistant Professor, Department of Radiation Oncology, University of Toronto, Toronto, Canada

Lisa Di Prospero MRT(T) BSc MSc
Manager, Research and Education, Radiation Therapy, Odette Cancer Center, Toronto, Canada
Assistant Professor, Department of Radiation Oncology, University of Toronto, Toronto, Canada

Craig Elith RTT BMRS(RT) BSc
Radiation Therapist, Fraser Valley Centre, British Columbia Cancer Agency, Surrey, Canada

John French RTT MSc FCAMRT CHE
Senior Director, Operations, Business and Strategic Planning, Radiation Therapy, Vancouver Centre, British Columbia Cancer Agency, Vancouver, Canada

Caitlin Gillan MRT(T) BSc MEd FCAMRT
Radiation Therapist, Radiation Medicine Program, Princess Margaret Cancer Centre, Toronto, Canada
Assistant Professor, Department of Radiation Oncology, University of Toronto, Toronto, Canada

Eric Gutierrez MRT(T) BSc CMD
Program Manager, Radiation Treatment Program, Cancer Care Ontario, Toronto, Canada

Nicole Harnett MRT(T) ACT BSc MEd
Director, Graduate Programs, Medical Radiation Sciences Program and Assistant Professor, Department of Radiation Oncology, University of Toronto, Toronto, Canada

Lori Holden MRT(T) BSc CCRP
Clinical Specialist Radiation Therapist and Vice Chair, Rapid Response Radiotherapy Program/Bone Metastases Clinic, Odette Cancer Centre, Sunnybrook Health Sciences Centre, Toronto, Canada
Assistant Professor, Department of Radiation Oncology, University of Toronto, Toronto, Canada

Shao Hui (Sophie) Huang MRT(T) MSc
Radiation Therapist, Radiation Medicine Program, Princess Margaret Cancer Centre, Toronto, Canada
Assistant Professor, Department of Radiation Oncology, University of Toronto, Toronto, Canada

Jaclyn Jacques MRT(T) BSc
Radiation Therapist, Windsor Regional Cancer Centre, Windsor, Canada

Katherine Jensen MRT(T) ACT BA
Clinical Instructor, Alberta School of Radiation Therapy, Tom Baker Cancer Centre, Calgary, Canada

Brian Liszewski MRT(T) BSc
Quality Assurance Coordinator, Odette Cancer Centre, Sunnybrook Health Sciences Centre, Toronto, Canada
Research Affiliate, Canadian Partnership for Quality Radiotherapy

Rosanna Macri MRT(T) BSc MHSc
Ethicist, Ontario Shores Centre for Mental Health Sciences, Whitby, Canada
Lecturer, Department of Radiation Oncology, University of Toronto, Toronto, Canada

Gunita Mitera MRT(T) BSc MBA PhD(c)
Quality Initiatives Specialist, Canadian Partnership Against Cancer, Toronto, Canada

Elizabeth Murray MA
Project Coordinator, Radiation Treatment Program, Cancer Care Ontario, Toronto, Canada

Cathryne Palmer MRT(T) MSc
Director, Medical Radiation Sciences Program and Assistant Professor, Department of Radiation Oncology, Unversity of Toronto, Toronto, Canada

Amy Parent MRT(T) BSc CMD
Radiation Therapist, Radiation Medicine Program, Princess Margaret Cancer Centre, Toronto, Canada

Tracey Rose RTT MSc
Radiation Therapist, Sindi Aluwahlia Hawkins Cancer Centre for the Southern Interior, British Columbia Cancer Agency, Kelowna, Canada

Emily Sinclair MRT(T) BSc MSc(c)
Clinical Specialist Radiation Therapist, Odette Cancer Centre, Sunnybrook Health Sciences Centre, Toronto, Canada
Lecturer, Department of Radiation Oncology, University of Toronto, Toronto, Canada

Michael Velec MRT(T) BSc PhD(c)
Radiation Therapist, Radiation Medicine Program, Princess Margaret Cancer Centre, Toronto, Canada

CASE STUDIES

Susan Awrey RN BScN
Paediatric Radiation Nurse Coordinator Princess Margaret Cancer Centre/The Hospital for Sick Children, Toronto, Canada

Susan Barker BA MISt
Digital Services and Reference Librarian, Faculty of Law, Bora Laskin Law Library, University of Toronto, Toronto, Canada
Adjunct Instructor, Faculty of Information (iSchool), University of Toronto, Toronto, Canada

Angela Cashell MRT(T) MSc
Clinical Educator, Radiation Medicine Program, Princess Margaret Cancer Centre, Toronto, Canada
Lecturer, Department of Radiation Oncology, University of Toronto, Toronto, Canada

Kitty Chan MRT(T) BSc MHSc
Clinical Specialist Radiation Therapist, Radiation Medicine Program, Princess Margaret Cancer Centre, Toronto, Canada

Rachel Harris MSc PgD PgCCE DCR(T) D Clin Res
Professional Officer for Research, Society and College of Radiographers, London, United Kingdom

Jane Higgins MRT(T) BSc CIA
Radiation Therapist, Radiation Medicine Program, Princess Margaret Cancer Centre, Toronto, Canada
Instructor, Department of Radiation Oncology, University of Toronto, Toronto, Canada

Tracey Hill MRT(T) BSc MEd
Radiation Therapist, Regional Cancer Care and Interprofessional Educator, Thunder Bay Regional Health Sciences Centre, Thunder Bay, Canada

Grace Lee MRT(T) BSc MHSc
Clinical Specialist Radiation Therapist, Radiation Medicine Program, Princess Margaret Cancer Centre, Toronto, Canada

Winnie Li MRT(T) BSc MSc(c)
Radiation Therapist, Radiation Medicine Program, Princess Margaret Cancer Centre, Toronto, Canada
Lecturer, Department of Radiation Oncology, University of Toronto, Toronto, Canada

Cheryl McGregor RTT ACT CTIC
Resource Therapist – Planning Module, Abbotsford Cancer Centre, British Columbia Cancer Agency, Abbotsford, Canada

Kathryn Moran RTT BSc CTIC
Radiation Therapist, Radiation Therapy Services, Nova Scotia Cancer Centre, Queen Elizabeth II Health Sciences Centre, Halifax, Canada

Tony Panzarella MSc PStat
Manager, Biostatistics Department, Princess Margaret Cancer Centre, Toronto, Canada

Sheila M. Robson MRT(T) ACT BSc
Manager and Head, Radiation Therapy Department, Odette Cancer Centre Sunnybrook Health Sciences Centre, Toronto Canada

Chelsea Soga RTT BSc MA(c)
Radiation Therapist, Prince Edward Island Cancer Treatment Centre, Queen Elizabeth Hospital, Charlottetown, Canada

Kristy M. Stanley RTT BSc BHSc
Radiation Therapy Graduate, Saint John Regional Hospital/University of New Brunswick – Saint John, School of Radiation Therapy Atlantic Health Sciences Corporation, Saint John, Canada

Angela Turner MRT(T) BA MHSc
Radiation Therapist, Odette Cancer Centre, Sunnybrook Health Sciences Centre, Toronto, Canada

REVIEWERS

Floortje Brus BSc
Radiation Therapy Student, Medical Radiation Sciences Program, the Michener Institute for Applied Health Sciences/University of Toronto, Toronto, Canada

Angela Cashell MRT(T) MSc
Clinical Educator, Radiation Medicine Program, Princess Margaret Cancer Centre, Toronto, Canada
Lecturer, Department of Radiation Oncology, University of Toronto, Toronto, Canada

Fiona Cherryman MRT(T) BSc MEd
Senior Chair, The Michener Institute for Applied Health Sciences, Toronto, Canada

Lorraine Clark RTT ACT BSc MEd
Program Head, British Columbia Institute of Technology, Burnaby, Canada

Dawn Danko MRT(T) MSc
Professor, Mohawk-McMaster Medical Radiation Sciences Program, Hamilton, Canada

Krista Dawdy MRT(T) BSc
Radiation Therapist and Clinical Educator, Odette Cancer Centre, Sunnybrook Health Sciences Centre, Toronto, Canada

Cynthia Eccles RTT RTMR BSc DPhil(c)
Research Radiographer, Gray Institute for Radiation Oncology and Biology, University of Oxford, Oxford, United Kingdom

Susan Fawcett MRT(T) BSc MA
Provincial Professional Practice and Academic Leader and Director, Alberta School of Radiation Therapy, Edmonton, Canada

Heather Fineberg MRT(T) BMRSc
Radiation Therapist, Carlo Fidani Peel Regional Cancer Centre, Mississauga, Canada

Rachel Harris MSc PgD PgCCE DCR(T) D Clin Res
Professional Officer for Research, Society and College of Radiographers, London, United Kingdom

Jane Higgins MRT(T) BSc CIA
Radiation Therapist, Radiation Medicine Program, Princess Margaret Cancer Centre, Toronto, Canada
Instructor, Department of Radiation Oncology, University of Toronto, Toronto, Canada

Bronwyn Hilder MRT(T) Dip App Sc (Ther Rad) BSc M Health Science M Health Man
Fellow of the Australian Institute of Radiography
Deputy Chief Radiation Therapist, Department of Radiation Oncology, Royal Hobart Hospital, Hobart, Australia

Tracey Hill MRT(T) BSc MEd
Radiation Therapist, Regional Cancer Care and Interprofessional Educator, Thunder Bay Regional Health Sciences Centre, Thunder Bay, Canada

Tessa Larsen MRT(T) BSc
Radiation Informatics System Specialist/Supervisor, Carlo Fidani Peel Regional Cancer Centre, Mississauga, Canada

Del Leibel RTT ACT BSc CTIC
Radiation Therapy Clinical Educator, Abbotsford Centre, British Columbia Cancer Agency, Abbotsford, Canada

Merrylee McGuffin MRT(T) MSc
Research Radiation Therapist, Odette Cancer Centre, Sunnybrook Health Sciences Centre, Toronto, Canada

Lyn Paddon MRT(T) ACT BSc MA(Ed)
Program Coordinator and Professor, Mohawk-McMaster Medical Radiation Sciences Program, Hamilton, Canada

Chelsea Soga RTT BSc MA(c)
Radiation Therapist, Prince Edward Island Cancer Treatment Centre, Queen Elizabeth Hospital, Charlottetown, Canada

Jill Sutherland RTT BSc MHS
Radiation Therapy Coordinator (Educational Programming), CancerCare Manitoba, Winnipeg, Canada

Kieng Tan MRT(T) BSc MEd
Academic Coordinator, Medical Radiation Sciences Program and Lecturer, Department of Radiation Oncology, University of Toronto, Toronto, Canada

Megan Trad RTT MSRS PhD
Assistant Professor, Texas State University, San Marcos, United States

Mona Udowicz MRT(T) MA
Director or Radiation Therapy, Community Oncology, Alberta Health Services, Calgary, Canada

Chris Zeller RTT ACT BEd MA
Radiation Therapy Manager, Education Services, CancerCare Manitoba, Winnipeg, Canada

LIST OF ABBREVIATIONS

AEC	Atomic Energy Commission
ANOVA	analysis of variance
ASCO	American Society of Clinical Oncology
ASRT	American Society of Radiologic Technologists
ASTRO	American Society for Radiation Oncology
CAMRT	Canadian Association of Medical Radiation Technologists
CARO	Canadian Association of Radiation Oncology
CBCT	cone-beam computed tomography
CEA	cost effectiveness analysis
CIHR	Canadian Institutes of Health Research
CMRTO	College of Medical Radiation Technologists of Ontario
COI	conflict of interest
CPQR	Canadian Partnership for Quality Radiotherapy
CRT	conformal radiation therapy
CTA	clinical trials application
CV	curriculum vitae
EBM	evidence-based medicine
FDR	Food and Drug Regulations
GCP	Good Clinical Practice
ICH	International Conference on Harmonization
HRQoL	health-related quality of life
HSR	health services research
IGRT	image-guided radiation therapy
IMRT	intensity-modulated radiation therapy
IP	intellectual property
JMIRS	Journal of Medical Imaging and Radiation Sciences
KT	knowledge translation
LYG	life years gained
MeSH	Medical Subject Headings

MRT(T)	Medical Radiation Technologist (Therapy)—abbreviation used for radiation therapists in regulated provinces (e.g., Ontario, Alberta)
NIH	National Institute of Health
NSERC	Natural Sciences and Engineering Research Council of Canada
NSCLC	non-small cell lung cancer
PDSA	plan, do, study (check), act
PI	principal investigator
PICO	population, intervention, comparison, outcome
QI	quality improvement
RCT	randomized control trial
REB	research ethics board
RTT	Radiation Therapist (Canadian abbreviation for those certified by the Canadian Association of Medical Radiation Technologists)
SBRT	stereotactic body radiation therapy
SoCRA	Society of Clinical Research Associates
SOP	standard operating procedures
SSHRC	Social Sciences and Humanities Research Council of Canada
TCPS/TCPS-2	Canada's Tri-Council Policy Statement
TQM	total quality management
VMAT	volumetric arc radiation therapy

FOREWORD

Radiation therapy has been the cornerstone of curative and palliative treatment for millions of cancer patients since its application to medicine in the early 1900s. Cancer treatment advances over the last century have resulted in steadily improving cure rates, but often at an unforeseen cost in late toxicity. Technological and biological advances hold much promise for improving the therapeutic ratio, but there is much to be done to harness this potential and bring it to the care team and to the patient. Radiation therapists are in a position to make unique contributions to the science of radiation medicine, working professionally at the interface of radiation oncologists and medical physicists, and daily at the interface of technology and the patient. This contribution can be elevated beyond competent patient care by personally embracing the notion of scholarship in day-to-day practice. This means learning to move beyond the "tell me what should I do" to the more difficult "why are we doing this?" and "could we be doing it better?" This contribution is further elevated through programmatic changes that acknowledge the need, and provide time and support, for the academic contributions of radiation therapy to the radiation medicine research teams. The leadership and vision of radiation therapists who have obtained advanced training in research and scholarship are the key to this evolution.

At the University of Toronto, we recognized in the late 1990s that this would be a long road but we have made steady progress. Firstly, with the opening of a BSc program (in collaboration with the Michener Institute) that provided an introduction to research and opportunities to undertake research. Secondly, with the opening of a radiation oncology research MSc and PhD stream in the Institute of Medical Science, open to all three radiation medicine disciplines. Thirdly, with the opening of a professional graduate degree in radiation therapy, the MHSc in Medical Radiation Sciences, to support the development of teaching, research, and advanced clinical care.

If radiation therapy is to take its rightful place academically in interprofessional radiation medicine teams, we need to see the profession build on a strong culture of clinical excellence and embrace the culture of research and scholarship. There is much to be done on many fronts, personally, at the hospital and university levels and within the professional organizations. The editors of this book are to be congratulated for their vision and leadership in putting this resource together, the first of its kind for radiation therapists by radiation therapists. It says a lot about how far the profession has come, and speaks volumes about the great things to expect in the future.

Pamela Catton MD MPHE FRCPC
Radiation Oncologist, Radiation Medicine Program,
Princess Margaret Cancer Centre, Toronto, Canada
Professor and Vice Chair, Department of Radiation Oncology,
University of Toronto, Toronto, Canada

September, 2013

PREFACE

This book represents a compilation of research expertise among Canadian radiation therapists (RTTs), and a collaboration of those at the helm of the evolution of the profession in this country. The content addresses a wide range of topics, from the principles of evidence-based practice to the process and dissemination of research to unique considerations such as clinical trials, patenting, and health services research. The case for evidence-based practice and a collaborative research culture is made, and the research process is presented in a practical and accessible manner by way of the scientific method. One of the more unique aspects of the scope of this project is the inclusion of chapters relating to the dissemination of knowledge, manuscript publication, and how to build an academic research program. As a whole, the book focuses on introducing RTTs to foundational principles, methodology, and terminology, and will highlight case studies of RTT research or experience to provide contextual examples and inspiration—RTTs around the country are successfully navigating the research world, contributing to their professional body of knowledge, and changing practice.

The book can be read cover-to-cover by students or novice researchers, to provide the foundational knowledge necessary to embark on a research journey for the first time. It can also be consulted as needed by more seasoned researchers looking for guidance in employing an unfamiliar methodology or approach to data analysis. Chapters focusing on research culture can be of benefit to administrators hoping to build a framework for supporting engaged RTTs in their departments.

There has been a noticeable shift from having other groups define the knowledge that guides radiation therapy practice to having the profession itself begin to drive and generate new therapy knowledge, truly defining radiation therapy as a profession in its own right. Our practice environment is unique, and requires unique considerations and approaches to research. It is hoped that this book will fill the identified need for a radiation therapy specific resource and serve as a valuable tool for those wishing to contribute to the growing wealth of radiation therapy research.

Caitlin Gillan MRT(T) BSc MEd FCAMRT
Lisa Di Prospero MRT(T) BSc MSc
Nicole Harnett MRT(T) ACT BSc MEd and
Lori Holden MRT(T), BSc CCRP

ACKNOWLEDGEMENTS

This project capitalized on a trait common among radiation therapists (RTTs)—collaboration. The combined expertise, time, and effort put forth by the authors who wrote the chapters and contributed their insight to the case examples, the reviewers who provided constructive feedback and perspective, and others who offered their administrative and motivational support, were invaluable to the realization of this project.

It goes without saying that those who were approached to author chapters for this book were people already juggling a demanding workload, and yet they realized the value of the initiative to their peers, their students, and even to themselves, and found the time to make it happen. Whether they tackled a chapter on their own or engaged a colleague to pool expertise or to provide a mentorship opportunity, the end result is an incredible mosaic of the knowledge base that has been built around this country relating to radiation therapy research.

Peer reviewers provided a fresh perspective on chapter drafts, and offered their own insight to ensure a comprehensive picture of the topic at hand. Operating on incredibly tight deadlines, they took drafts with them on summer vacations and made notes in margins and dug up key references to provide guidance and support to the authors. Worthy of a special mention is Floortje Brus, a clinical radiation therapy student in the Medical Radiation Sciences Program at the Michener Institute for Applied Health Sciences and the University of Toronto, who powered her way through the entire book draft and offered her "end-user" perspective on the content. If the book provided her information that proves to be of benefit as she completes a clinical research project, and encourages her to stay involved in research as a practicing RTT, we have all done our jobs!

Another person who does not fit neatly into any of our categories of acknowledgements (she never does!) is Olive Wong. A recent graduate of the same program as Floortje, and a newly minted RTT, Olive may not have known what she agreed to when she took on a job as a summer research assistant at the Princess Margaret Cancer Centre. She jumped wholeheartedly into our book project and spent endless hours organizing, editing, proofreading, referencing, formatting—and chasing—the work produced by the dozens of authors and reviewers. Olive is truly an example of the future breed of RTT, and the editors are looking forward to sitting back and watching her shine!

Finally, we would be remiss if we did not articulate our appreciation for the University of Toronto's Department of Radiation Oncology (UTDRO), and its affiliated clinical sites where we are employed—Caitlin and Nicole at the Princess Margaret Cancer Centre and likewise Lisa and Lori at the Odette Cancer Centre at Sunnybrook Health Sciences Centre. The UTDRO was supportive and encouraging of this book initiative, as it represents the departmental legacy and vision of collaboration and empowerment of RTTs. The majority of the contributors to this project are in some capacity the product of this legacy and vision, and under the guidance of the UTDRO Chair, Fei-Fei Liu, and the Vice-Chair, Education, Pamela Catton, we are confident that we will continue to lead the further evolution of our profession.

INTRODUCTION

"If we knew what it was we were doing, it would not be called research, would it?"

—Albert Einstein

An interesting conversation took place on the Facebook page of the open group "World Wide Radiation Therapist." It started with a post from the United States requesting insight on practices relating to the use of deodorant or alternatives for patients receiving breast radiotherapy. The comments that emerged were supportive and insightful, but varied. Some spoke of "tried and true" alternatives such as natural antiperspirants, corn starch, or avoiding use of anything at all. Others quoted published research that found no impact on skin reaction with the use of regular deodorants or antiperspirants (see McQuestion[1]). This exchange, with contributions from around the world, suggests two things with regards to the state of aspects of practice in radiation therapy. First of all, it demonstrates the emergence of an understanding of the value of professional communities of practice, and secondly a desire on behalf of radiation therapists (RTTs) to gather information to inform clinical decisions and practices. The use of social media as a forum to request insight from others within the profession is not unique to radiation therapy, but is nonetheless reflective of a more inquiry-based culture than has been the norm in the past. This series of Facebook posts also demonstrates that regardless of the desire for information, there is a continued reluctance of many to adopt evidence-based practice. Even when presented with published data that contradicts a long-standing practice, some RTTs would prefer to stick with what they have "always been taught." Thus, while great strides are being made in encouraging RTTs to be aware of and engaged in striving for evidence-based practice, the culture will not evolve overnight and will require continued emphasis, informed champions, and availability of necessary resources.

It is from this desire to provide RTTs the tools to support an evidence-based practice and professional culture that this book project has emerged.

This book is about opportunity—the opportunity for expert RTTs from across the country to come together for a common purpose; the opportunity for members of the profession to contribute a valuable resource to their growing scope of practice; and the opportunity to build research capacity within the profession, by facilitating further growth and evolution in the field.

Be it the development and implementation of a patient satisfaction survey within a single department or a multicentre clinical trial investigating the relative value of a novel radiation therapy fractionation schedule, the research conducted today will form the foundation of future practice. As RTTs work to carve their own niche in the field of radiation medicine, it is important that they build this foundation. As new knowledge is created, it is also imperative that it be appropriately disseminated and subsequently adopted by those at the front lines, to ensure the provision of the most informed and highest quality care for patients. The practical research principles and concepts addressed in this book can serve to provide the tools necessary to create, disseminate, and interpret new knowledge, and to stimulate those in a position to foster and support a research culture.

From a Facebook conversation to a departmental staff meeting to a peer-reviewed publication in the *International Journal of Radiation Oncology, Biology, Physics (IJROBP)*, RTTs are engaging in valuable knowledge exchange and steadily establishing a solid research presence. It is hoped that the insight and knowledge compiled by expert RTT researchers around Canada will help to equip others to begin addressing their own unanswered questions, and further contribute to evidence-based practice.

Caitlin Gillan MRT(T) BSc MEd FCAMRT
Lisa Di Prospero MRT(T) BSc MSc
Nicole Harnett MRT(T) ACT BSc MEd
Lori Holden MRT(T) BSc CCRP
Toronto, September 2013

REFERENCES

1. McQuestion, M., Evidence-Based Skin Care Management in Radiation Therapy: Clinical Update. *Seminars in Oncology Nursing* **2011**, *27(2)*, e1–e17.

PART 1

MAKING A CASE FOR RESEARCH

CHAPTER 1

EVIDENCE-BASED MEDICINE AND THE SCIENTIFIC METHOD

LORI HOLDEN MRT(T) BSc CCRP

Clinical Specialist Radiation Therapist & Vice Chair, Rapid Response Radiotherapy Program/Bone Metastases Clinic, Odette Cancer Centre, Sunnybrook Health Sciences Centre, Toronto Canada
Assistant Professor, Department of Radiation Oncology, University of Toronto, Toronto Canada

CONTENTS

"Why do research?"
"What's in it for me?"
"How does it put me ahead in my career?"
"What is evidence-based medicine?"

These types of questions circle in the heads of many radiation therapists (RTTs) when discussing research. This introductory chapter aims to address these and other fundamental questions about the nature and importance of research.

The need for research-based evidence in radiation therapy practice parallels other healthcare disciplines. In the last 10 years, there has been a proliferation in the number of published articles in the field of radiation medicine. Patients are also able to access a vast array of information from on-line resources. With the combination of an insurmountable volume of literature and new knowledge, and expectations of the patients for the best possible care, RTTs are faced with the continued challenge of remaining current and up-to-date with scientific findings to make informed clinical decisions.

The problem remains, however, that many RTTs have limited spare time to be combing through data and trying to differentiate between a valid paper and one that is perhaps not useful. This is where the evidence-based decision-making process proves crucial.

1.1 EVIDENCE-BASED DECISION-MAKING PROCESS

The concept of evidence-based medicine (EBM) was originated in 19th century France, though it has been championed in some areas for thousands of years, and was not formalized until the evolution of the field of clinical epidemiology.[1] The evidence-based decision-making process (an extension of EBM) is the systematic process that allows for "the conscientious, explicit, and judicious use of current best evidence in making decisions about the care of individual patients.[1]" In the past, judgments and decisions regarding treatment were often based on previous clinical practice, experience, and opinions. However, in this new era, the practice of EBM means "integrating individual clinical expertise with the best available external clinical evidence from systematic research.[1]" EBM seeks to assess the strength of the evidence of risks and benefits of treatments (including lack of treatment) and diagnostic tests, assessing the risk versus benefit to the patient.[2,3] With the huge influx of information and studies, healthcare providers have no choice but to follow the principles of EBM. By relying on and integrating EBM in their clinical practice, it can be ensured that patients are being offered the best and most up-to-date care possible. In the 20 years since the term was coined, the evolution of EBM has really come to the forefront in the radiation medicine disciplines. If one were to do an online search of radiation therapy, a vast abundance of articles would be returned pertaining to all aspects of medical radiation science. As front-line healthcare providers, there is an inherent responsibility to be able to translate new discoveries, treatments, and technologies into value to the patient – in essence, to practice evidence-based medicine. Clinical leaders in large centres can also cull the literature to seek insight to guide practice change. By implementing EBM into their clinical practice, RTTs can:[4]

- remain current with the literature and evidence
- contribute to the creation of systematic reviews
- reduce variability in practice
- close the gap between knowledge and practice
- improve quality of care for patients
- impact cost and cost-effectiveness
- improve patient outcomes

The challenge remains, however, that many are reluctant to enter the world of EBM due to a variety of barriers. On a departmental level, the research culture itself can be a barrier (*see* Chapter 14: Getting Started: Building a Research and Evidence-Based Culture). Reeves identified that the "overall research culture within radiology is low and the same is currently true of radiography.[5]" This can then be extended to the realm of radiation therapy. Fauber further states that "the profession must seek to overcome attitudinal and environmental barriers that inhibit research productivity.[6]" Other obstacles and barriers encountered by other departments and individuals have included a lack of time, lack of funding, inadequate research skills, lack of mentors and lack of authority to change practice.[4,7,8]

There has been a slight paradigm shift in recent years. Centres are now recognizing the value of academic activity, raising the profile of research in their clinical departments, and viewing it as an integral and necessary feature (*see* Chapter 13: Academia and Scholarship).[9] In addition, there is recognition of the large untapped intellectual capital in the RTTs of their departments. In Ontario, a recently created Master of Health Science in Medical Radiation Sciences program was developed to provide and encourage higher learning for those interested, incorporating courses on research and evidence-based medicine in the curriculum. As well, in 2004, in collaboration with Ontario's Ministry of Health and Long Term Care, the Clinical Specialist Radiation Therapist Project began in that province, serving as an exploration of the potential for advanced practice radiation therapy roles. Throughout the subsequent years, with the continued support and approval of the Ministry, these roles have proven to be very useful and beneficial to their respective departments. The roles provide autonomy of practice to the incumbent, as well as the requirement to build strong research and clinical portfolios.[9–10] Many of these individuals are involved in the creation and implementation of new models of care, thus imploring them to be aware of the best evidence available to apply to their clinical practice.

Lack of knowledge of the entire process, though, remains a deterrent encountered by many. "What makes a good question?" "How do I do a literature search? What makes a good article? How do I ensure they are collecting robust data?" It has only been in the last five years or so that research methodology courses have consistently been made an integral component of the medical radiation sciences degree programs. Even so, these are often an elective course and not assigned importance within the overall curriculum. So, not only does the thought of practicing EBM remain daunting to many, so does the thought of actually performing one's own research.[11] However, gaining an understanding of the steps involved in conducting research, known as the scientific method, lends itself to actually practicing EBM. The steps involved in both processes are very similar, and understanding one makes it easier to translate to the other.

1.2 THE SCIENTIFIC METHOD

In order to conduct scientifically sound research, one should follow the steps of the scientific method (research process).[12,13] They are as follows:

1. Define a broad question

2. Search the literature
3. Narrow the question (and often develop a hypothesis)
4. Define the study design
5. Operationalise the outcome measures
6. Conduct the experiment
7. Analyse the data
8. Reach conclusions (and disseminate new knowledge)

HOT TIP

The scientific method is often presented in more fundamental terms, as the question, the hypothesis, the methods, the results, and the conclusion. While these suggest the basic steps in undertaking research, they assume each investigation to be independent of existing knowledge or systems or the need to communicate results and translate findings into practice. Research must instead be seen to be a part of a broader and continuous mechanism of inquiry, investigation, and change in practice, such as with the Deming Cycle (see Chapter 9: Health Services Research and Program Evaluation).

Most of the steps above are covered in great detail throughout the subsequent chapters within this book, and have in fact provided the structure according to which the different chapters are presented. An important exception is the development of a focused and feasible research question. The research question forms the foundation of a successful investigation and warrants further attention here.

1.2.1 DEVELOPMENT OF A RESEARCH QUESTION

All research begins with an idea, and generating a research question related to that idea should be a creative and informed process. The most valuable research questions often emerge from observations made by the researcher in the course of daily practice or activity or by a question or gap in the literature identified by a seasoned consumer of that body of literature. This further suggests the importance of having radiation therapists (RTTs) engage in research, as it is often more likely for an RTT to recognize the potential for a valuable research investigation in his or her own environment than it is for someone else to do so from an outside perspective. A question may be grounded in any number of observations, concerns, or queries, including the following:

- the recognition of a gap or inefficiency in practice
- an observation that is not readily explained by available evidence or knowledge (such as an unusual side effect, an unexplained belief or behaviour amongst a group of patients, a deficiency in the knowledge base of a new cohort of students in the clinical environment)
- uncertainty about the value of a planned or newly implemented technique, curriculum, resource or other program or initiative
- an idea discussed informally amongst staff that could have merit but has never been operationalised
- an emerging concern about the value or appropriateness of a longstanding practice or approach

HOT TIP

FINER Criteria for Developing a Good Research Question:

When developing a research question, it is beneficial to keep the FINER criteria in mind, to maximize the likelihood that the ultimate question and study design will be something that can be realistically pursued and realized.

F – **F**easible

I – **I**nteresting

N – **N**ovel

E – **E**thical

R – **R**elevant

Research initiatives can serve many purposes, and it is important to keep the end goal in mind when developing the question, as this can inform the scope, context, and eventually the methodology used to answer the question. Research can be broadly categorized as either exploratory, descriptive, or explanatory.[14]

Exploratory research: provides initial insight into a topic, to distil the key issues at hand that can guide further research initiatives

Descriptive research: serves to outline a clear picture of a phenomenon, process, or relationship

Explanatory research: builds on descriptive elements to establish the underlying mechanism that can support, contradict, or generate a theory or principle

Once the foundation for a broad research question has been distilled, the researcher can then embark on the subsequent steps in the research process. The nature of the developing question will both inform and be informed by the available information, resources, methodological approaches, and timelines, and will thus likely be reworked and refined many times before being finalized. Case example 1.1 provides an example of the generation of a research question by a clinical RTT student in Saint John, New Brunswick.

CASE EXAMPLE 1.1

Development of a Relevant and Feasible Research Question: a Student's Experience in Saint John

Kristy M. Stanley RTT BSc BHSc
Radiation Therapy Graduate, Saint John Regional Hospital and University of New Brunswick – Saint John, School of Radiation Therapy, Atlantic Health Sciences Corporation, Saint John, Canada

As a radiation therapy student, I was provided with unique insight into the path of a cancer patient's treatment journey. I often found myself able to follow in a patient's footsteps as I gained experience in each area of the radiation therapy department. Early in my time as a student, I began to notice that for some patients, information gaps existed, which led to detrimental consequences like increased anxiety and distress. With these patients, I saw this translate into poor adherence to treatment regimes, physical manifestations of stress, and difficulties with coping – all appearing to decrease quality of life. These observations led me to formulate the question: "Does an educational intervention set forth before a patient begins their treatment journey reduce stress and anxiety to improve self-efficacy, and, most importantly, improve a cancer patient's quality of life?"

As a student, I was given the opportunity to address this question formally through a clinical research project. I felt that to provide the highest level of quality care, preparatory patient education was an area where a resolution is highly worthy of investigation. Due to resource constraints and limited time as a student to conduct my own in-house study, I chose to complete an integrative review to answer my question. Selecting the appropriate methodology was important to ensure that it was feasible and likely to generate useful results. This methodology afforded me the opportunity to find an answer based on up-to-date, high quality, and evidence-based research. I was then able to creatively construct a research agenda for future study from both piecing together strengths and highlights from the studies analyzed and adding my own personal insight.

Preparatory educational interventions are currently not a standard of care in some radiation treatment programs and are an emerging area of research focus. I found that they can provide a novel approach to optimizing the patient's experience within the cancer centre, better humanizing the technology, and reducing anxiety and distress: ultimately leading to an enhanced quality of life.

A strategic and open-minded approach to the generation of a research question may allow the researcher to explore new and different ways of approaching and studying the topic. Cryer suggests the following strategies for generating creative ideas:[15]

- talk things over
- keep an open mind
- view the problem from imaginative perspectives
- view the problem from the perspective of another discipline
- brainstorm

- negative brainstorm (consider the possible ways in which a particular question or research methodology could fail to achieve its purpose, to encourage a proactive approach to mitigating wasted effort)
- concentrate on anomalies and focus on byproducts (be willing to consider the peripheral aspects of a research question that might otherwise be too easily dismissed as irrelevant, but that could form the basis of a valuable question that might never have been addressed)

It is interesting to observe how the steps in the scientific method parallel the EBM process. It is the scientific data that is collected using the scientific method that are collectively analyzed in the following steps, to ascertain the best possible evidence. By following these basic steps, one can successfully appraise and integrate evidence-based medicine.

1.3 THE FIVE STEPS OF EVIDENCE BASED MEDICINE

The literature commonly reports five steps to the EBM process, however some report seven steps, as below, with steps 0 and 7 being extraneous but contributory:[16,17]

STEP 0: FOSTERING A SENSE OF INQUIRY

Do not be afraid to question anything. Without this spirit, the next steps are unlikely to occur.

STEP 1: ASKING AND DEVELOPING A CLINICAL QUESTION

This is a very crucial and fundamental step. It is often time-consuming; however, it is imperative that effort be put into the development of a good clinical question, as it dictates the subsequent design of the trial. When composing the question, one should apply the PICO principles, taking into account:

- **P**opulation being studied: is it a particular group of patients? Students? RTTs?
- **I**ntervention being assessed – what will be done to the population?
- **C**omparison intervention or group – what is the alternative (should be specific and limited)?
- **O**utcome – what will be effected (should be measurable)?

A well-designed question helps drive a successful research endeavour.[4,17]

STEP 2: SEARCHING FOR THE BEST EVIDENCE

By formulating and searching a proper PICO-based question, the search of the literature should provide only relevant articles. Evidence is "the product of well-designed and well-controlled research investigations.[16]" It is the compilation of an argument based on a spectrum of previous findings that constitutes the evidence for a clinical question. There are different sources of evidence and its hierarchical order is based on a study's internal validity (as well as statistical validity, clinical relevance, and peer-reviewed acceptance), the notion of causation and need to control for bias (*see* Chapter 7: Survey Methodologies and Analysis) for more information about validity). Figure 1.1 illustrates the different study designs conducted to answer clinical questions.[17] The top of the pyramid is considered the gold standard, with meta-analyses and systematic reviews representing the highest level of evidence, often hard to refute. Working down through randomized control trials, and finally ending in expert opinion, generally considered the lowest level of evidence and with the greatest chance of bias. Specifics regarding the actual study types listed within the pyramid will be described in greater detail in later chapters, however it is important to understand where each fits in the diagram and how it also relates to strength of evidence.

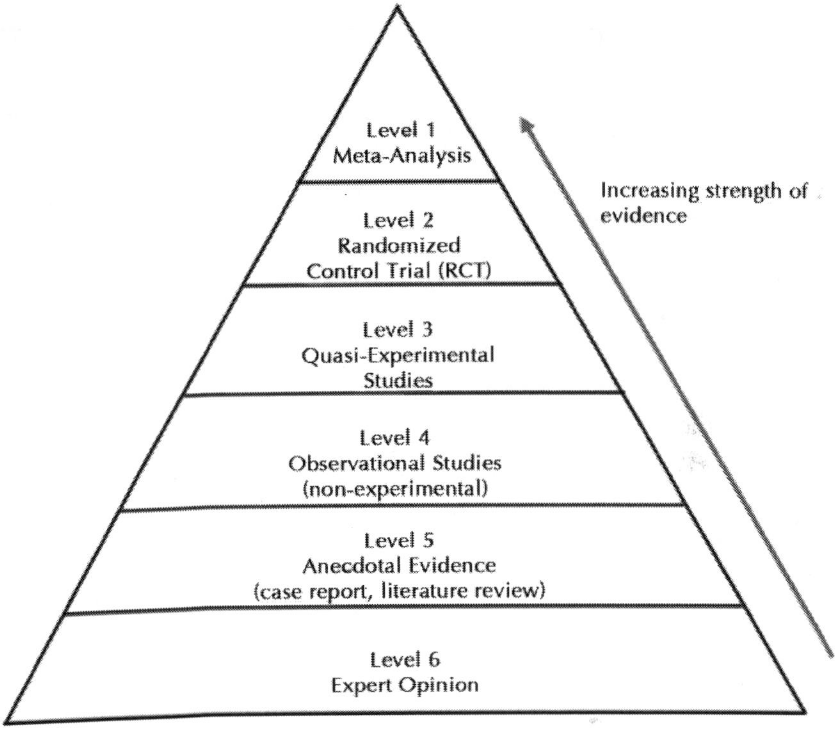

FIGURE 1.1 Levels of Evidence.

Table 1.1 further differentiates between the different levels of evidence, breaking them down with respect to research design.[19]

TABLE 1.1 Definitions of Levels of Evidence.

Level	Category of Evidence
1a	Systematic review with correlation of randomized control trials
1b	Individual randomized control trial with a narrow confidence interval
1c	"All or none"—related outcome

TABLE 1.1 *(Continued)*

Level	Category of Evidence
2	Systematic review with homogeneity of cohort studies
3	Individual cohort study (including low-quality randomized control trials, i.e., <80% follow up)
2c	Outcomes research; ecological studies
3a	Systematic review with homogeneity of case-control studies
3b	Individual case-control study
4	Case series (and poor-quality cohort and case-control studies)
5	Expert opinion without explicit critical appraisal, or based on physiology, bench research or "first principles"
Grades of Recommendation	
A	Consistent level 1 studies
B	Consistent level 2 or 3 studies or extrapolations from level 1 studies
C	Level 4 studies or extrapolations from level 2 or 3 studies
D	Level 5 evidence or troublingly inconsistent or inconclusive studies of any level

STEP 3: CRITICALLY APPRAISING THE EXISTING EVIDENCE

In this step, articles are appraised for their internal and external validity, their impact, reliability and applicability to the clinical question. Often this is an arduous task, but by answering the following three basic questions, the process can be accelerated:[17]

- Are the results of the study valid?
- What are the results and are they important?
- Will the results help me care for my patients?

STEP 4: INTEGRATING THIS NEW EVIDENCE WITH CLINICAL EXPERTISE AND PATIENT PREFERENCES AND VALUES

STEP 5: EVALUATING THE OUTCOMES BASED ON EVIDENCE

STEP 6: DISSEMINATING THE RESULTS

Steps 4–6 above can be considered as one, and there are in fact several different avenues through which EBM can be disseminated and integrated into practice. The development of evidence-based guidelines and care pathways is just one example of the use of systematic evidence-based analysis. Their development is grounded in EBM, relying on a systematic review of all published research studies about that subject, placing stronger emphasis on the randomized controlled trial (RCT). This type of systematic review – a meta-analysis (*see* Chapter 2: Literature Reviews) has become the gold standard, as it is more likely to inform us and less likely to mislead us.[1]

One of the most renowned and respected examples of the systematic review is the Cochrane Collaboration.[20] With more than 50 review groups, it is able to collect and assess the best evidence, categorize the evidence as being either beneficial, harmful or neither, and thus evaluate a particular treatment or intervention. The Cochrane Collaboration, along with other major organizations such as the Centre for Evidence Based Medicine, has adopted the definition and principles of EBM.[20] Cancer Care Ontario, the American Society of Therapeutic Radiation Oncology (ASTRO), the American Society of Clinical Oncology (ASCO) and many other organizations have also adopted and strongly support the concept of EBM. They have each developed a type of quality practice initiative and an extensive set of practice guidelines and expert opinions for an expansive topic list, based on current available scientific evidence. The importance of these guidelines cannot be undervalued, as clinicians often refer to these guidelines as they aid in providing continuity of care, the highest quality of care, and the best outcomes for the patients.

With a brief introduction of the steps involved in the scientific research process, hopefully the curiosity of the reader has been piqued, imploring

RTT researchers to continue to read on and gain further knowledge and insight in each of these concepts. Having confidence in conducting one's own research can lead to improved clinical care, job satisfaction, and improved professional profile, amongst other benefits. Being able to critically evaluate existing and emerging scientific literature is key to this. To systematically synthesize a collection of literature to make up-to-date and relevant decisions regarding a clinical situation is imperative. With the continued ease with which patients are able to obtain information from the Internet and other resources, it is important that healthcare providers be able to sift through and evaluate their usefulness or validity of a given piece of information. Utilizing information contained in this chapter and throughout the rest of this book, it is hoped that the reader gains an understanding that neither process – either evaluating the research or conducting one's own research – should be prohibitively daunting or unmanageable. There are steps that guide both processes.

The concept of evidence-based medicine is not going away. It is here to stay and it is incumbent on RTTs to be able to contribute to or practice with this evolving practice paradigm.

KEYWORDS

- Evidence-based medicine
- Scientific method
- Levels of evidence
- Research question

REFERENCES

1. Sackett, D. L.; Rosenberg, W. M.; Gray, J.; Haynes, R. B.; Richardson, W. S. Evidence based medicine: what it is and what it isn't. *BMJ.* **1996,** *312(7023)*, 71.
2. Elstein, A. On the origins and development of evidence-based medicine and medical decision making. *Inflamm. Res.* **2004,** *53(2)*, S184–S189.

3. Atkins, D.; Eccles, M.; Flottorp, S.; Guyatt, G. H.; Henry, D.; Hill, S.; Liberati, A.; O'Connell, D.; Oxman, A. D.; Phillips, B. Systems for grading the quality of evidence and the strength of recommendations I: critical appraisal of existing approaches The GRADE Working Group. *BMC Health Serv. Res.* **2004**, *4(1)*, 38.
4. Gilbert, R.; Fader, K. Evidence-based decision making as a tool for continuous professional development in the medical radiation technologies. *Can. J. Med. Radiat. Technol.* **2007,** *38(1)*, 39–44.
5. Reeves, P. J. Research in medical imaging and the role of the consultant radiographer: A discussion. Radiography. **2008,** *14*, e61–e64.
6. Fauber, T. L.; Legg, J. S. Perceived research needs and barriers amongst RT educators. Radiologic technology. **2004,** *76(1)*, 19.
7. Russell, W.; McNair, H. A.; Heaton, A.; Ball, K.; Routsis, D.; Love, K.; Miles, E. Gap analysis of role definition and training needs for therapeutic research radiographers in the UK. *Br. J. Radiol.* **2007,** *80(957)*, 693.
8. Halkett, G.; Scutter, S. Research attitudes and experiences of radiation therapists. *The Radiographer*. **2003,** *50(2)*, 69.
9. Bolderston, A.; Harnett, N.; Palmer, C.; Wenz, J.; Catton, P. The scholarly radiation therapist. Part two: developing an academic practice—the Princess Margaret Hospital experience. *J. Radiother. Pract.* **2008,** *7(2)*, 105–111.
10. Harnett, N.; Palmer, C.; Bolderston, A.; Wenz, J.; Catton, P. The scholarly radiation therapist. Part one: charting the territory. *J. Radiother. Pract.* **2008,** *7(2)*, 99–104.
11. McAlister, F. A.; Graham, I.; Karr, G. W.; Laupacis, A. Evidence-Based Medicine and the Practicing Clinician. *J. Gen. Intern. Med.* **1999,** *14(4)*, 236–242.
12. Holden, L.; Stanford, J.; Barker, R. Clinical Research Made Easy—A Guide for Research in Radiation Therapy. *J. Med. Imag. Radiat. Sci.* **2009,** *40(4)*, 160–164;
13. Roxburgh, M. An exploration of factors, which constrain nurses from research participation. *J. Clin. Nurs.* **2006,** *15(5)*, 535–545.
14. Brotherton, B. In: Researching Hospitality and Tourism. Sage Publications: Thousand Oaks, CA, 2008.
15. Cryer, P. In: The Research Student's Guide to Success, 2nd ed.; Open University Press: Buckingham, UK, 2000.
16. Forrest, J. L.; Miller, S. A. Evidence-based decision making in action: Part 1—Finding the best clinical evidence. *J. Contemp. Dent. Pract.* **2002,** *3(3)*, 10–26.
17. Melnyk, B. M.; Fineout-Overholt, E.; Stillwell, S. B.; Williamson, K. M. Evidence-based practice: step by step: the seven steps of evidence-based practice. *Am. J. Nurs.* **2010,** *110(1)*, 51–53.
18. Centre for Evidence-Based Management. What are the levels of evidence? http://www.cebma.org/frequently asked-questions/what-are the-levels-of-evidence/ (accessed August 12, 2013).

19. Oxford Centre for Evidence-based Medicine. Levels of Evidence. http://www.cebm.net/?o=1025 (accessed August 30, 2013).
20. The Cochrane Collaboration. Evidence-based health care and systematic reviews. http://www.cochrane.org/about-us/evidence-based-health-care (accessed August 30, 2013).

CHAPTER 2

LITERATURE REVIEWS

CAITLIN GILLAN MRT(T) BSc MEd FCAMRT

Radiation Therapist, Radiation Medicine Program, Princess Margaret Cancer Centre, Toronto Canada
Assistant Professor, Department of Radiation Oncology, University of Toronto, Toronto Canada

JACLYN JACQUES MRT(T) BSc

Radiation Therapist, Windsor Regional Cancer Centre, Windsor Canada

CONTENTS

As discussed in Chapter 1, a well-conducted literature review can serve as the foundation of a solid research question, provide context in which to interpret the results of a research project, and may even constitute research in itself. Whether approached as a formal and systematic assessment of the state of knowledge on a topic, or an informal perusal of a few key peer-reviewed articles to inform future work, the ability to access and assess relevant and reliable information is critical to the conduct and interpretation of research.

With the advent of the Internet and the resultant phenomenon known as the Information Age, the volume of medical information and literature has grown exponentially over the past few decades. It is more readily available to healthcare professionals, patients, and the general public.[1] Interestingly, the same mechanisms that have facilitated the increase in quantity have necessitated a more critical approach to assessing the quality. It has been said that "finding useful clinical information in the 2000s is like finding a specific grain of sand in a four meter tidal wave as it crashes onto the beach.[2]" A literature review should encompass not only a navigation of the available information, but also the appraisal of the value of the results to current knowledge and future research directions.[3]

A literature review can serve the following purposes:

- assist in developing and refining a research question
- identify whether a research question has been previously posed or answered
- suggest the most appropriate methodology to address a given question
- highlight areas of controversy or continued debate that might require attention through future investigation
- provide insight on limitations in past research that could be avoided moving forward
- contribute to the state of knowledge in a given area through compiling and analyzing multiple sources of data
- inform evidence-based practice (development of standards and practice guidelines)

2.1 TYPES OF LITERATURE REVIEW

Depending on the intended purpose and resources available, a review can be approached in many ways, with varying degrees of rigour and comprehensiveness. Systematic reviews follow the most formal guidelines. Results of a systematic review can be approached and reported qualitatively (narrative synthesis) or quantitatively (meta-analysis).[4–6] Scoping reviews can serve as an exploratory or preliminary approach when feasibility precludes a systematic review or when the intent is solely to identify key concepts or gaps in the state of knowledge on a topic.[6,7] Below is an overview of the various approaches to literature reviews.

2.1.1 SYSTEMATIC LITERATURE REVIEWS

By undertaking a systematic review of the literature, information from a variety of sources can be integrated to determine consistency in findings and generalizability across populations, jurisdictions, settings, and variations in intervention.[8] Synthesizing an otherwise unmanageable amount of data into a summary of the state of knowledge on a topic can inform evidence-based practice and guide further research.[9] As acknowledged by Mulrow in an article on systematic reviews in the *British Medical Journal*, "through critical exploration, evaluation, and synthesis the systematic review separates the insignificant, unsound, or redundant deadwood in the medical literature from the salient and critical studies that are worthy of reflection.[8]"

2.1.2 NARRATIVE SYNTHESIS

The narrative synthesis is primarily a qualitative approach to reporting the results of a systematic review. Traditionally, it would include the categorization of studies into thematic categories according to study design, context, or outcome to guide analysis and interpretation both within and between studies.[6] This can be compared to a formalized and comprehensive literature review, reporting on all published information that fits within a defined scope.

2.1.3 META-ANALYSES

A meta-analysis is a type of systematic review, more specifically a statistical tool used to compile and report results of quantitative studies that address the same research question.[10] It constitutes the highest level of evidence (*see* Chapter 1: Evidence-Based Medicine and the Scientific Method), through a pooling of results to increase statistical power over individual empirical studies.[2,8] Comparative effectiveness reviews (CERs) are meta-analyses that compare healthcare interventions and can thus be undertaken to guide clinical decision making.[11] For example, Warde and Payne conducted a meta-analysis of 11 published randomized trials to determine the relative value of including thoracic irradiation in addition to systemic chemotherapy in the treatment of small-cell lung cancer.[12]

2.1.4 SCOPING REVIEW

A scoping review is an exploratory search, often conducted as a precursor to a full systematic review. It is designed to determine the amount of information available on a topic and the key findings and gaps. While the steps in the process might be the same as in a more rigourous systematic review, the intent is not to be as comprehensive in scope or all encompassing in quantity. In other words, it is an attempt to take the pulse of the literature on a given topic, and can be used to lend insight to research or grant proposals (*see* Chapter 3: Research Proposals), guide novel research, or simply to inform or reinforce practice.[6]

2.2 STEPS IN A LITERATURE REVIEW

The steps in a systematic review are the same steps as those that might be applied to a less formal review of available information, but it is the methodical and comprehensive approach to each step that establishes the systematic review as methodology unto itself.

A literature review can be broken down into seven main steps:[9,13]

1. Define the research question
2. Determine the search strategy
3. Conduct the search
4. Apply inclusion and exclusion criteria
5. Perform data extraction or abstraction
6. Critically appraise and evaluate data
7. Compile results
8. Interpret and report findings

It is important to acknowledge that this process is often an iterative one. Various steps must be revisited as the question and criteria are refined to better address the goal of the review. This might apply most readily to the first three steps in the process. A preliminary question can guide an initial search of the literature, and the results might suggest the need to refine the scope or focus of the question.[9,14] The development of a solid research question has been covered in Chapter 1 (Evidence-Based Medicine and the Scientific Method). The remaining steps in the review process will be addressed here.

2.3 SOURCES

The choice of a search strategy must take into consideration the types and scope of information source to be considered. This, in turn, depends on the information sought. Novel research to guide evidence-based practice might be most readily found in scientific journals, while government reports and white papers might provide standards and benchmarks to inform departmental policies and performance indicators. A given search technique can be used to identify several types of source, but it is important to interpret and employ each appropriately.

2.3.1 PEER-REVIEWED SCIENTIFIC JOURNALS AND TEXTBOOKS

Sources can most broadly be categorized according to whether or not they have undergone peer review. Peer review is the independent evaluation of work prior to publication.[14–15] A "peer" is often a volunteer with subject matter expertise in the content area, who is entrusted to provide a reasonable assurance that the work represented was undertaken in an ethical and scientifically rigourous manner and that the conclusions reflected the results. Work published in scientific journals is the most common example of peer-reviewed material (refer to Appendix for a list of relevant journals and associated information). Journal articles include reports of primary research, review articles analyzing and evaluating the findings of several research reports, and descriptive articles summarizing the current state of understanding on a topic.[9,14]

It is important to note that not all articles in respected journals are subject to review, such as opinion pieces, yet this does not necessarily invalidate their content.[2,9] While peer review can ensure a high standard of quality, non peer-reviewed sources are important to consider in certain contexts, and can also provide an introduction for the novice researcher looking for an overview on a topic prior to delving into the peer-reviewed literature.[9,14]

Textbooks are also valuable information sources. However, while useful to provide an overview of factual data on a topic, the information can become outdated with time after publication depending on the topic and information being presented.[14]

2.3.2 GREY LITERATURE

Depending on the definition used, most other information sources are considered "grey literature." In a definition developed at the Grey Literature Conference in 1999, this spectrum of source is considered to include "that which is produced on all levels of government, academics, business, and industry in print and electronic formats, but which is not controlled by commercial publishers.[16]" This would thus include conference proceedings, clinical trial registries, professional association or group websites, dissertations, theses, government reports, and committee reports, and can often be difficult to locate, interpret, or appraise, though often valuable.[3,9,16]

A thesis is an in-depth exploration of a given topic, often performed in the course of completing a graduate degree. Published and made available by the university where the thesis was undertaken, it is considered as reference work, though not strictly peer-reviewed. Government documents might include reports or standards on system performance metrics, conducted by government agencies or departments. For example, the Canadian Institute for Health Information's *Medical Radiation Technologists in Canada, 2011* report would be a valuable and reliable source of information on national and provincial data on the radiation therapy workforce.[17]

2.3.3 WHITE PAPERS

White papers are authoritative reports or guidelines on a given topic, often compiled by government agencies, experts in a field, or by a task force on behalf of professional groups or associations. Although they originated in government and are generally considered grey literature, white papers can also be published in peer-reviewed journals. They can serve to guide or standardize practice, often framed as a "call to arms" to those in a position to lead or contribute to change. Two landmark radiation medicine white papers in recent years were the American Society for Radiation Oncology (ASTRO)'s *Safety is no accident: a framework for quality radiation oncology and care* and the American Society of Radiation Technologists (ASRT)'s *Advanced Practice in Radiation Therapy.*[18,19]

2.3.4 PUBLIC SOURCES

Websites and newspapers can also be sources of information, but any statements or data should be considered with caution if a reliable reference is not provided. Certain information is actually best sought from a website, such as mission or vision statements for professional associations or agencies. It is also important to remember that while the most accessible sources of information – such as websites and newspaper articles – are not necessarily the most accurate, they are often the primary resource for patients and the general public and can provide insight to their perceptions and interpretations of health-related information.[2]

2.3.5 *PROFESSIONAL EXPERTISE*

Personal communication is a means used to convey information and expertise on a given topic amongst peers, colleagues and experts. It can either be in person, over the phone, or over email. This type of knowledge sharing can be a valuable source of information that is specific to the context of research being sought. It often allows the researcher to solicit specific insight to answer an individual research question. These sources can provide time-sensitive information, which can sometimes be challenging to find in published data due to delays in the publishing process.

2.4 SEARCH STRATEGIES AND TECHNIQUES

There are many search strategies available. The most common is a keyword search of an online database. Other techniques, such as snowballing and citation tracking, can be used to pursue a particularly valuable path or to provide another option if a keyword search does not prove fruitful.

2.4.1 *KEYWORD SEARCH*

Online databases, consisting of peer-reviewed articles, textbooks, and often other sources, can be a goldmine of information, but it is important to approach the search in a strategic manner to ensure valuable results. This relies on the use of keywords to search the databases.

The process of defining keywords should flow in a linear fashion, first selecting terms and then conducting the search. Before selecting the keywords for a search, a working topic must be defined. A working topic is a preliminary idea of a research question, a theory, or a statement used for a thesis. Using this working topic, the researcher can then list words or phrases that describe the concept. The more concise the terms, the more likely it becomes to identify appropriate literature.[20] It is often valuable and even necessary to revisit the search strategy and refine keywords based on findings from initial searches.[21] Following the iterative process discussed previously, evaluation of keywords on the topic should include:

- Common phrases and terms
- Recurring keywords
- Synonyms or acronyms of the keywords
- Alternative spellings (for example: pediatric/paediatric)
- Alternate Medical Subject Headings (MeSH) terms

The MeSH system acts as a built-in thesaurus within a database. This system is used to assign index terms to research articles for content and subject. Each article is assigned up to 20 index terms to help researchers identify the relevancy of the article to the topic being searched in the database.[20,22]

Using the list of generated key concepts and terms, it is important to understand how to phrase or combine them in a way that can facilitate interpretation by a database search engine. Databases use a set of rules called Boolean logic for this interpretation.[21,22] The three main Boolean operators are AND, OR and NOT (Table 2.1). These can be used individually or in combination between the keywords in the search box to define and specify exactly what is sought. Databases also recognize two additional tools to expand search terms: truncation and wildcards. Truncation allows the researcher to identify the main base of any keyword through use of an asterisk (*). For example: entering the term radi* would include terms like radiation, radiotherapy, etc. The wildcard is identified with a question mark (?) to represent a letter that can be exchanged for another in the search results. For example: wom?n would include results like women and woman.

TABLE 2.1 Boolean Operators.

Boolean Operator	Use	Example
AND	identify terms that must appear in the results. Useful when combining terms that include truncated or wildcards. This term will narrow results	Handwash* AND complian* AND nurs* This would return results that include all three terms in any truncated form
OR	broaden the search by indicating that any of the listed terms are acceptable in the results. Using OR will allow many different synonyms to be linked together	Handwash* OR hand wash* OR hand hygiene

TABLE 2.1 *(Continued)*

Boolean Operator	Use	Example
NOT	narrow the search by identifying a term that is excluded from the results	Handwash* NOT alcohol gel These results would include articles on hand washing but would exclude those where alcohol gel was used.
AND plus OR	using both these term in combination can be great time savers. Using them together they must be grouped into brackets for many internet and database searches	(Handwash* OR hand wash* OR hand hygiene) AND (complian* OR non-complian*) AND nurs*

2.4.2 SNOWBALLING

"Snowballing" refers to the process of scouring the reference list in a key article that proved relevant. In reviewing the references used in writing this article, other valuable articles might be identified. This process could be repeated for these articles, and so on, hence the concept of an exponentially growing, or snowballing, pool of potentially valuable sources.[23]

2.4.3 CITATION TRACKING

Citation tracking is essentially the reverse of snowballing, and requires the use of online tools or functionalities, which are often available through searchable databases. Rather than looking retrospectively at sources that informed a key reference, this technique seeks to identify other subsequent articles or research that made reference to the initial source. Articles that referenced the identified key article within their work can be identified and further investigated for usefulness.[23]

2.4.4 HAND-SEARCHING AND POWER-BROWSING

Hand-searching, or power-browsing, is an extended search technique used by trained persons to review a journal volume in a "cover-to-cover" fashion.[24]

By reading each article individually, possible errors in indexing can be highlighted and potentially relevant articles identified that may have been excluded from search terms used in previous searches. This can be increasingly challenging in the digital era with the decreased emphasis on print material, but is still possible in online publications.

2.5 INCLUSION AND EXCLUSION CRITERIA

Once the researcher is ready to begin searching the literature, it is important to brainstorm some specifics of the topic of interest. Using inclusion and exclusion criteria will give the search a framework to respect throughout the process, helping the researcher collect articles that have valuable commonalities. Inclusion criteria determine the minimum characteristics that would warrant an article to be considered, and exclusion criteria suggest characteristics that would eliminate an article, regardless of whether it met inclusion criteria, basically setting the boundaries on the literature search. Furthermore, identifying additional limiting factors and filters will help decrease the volume of returned search results, creating a collection of articles that are more manageable and relevant to the needs of the literature search itself.[20,22] Table 2.2 provides examples of common limiting factors.

TABLE 2.2 Limiters (Inclusion and Exclusion Criteria).

Limiter	Example
Publication Dates	For searches on current clinical practice, publications less than 5 years old are best suited. Assess the date and content critically to determine if the findings are applicable to current practices. Is the technology discussed up to date?
Study Subject	Consider subject age, sex, and species. Some studies report results on animal subjects and some on human subjects.
Language of Publication	Is there a full-text option in English? Sometimes only abstracts may be translated.
Geographic Area	For human studies, which geographic population was included?
Document Features	Is full-text available?
Document Types	Primary or secondary source?

Each different database or search engine handles limits differently. Most search databases have tutorials available within the search engine and viewing these tutorials will help the researcher become familiar with how the search engine interprets and defines advanced limits.

2.6 DATABASES AND ACCESS

A database is a virtual space containing a variety of documents. Some databases are available free of charge, called open access, and others will require a subscription to access documents (*see* Table 2.3). Some helpful databases include Google Scholar, PubMed and the Cochrane Library, some providing free access to articles and others having an associated cost for access. Google Scholar is academically based and can help the researcher locate abstracts, books, technical reports, theses and peer-reviewed journals. Universities, academic institutions and hospitals may also hold subscriptions to different databases deemed relevant by the organizations. Students, alumni, and staff will be entitled to privileges to access these databases either independently or through the assistance of a librarian.

TABLE 2.3 Valuable Open-Access and Subscription Searchable Databases (modified from Czaplewski, 2012)[20]

Open Access	Subscription
Cochrane Library	Alt Healthwatche
Google Scholar	CINAHL / CINAHL Plus
Knowledge Finder	EMBASE
MEDLINE	Scopus
PubMed	Web of Knowledge

Another important online source is the Cochrane Library. The Cochrane Collaboration performs highly structured systematic reviews and publishes findings to support evidence-based decision making among professionals in health fields. Their work is recognized internationally and provides a great wealth of insight through the review and compilation of findings from numerous primary sources.[25] Reviewing the published articles from the Cochrane Collaboration is an ideal way to integrate findings from primary sources into evidence-based clinical decisions in a timely manner; however each systematic review is formulated around one very specific clinical question chosen by the collaboration groups.[25] While it is very helpful in the clinical setting, applying these findings to a specific literature review can be more challenging than referencing primary sources directly, as each Cochrane review represents multiple individual publications and covers each in lesser detail than the primary source.

2.6.1 ACCESSING SUBSCRIPTION-BASED DATABASES

Using free or open-access databases for searching, the researcher can first access the abstracts and may wish to pursue articles that are of interest. Chosen articles can be sought either through the open-access options, or, if unavailable, through restricted databases, for a fee. Comprehensive subscriptions to restricted databases are costly and are often held by hospitals, governmental agencies, professional associations, and academic institutions like universities and colleges.[20] If not directly accessible through the Internet, the researcher should explore gaining access via alumnus, member, or employee status with any of these organizations. Contacting these groups could also be beneficial if a certain journal or reference emerges as having great value but is not subscribed to by an organization that might benefit from its content.

2.6.2 MANAGING CITATIONS

Searches can sometimes yield a suboptimal number of citations for the researcher to review. Having too many results can be very overwhelming, however, insufficient results will not support the research topic (*see* Case example 2.1).

2.6.2.1 WHEN A SEARCH YIELDS TOO MANY RESULTS

This can be a sign that further care is needed to narrow down citations to a manageable number. Reviewing results and identifying necessary changes in strategy can help narrow down search results to relevant documents. Beginning with the original keywords and concepts for comparison, this is the time to use the iterative process. Modifying keywords, adding Boolean operators AND or NOT and removing truncations will aid with the process of narrowing search results. Reviewing and revising inclusion and exclusion criteria based on irrelevant citations being returned in a search can help to narrow the focus. This might include restricting the date range that is being searched, especially as it might be considered more valuable to focus on more recent work. Other examples of exclusion and inclusion criteria can be found in Table 2.2.

HOT TIP

How old is too old?

A general rule of thumb is to focus on literature published within the past five years. This can be extended to ten years if the topic is more obscure (meaning there is less likely to be sufficient literature within a five-year window). The nature of the topic is also a consideration: technology and treatment techniques evolve more quickly than patient education approaches, for example, and research will become outdated more quickly. Even with these date ranges in mind, there are instances where an older reference is valuable – either as a seminal or classic work in a given area, or to provide evidence of a past practice or state.

2.6.2.2 WHEN SEARCH RESULTS YIELD TOO FEW RESULTS

Completing document searches with little to no insight to previous evidence can be discouraging. Removing limits, introducing the Boolean operator OR and using truncation can help to broaden the search. It might also be helpful to rely on a database thesaurus to identify additional MeSH terms to be included in the key terms.

2.7 ENGAGING A LIBRARIAN

Librarians are informed professionals who work with databases and academic documents on a regular basis. A librarian can add insight and expertise to many phases of the search process and is a very valuable resource to the researcher. Most hospitals and academic institutions rely on these professionals to provide research guidance. In the hospital setting, librarians can help locate evidence-based research and protocols to increase the quality of care and decision making information. This expertise is also supported by the Board on Health Care Services as a standard to ensure scientific validity in systematic reviews.[26]

When engaging the help of librarian, care should be taken to provide the most accurate information following the same requirements for any search. Defining and requesting a search will vary by institution. In some instances a predetermined search form may be available outlining exactly what is required from the researcher for the librarian to have the necessary information to perform the search. Case example 2.1 provides the perspective of a librarian on her role in the collaborative research process.

CASE EXAMPLE 2.1

A Librarian's Perspective on Research Collaboration

Susan Barker BA MISt
Digital Services and Reference Librarian, Faculty of Law, Bora Laskin Law Library, University of Toronto, Toronto, Canada
Adjunct Instructor, Faculty of Information (iSchool), University of Toronto, Toronto, Canada

When embarking on any journey or voyage, you would never set out knowing nothing more than the direction of your destination. You need information: maps, resources and a trusted guide to help you navigate. The same applies when you are starting your research; here too, you need maps, resources and a trusted guide – your librarian – to help you on your way. Here's a cautionary tale to illustrate why.

I attended a conference of librarians where the plenary speaker recounted the sad story of the death of Ellen Roche. In 2001, Ellen volunteered to participate in an asthma research study at Johns Hopkins University. The study involved the inhalation of hexamethonium, essentially to induce an asthma attack, to evaluate how healthy lungs would respond to such an attack. The day after being given hexamethonium to inhale, Ellen became severely ill with a reduced lung capacity. Within a month, she was dead.
Now, I can imagine you are asking yourself. "What does this possibly have to do with librarians?"

While there were several factors at play in Ellen's death, the one which is relevant here is that the researcher's literature search did not locate articles identifying the potential dangers of the use of hexamethonium. In hindsight, it is fairly clear that the research was inadequate: only current editions of a limited number of textbooks were consulted and a quick PubMed search was conducted. Additional searches in Google and other search engines were made. Some articles were found, but none of them indicated the dangers of using hexamethonium in this way. In addition to the limited research, one of the problems was that PubMed, at that time, only included articles back to the mid 1960s. In fact, there were articles describing potential dangers of hexamethonium written in the early 1960s and the 1950s, as well as commentary in older texts, which was missed.

Because medical librarians are professionals – usually holding a masters degree in library science or information studies and also having an undergraduate or perhaps even a graduate degree in the sciences – they are experts in medical literature and medical information resources such as PubMed. A medical librarian would have known of the limitations of the database and likely recommended further research in other databases and print resources.

> Never hesitate to ask your librarian! We are happy to consult with you on your research, to offer guidance on formulating search strategies, to identify the best resources available and to train you on the use of these resources. While it might be overstating to claim that asking a librarian for assistance could have prevented Ellen's death,[27] it is certainly not overstating to say that it is wise to make use of your librarian's expertise and experience to guarantee the best research results.

2.8 CRITICAL APPRAISAL

Not all research is created equal. The information and data acquired through a literature review, even if pertinent to the topic at hand, cannot simply be taken at face value. It is important that anyone undertaking a review have a basic understanding of how to weigh the respective value of various sources, methodologies, and levels of evidence, and how to determine if appropriate conclusions were drawn from investigational data. This is often referred to as the critical appraisal of the literature.

2.8.1 *METHODOLOGICAL RIGOUR*

The methodology used to conduct a study can often provide the clearest picture of the value of certain data. In fact, if the methods used to conduct the study are not clear, this is an indicator that the results should be questioned. It is often said that an investigation's methods should be reported in sufficient detail such that an independent investigator could replicate the study, and if completed within a similar setting, could expect the same results.[2]

The nature of the population included in the study should be reviewed; the appropriateness of the inclusion and exclusion criteria, the study population, and the sample size and its generalizability to any broader population being studied.[3–6] The study design itself should be evaluated, including the nature and duration of any intervention, the setting, and timing (e.g., prospective versus retrospective).[3–6] The inherent strength of various methodologies is an important factor to consider, as identical results from a case study and from a randomized control trial cannot be weighed as equivalent. For more information on levels of evidence, please refer to Chapter 1 (Evidence-Based Medicine and the Scientific Method). Measures of outcome and methods of analysis are also determinants of the quality of a study, as important outcomes might not be detected if the measures or analysis are not sensitive to the magnitude of a difference or are not designed to assess a certain outcome at all. For example, reporting the number of reported treatment incidents at two centres will not suggest, which centre is safer, unless such considerations as number of treatments delivered, criteria for classification as incidents, and the culture of reporting are taken into account. The objectivity of decision making in this area should be reinforced by investigators, and the strengths and limitations of a given methodology should be presented.

2.8.2 INFERENCE

After making an assessment of the strength, validity, and generalizability of the results, it is important to think critically about whether the investigators have drawn the appropriate conclusions based on this assessment. Conclusions should be specific and made in the context of the results.[2] Specifically, they should answer the research question. The lack of a clear question at the outset of a study is in and of itself a sign of a poorly designed investigation. Any inferences made by investigators should not extend beyond what is supported directly by the results, including when outlining the implications of results for practice and decision making.[2,8] The above example about incident reporting can be considered here as well. Weaknesses in the data that preclude stronger conclusions should be highlighted and suggestions for future research that might address such weaknesses should be made.[13]

2.8.3 *BIAS*

The potential for bias should be kept in mind when reviewing a body of literature on a given topic. First of all, positive results are often more likely to be published, meaning that researchers can be biased towards pursuing publication if their results suggest that an intervention or change in care had a positive outcome.[4] Research sponsored by someone with a vested interest in the results, such as a pharmaceutical company or the vendor of a particular technology, can be particularly subject to this bias. While the reputation of the authors and the institution where the research was conducted are both important considerations in appraising an article, these do not single-handedly assure the rigour of the methodology or the appropriateness of the conclusions.[4] While bias is not always avoidable, it should be acknowledged and minimized where possible.[3–6]

It should be noted that just because a strong critique of a given article or source of information might suggest that its results should not be considered with much weight, it does not mean that familiarity with the work is not important. The more easily accessible information is, and the more superficially valid its results might seem, the more likely it is to be quoted and considered by lay people, especially the media and patients who are often seeking information without the appropriate tools to critique and evaluate it.[4] Being familiar with recent and prevalent literature can facilitate conversations with patients, and can help the clinical radiation therapist engage in a balanced discussion with patients about their own information-seeking.

2.9 MANAGING REFERENCES

Maintaining organization of the many references is an important step for compiling the final product of the literature search. There are several software options available to build a personal databank of articles and relevant referencing information.

Endnote® is a flexible but complex program installed directly onto the computer and interlinked with a word processor. This software must be purchased and installed on a specific computer. RefWorks is another reference software that is sometimes offered free-of-charge, especially in academic institutions. This program works by storing inputted references online, allowing access to ongoing work from any computer with Internet access.[28]

The annotated bibliography can be a helpful way to maintain notes on research articles. This involves creating a condensed version of the article, in the researchers' own words that address the following: the objectives of the article, the main methods of the study and the main conclusions. It often also includes notes about the reputation of the work of the principal author or the journal, and other factors in considering the relative importance of the resource. Such summaries are valuable when referenced as a group at a later date, to remind the researcher of key points and commonalities, distilled down to a manageable compilation.[29]

HOT TIP

While using software to manage referencing can be very helpful, not all research requires it. Some researchers may have limited access to these types of programs but organization does not need to be compromised! Keeping a set of index cards with source information and important details about each reference will help to keep things organized!

2.10 SEARCH REPORTING

Just as the importance of detailed and rigourous methodology has been stressed in the evaluation of literature amassed in a review, it is equally as important to report the methodology used in a literature review if it is to be used as more than information gathering to guide other work. Throughout the process of conducting a systematic literature review, a record should be kept of the search strategy and methodology. As acknowledged earlier, another researcher should be able to replicate the search and review based on the reported methods, and come up with similar results. This methodology should include a list of the inclusion and exclusion criteria and the rationale for decisions made here, including language, year of publication, and specific study designs, populations, and settings.[13] The process of reviewing search results requires an explanation of the stage at which returned results are reviewed (title, abstract, and full text), and how independent assessments are conducted to reduce bias and judgment differences, including any arbitration or consensus exercises to address disagreements in categorization.[13] A flow chart is often used to provide a clear picture of the process, with numbers of results reflected at each stage. Case example 2.2 highlights a systematic literature review undertaken to identify barriers to access to radiation therapy in Canada.

CASE EXAMPLE 2.2

Barriers to accessing radiation therapy in Canada: a systematic review

In efforts to determine and classify barriers to access to radiation therapy in Canada, Gillan et al. undertook a systematic review of the literature.[30] MEDLINE, CINAHL and EMBase databases were used to search keywords relating to barriers to access or utilization of radiation therapy, using a search strategy built with the aid of a librarian.

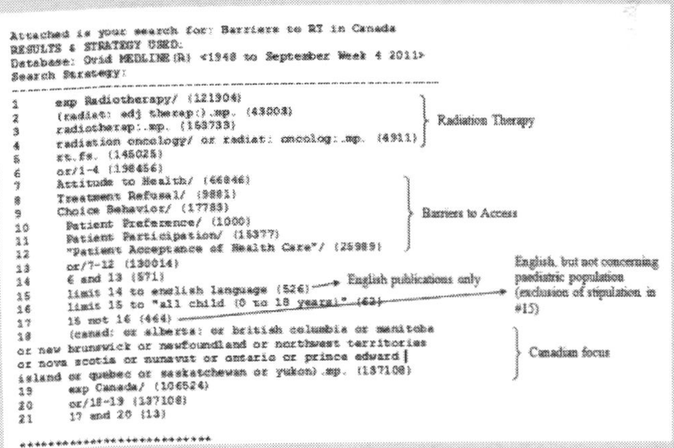

```
Attached is your search for: Barriers to RT in Canada
RESULTS & STRATEGY USED:
Database: Ovid MEDLINE(R) <1948 to September Week 4 2011>
Search Strategy:
--------------------------------------------------------------------------------
1     exp Radiotherapy/ (121304)
2     (radiat: adj therap:).mp. (43003)
3     radiotherap:.mp. (153733)
4     radiation oncology/ or radiat: oncolog:.mp. (4911)
5     rt.fs. (145025)
6     or/1-4 (198456)
7     Attitude to Health/ (66846)
8     Treatment Refusal/ (9881)
9     Choice Behavior/ (17783)
10     Patient Preference/ (1000)
11     Patient Participation/ (15377)
12     "Patient Acceptance of Health Care"/ (25989)
13     or/7-12 (130014)
14     6 and 13 (571)
15     limit 14 to english language (526)
16     limit 15 to "all child (0 to 18 years)" (62)
17     15 not 16 (464)
18     (canad: or alberta: or british columbia or manitoba
or new brunswick or newfoundland or northwest territories
or nova scotia or nunavut or ontario or prince edward
island or quebec or saskatchewan or yukon).mp. (137108)
19     exp Canada/ (106524)
20     or/18-19 (137108)
21     17 and 20 (13)

****************************
```


FIGURE 2.1 Preliminary search strategy for literature review.

Inclusion criteria were that articles were conducted within the Canadian context, and specifically referred to barriers to radiation therapy as opposed to other modalities of treatment. Restriction to publication after 2000 was introduced at a later point. Collected abstracts were reviewed independently. The search was refined based on initial results, and the final search was managed using Endnote. To provide clarity to the reader, the process was reported using the flowchart below. This involved initial abstract review and categorization into perceived relevancy, retrieval of full-text articles and review. The final phase extended to the categorization of barriers found as a result of the search. Barriers identified in relevant articles were categorized as relating to the health systems, patient sociodemographic, patient factors, or provider factors, contexts and thematic analysis performed for each context. The detailed reporting of the steps in the search process should permit another researcher to distil the same final set of articles (and instruments) if approached in the same way.

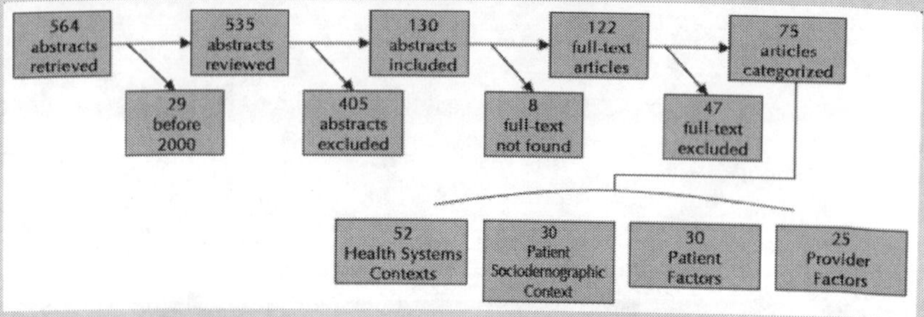

FIGURE 2.2 Flowchart of review and categorization process.

As a result of this systematic literature review, 535 unique abstracts were collected, and from it 75 met inclusion criteria and 46 (61.3%) addressed multiple themes. The most cited barriers to accessing radiation therapy when indicated were patient age (n=26, 34.7%), distance to treatment centre (n=23, 30.7%), wait times (n=22, 29.3%), and lack of physician understanding about the use of RT (n=16, 21.6%). The role of provider factors and the lack of attention in the literature to patient fears and mistrust as potential barriers were unexpected findings demanding further attention through future research initiatives.

By recording the search strategy and the tallies of sources included and excluded at various stages, it becomes easier both to keep track of decisions being made by the reviewers and also to summarize for the purposes of reporting. This might include the following:

- an outline of the search and review stages
- a record of any search terms and included databases
- an ongoing tally of references included and excluded at each stage and for what reasons
- the nature of the source type and type of research reported[14]

Literature reviews are a valuable source of information, but require a strategic approach and a critical eye for the information to be used and interpreted responsibly. While not all research questions or topics lend themselves to a formal systematic review, it is nonetheless important to be comfortable navigating the literature. Research conducted in isolation from what is known on a subject is bound to be flawed, and needless effort may be wasted in repeating mistakes that have been flagged through previous research, or in attempting to answer a question that has already been addressed definitively. Armed with a clear understanding of where gaps in knowledge might exist and with methodological insight from previous work, the researcher can begin to define the novel research initiative and be confident that it will be well grounded.

KEYWORDS

- Systematic review
- Meta-analysis
- Critical appraisal
- Peer review
- Grey literature
- Keyword

REFERENCES

1. Cline, R. J.; Haynes, K. M. Consumer health information seeking on the Internet: the state-of-the-art. *Health Educ. Res.* **2001**, *16(6)*, 671–692.
2. Rosser, W. W. Looking right down to the pores: why it is important to learn how to read journals. In: Information Mastery: Evidence-Based Family Medicine 2nd ed; Rosser, W. W.; Slawson, D. C.; Shaughnessy, A. F. Ed.; BC Decker Inc: Hamilton, 2004; pp. 76–82.
3. Keary, E.; Byrne M.; Lawton A. How to conduct a literature review. The Irish Psychologist. **2012,** *38(9–10)*, 239–245.
4. Rosser, W. W. Using Systematic Reviews and the appropriate meta-analysis. In: Information Mastery: Evidence-Based Family Medicine 2nd ed; Rosser, W. W.; Slawson, D. C.; Shaughnessy, A. F. Ed.; BC Decker Inc: Hamilton, 2004; pp. 113–116.
5. Centre for Reviews and Dissemination. Systematic Reviews: CRD's guidance for undertaking systematic reviews. University of York: York, UK, 2009.
6. Grimshaw, J. A Knowledge Synthesis Chapter; Canadian Institute of Health Research. (Online) http://www.cihr-irsc.gc.ca/e/documents/knowledge_synthesis_chapter_e.pdf (accessed April 17, 2013).
7. Davis, K.; Drey, N.; Gould, D. What are scoping studies? A review of the nursing literature. Int. *J. Nurs. Stud.* **2009**,*46(10)*, 1386–1400.
8. Mulrow, C. D. Rationale for systematic reviews. *BMJ.* **1994**, *309(6954)*, 597–599.
9. Bolderston, A. Writing an effective literature review. *J. Med. Imag. Radiat. Sci.* **2008**, *39*, 86–92.
10. Field, A.; Gillett, R. How to do a meta-analysis. *Br. J. Math. Stat. Psychol.* **2010**, *63(3)*, 665–694.
11. Agency for Healthcare Research and Quality. Methods Guide for Effectiveness and comparative effectiveness reviews. (Online) **2013** http://effectivehealthcare.ahrq.gov/ehc/products/60/318/CER-methods-guide-130916.pdf (accessed September 10th, 2013).
12. Warde, P.; Payne, D. Does thoracic irradiation improve survival and local control in limited-stage small-cell carcinoma of the lung? A meta-analysis. J. Clin. Oncol. **1992,** *10(6)*, 890–895.
13. University Health Network Libraries. Systematic Review Gateway. http://documents.uhn.ca/sites/uhn/VL/Guides/UHNLibraries_Systematic_Review_Gateway.pdf (accessed May 15, 2013).
14. Timmins, F.; McCabe, C. How to conduct an effective literature search. Nurs. Stand. **2005**, *20(11)*, 41–47.
15. Buchsel P. C. Researching and referencing. *Clin. J. Oncol. Nurs.* **2001**, *5(3)*, 7–11.
16. Grey Literature Network Service. Fourth International Conference on Grey Literature: New Frontiers in Grey Literature, Washington DC, 1999.
17. Canadian Institute for Health Information. Medical Radiation Technologists in Canada, 2011; Ottawa, 2011.
18. American Society for Radiation Oncology. Safety is No Accident: a framework for quality radiation oncology and care; American Society of Therapeutic Radiation Oncology; 2012.

19. Martino, S.; Odle, T. G. Advanced Practice in Radiation Therapy; American Society of Radiation Technologists: Albuquerque, NM, 2007.
20. Czaplewski, L. M. Searching the literature: a researcher's perspective. *J. Infus. Nurs.* **2012**, *35(1)*, 20–26.
21. Harvard, L. How to conduct an effective and valid literature search. *Nurs. Times.* **2007**, *103(45)*, 32–33.
22. Ebbert, J. O.; Dupras, D. M.; Erwin, P. J. Searching the medical literature using PubMed: a tutorial. *Mayo Clin. Proc.* **2003**, *78(1)*, 87–91.
23. Greenhalgh, T.; Peacock, R. Effectiveness and efficiency of search methods in systematic reviews of complex evidence: audit of primary sources. *BMJ* **2005**, *331(7524)*, 1064–1065.
24. Giustini, D. Hand-searching. http://hlwiki.slais.ubc.ca/index.php/Hand-searching (accessed April 4, 2013).
25. The Cochrane Collaboration. www.cochrane.org/cochrane-reviews (accessed July 26, 2013).
26. Eden, J.; Levit, L.; Berg, A.; Morton, S. Finding what works in Health Care: standards for systematic reviews. Institute of Medicine, 2011.
27. Perkins, E. Johns Hopkins' Tragedy: could librarians have prevented a death? http://newsbreaks.infotoday.com/nbreader.asp?ArticleID=17534 (accessed September 16, 2013).
28. Manage Your References. http://www.dartmouth.edu/library/leo/refmanagement/ref_man.html (accessed April 21, 2013).
29. Knott, D. Writing an Annotated Bibliography. http://www.writing.utoronto.ca/advice/specific-types-of-writing/annotated-bibliography (accessed April 21, 2013).
30. Gillan, C.; Briggs, K.; Goytisolo Pazos, A.; Maurus, M.; Harnett, N.; Catton, P.; Wiljer, D. Barriers to accessing radiation therapy in Canada—A systematic review. *Radiat. Oncol.* **2012,** *7,* 167.

CHAPTER 3

RESEARCH PROPOSALS

EMILY SINCLAIR MRT(T) BSc MSc(c)
Clinical Specialist Radiation Therapist, Odette Cancer Centre, Sunnybrook Health Sciences Centre, Toronto Canada
Lecturer, Department of Radiation Oncology, University of Toronto, Toronto Canada

CRAIG ELITH RTT BMRS(RT) BSc
Radiation Therapist, Fraser Valley Centre, British Columbia Cancer Agency, Surrey Canada

TRACEY ROSE RTT MSc
Radiation Therapist, Sindi Aluwahlia Hawkins Cancer Centre for the Southern Interior, British Columbia Cancer Agency, Kelowna Canada

CONTENTS

The preceding chapters in this book established the concept of the scientific method, the development of a research question and how to perform a literature review. This chapter will discuss how each of these components can bring to bear on the research proposal that will be used for presentation to the team, to the leadership, to the funding agency, and to the ethics board. More importantly, the proposal will be a key record of intended plan for the research study that can be referred to throughout the project as a check to ensure that the work is on course. It ensures the team has considered all stages of the research process – in essence that due diligence has been done.

3.1 INTENT AND RATIONALE

A research proposal can be compared to a company stating a business case. The proposal must convince researchers, funding agencies, organizations, stakeholders, and administration that the research is worth investment – of both time and money – and support.[1] A poorly written proposal may result in denial of funding, lack of support by a clinical department, prolonged deliberation at the institutional or ethics review board, or result in the actual research project getting off track.[2]

In the broad sense, the research proposal is a detailed statement of intent to carry out a piece of research. It must be formal, clear, and concise. The text should include as little technical jargon as possible, and should be understood by the lay reader if possible, as the review board may not necessarily include experts in the individual topic area of the research. The proposal is also where the first impression is made, so it needs to make an impact. If it is not well presented (either in flow, clarity, or grammar), then the reviewers may just pass it by, even if the subject matter is worthwhile.

HOT TIP

Always have your research proposal read by an individual not familiar with the work – if it is written well, the proposal's intent should be clear. Do not assume that the reviewer will understand what you are trying to say – be explicit but concise.

A prerequisite to the research proposal is defining the research question (*see* Chapter 1: Evidence-Based Medicine and the Scientific Method). The research question will drive the subsequent components of the proposal. As the proposal is being written, frequent referral back to the actual question should be conducted. This provides an iterative quality assurance process to ensure the proposal is built around what exactly was set out to be defined.

3.2 THE RESEARCH TEAM

Traditionally, the researcher who develops the research question and plans to steer the project's course will self-identify as the principal investigator (PI). The PI assumes responsibility for the research project and accountability for the work. In addition to the initial proposal, the PI is responsible for realization and reporting of the final outcome, defined as achieving the deliverable and dissemination of the work. This is accomplished by careful orchestration and management of the progression of the research, such as within well-defined timelines. The PI is also accountable for strict adherence to methodology, ethical conduct in all areas of the research, authenticity of the data, and in the case of a funded project, for the finances.

HOT TIP

Most research is subject to an ethics review process, and all projects seeking formal funding may also be subject to interim review by the funding body. No matter how small the project is, the team involved must ensure transparency of the work, even after publication, as research can be questioned and data reviewed at any time. A solid proposal with routine, scheduled checks will help to ensure that a review will cause little disruption to the project.

Additional members of the research team that take responsibility for the work are often referred to as coinvestigators (CI), and have similar responsibilities to the PI. The CIs are likely the main instigators of the research, along with the PI. The PI should both collaborate with and delegate tasks to the CIs as necessary. Chapter 8 (Clinical Trials) provides greater insight into the division of responsibilities within a research team, including the use of a Task Delegation Log. In addition to the PI and CIs, other research team members can provide expert consultation and assistance with various phases of the work. These individuals are identified as "collaborators," and may include members of other disciplines, such as a librarian or a biostatistician (these are discussed further in Chapters 2 (Literature Reviews), 5 (Quantitative Methodologies and Analysis), and 14 (Getting Started: Building a Research and Evidence-Based Culture)).

When writing the research proposal, the PI is encouraged to initiate a discussion with the CIs and collaborators early in the project about who will be part of the authorship team as well as the order of authorship. Overall, authorship should credit contribution to the study itself and can be reexamined during various stages of the work, as circumstances can change based on timelines, competing commitments, changing interests, and engagement in the work. Chapter 12 (Preparing and Submitting a Manuscript for Publication) goes into greater detail about the criteria and considerations regarding authorship.

HOT TIP

The PI should discuss the authorship and responsibility of each team member. It is important to establish the role and responsibilities of each collaborator early on in the project. People are often excited with the prospect of being part of the research; however, they may change their minds if the workload becomes heavy.

3.3 COMPONENTS OF A RESEARCH PROPOSAL

A well-written proposal comprises many elements. The elements may vary slightly depending on the intent of the proposal, for example, whether the proposal is for an Ethics Board review (*see* Chapter 4: Research Ethics Applications), or a proposal for funding. The following is a list of components common to most research proposals.

3.3.1 TITLE PAGE AND FORMATTING

Every proposal should begin with a title page. Although basic, this is the first impression of the work that will be imparted to the reader. Instructions for submission of any proposal will either include or exclude a title. If no recommendations are indicated, a standardized format should be followed for all proposals. The full title, being the most integral part of the proposal, should be aligned, halfway down the page. Generally the PI should also be listed, as well as his or her professional credentials, institutional affiliation, contact information, and date of submission. Each subsequent page should be numbered and include a header, usually a shortened version of the title called a "running head."

HOT TIP

The title of the work should be clear and concise so that the reader knows exactly what you are investigating – however, add some "jazz" to the title. This will pique interest.

3.3.2 ABSTRACT OR SUMMARY

The proposal requires an abstract or summary of the proposed study. This should be a concise synopsis of the research proposal. The research problem should be stated, along with a brief rationale of the value in addressing the problem. The proposed research methodology can be briefly outlined and justified, with reference to plans for data analysis. Suggesting the intended outcomes and hypothesized significance of the findings will further highlight the gap in knowledge or practice to be filled with the proposed work. The abstract does not generally include references; however, the rationale should provide key insight to frame the research question for the reader.

3.3.3 RATIONALE AND AIM

The rationale is framed by the literature review and should include a statement of why the research is important. More specifically, the rationale should include a brief explanation of how the study will contribute to the existing knowledge on the subject and how the findings might make an impact locally or on a broader scale. As part of the rationale, the primary and secondary objectives need to be stated. Primary objectives describe how the research is going to answer the question being asked – this is referred to as the principal aim. Secondary objectives are "by-products" of the primary objective and could be findings that occur as a result of other measures that are being collected. Both primary and secondary objectives should be measurable. Case example 3.1 defines objectives for a study relating to patient satisfaction.

CASE EXAMPLE 3.1

A research team wanted to determine if patients are satisfied with the service they are receiving at the cancer centre. The primary objective of the patient satisfaction survey was to determine how satisfied the patients were with the check-in process at the front desk. This was measured by how long they had to wait to be checked in and the friendliness of the staff (determined through the patient's own perception).

The aim was thus: "To assess patient satisfaction with the check-in process."

The secondary objective of the study was to capture the time of day that the patient checked in so that the team could assess any relationships between satisfaction and time.

The secondary objective thus became "To determine if any relationships exist between satisfaction and time of check-in."

3.3.4 LITERATURE REVIEW

In a literature review, the researcher is able to indicate where the proposed study will fit into the current body of evidence and distinguish the novel work from what is currently published, providing incremental value to the knowledge base. While a critique of the available literature is necessary, the review should focus on the major areas of disagreement, or gaps, in the work that provide the platform for the proposed research. The literature review does not need to be lengthy. It requires thoroughness that demonstrates an understanding of the research topic as well as an awareness of the published material already available on the subject (*see* Chapter 2: Literature Reviews). It is rarely beneficial to explain individual studies in detail, but is instead important to focus on the cumulative state of knowledge on the subject. Multiple references might be used to support a single statement, and two or three key papers might be discussed in greater detail, depending on guidelines for the length and scope of the background review.

HOT TIP

In reading the literature review, it should be clear as to what information is already out there, what is missing, and how your proposed study will address the "missing" piece. If you are unable to clearly identify these three elements – reevaluate!

HOT TIP

Researchers should be cognizant of plagiarism in writing a research proposal. Follow guidelines as they pertain to referencing work of others. Quotation marks must be used when copying text verbatim. As work is cited and incorporated into your proposal, be sure to restate it in your own words. Even the restatement of another's findings or thoughts does require reference to the original work!

3.3.5 THE RESEARCH QUESTION

In Chapter 1 (Evidence-Based Practice and the Scientific Method) the formulation of a concise and valid research question was discussed, demonstrating its importance as a taxing but critical exercise. A good research question forms the basis of research because it allows researchers to identify what they want to know. It is the foundation for the rationale and aim. While the process of defining a question has already been addressed in Chapter 1 (Evidence-Based Medicine and the Scientific Method), it is important to incorporate it clearly into the proposal. This may or may not be achieved in the form of a question. In fact, a statement in the form of a question is often not the most appropriate way to define the intended research, but the research focus should build naturally out of the literature review and be clearly identifiable as the problem to be addressed.

The question should also be directly linked to the methodology and how the data will be collected and analyzed. In developing a methodology, the researcher should keep the research question in mind to ensure that the methodology will answer the question. The more general the question, the more difficult it will be to focus in on a measurable outcome. Case example 3.2 suggests some of the challenges in framing a good research question. Other considerations are discussed in Chapter 1 (Evidence-Based Medicine and the Scientific Method).

CASE EXAMPLE 3.2

"Do wait times for appointments negatively impact patients?"

This is a poorly framed research question, as both the nature of the appointments and the scope of "negative impact" are not defined. Instead, identifying what should be measured can better suggest to the reader what information is being requested and how it would be informative. A more appropriate question might be "Does waiting for a radiation therapy consultation appointment increase patient anxiety?" In focusing the question, the researcher is looking at anxiety levels along with wait times. In this example, the second question is much easier to research and focus. The research now has clearly identified that anxiety levels will be measured. It is then important that the measures and methodology chosen will ensure that anxiety levels are indeed what is assessed.

HOT TIP

Revisit the research question occasionally, and repeat literature reviews of the project, as new evidence may be published that may redirect the work.

3.3.6 METHODOLOGY

The study methodology is the means by which the question is proposed to be answered. Within the methodology, the researcher should state how the data will be collected and how it will be analyzed as it relates to the research question. The researcher must demonstrate that the process is systematic and rigourous, with adherence to a strict set of rules, which can be evaluated and reproduced by an independent investigator.[3] Explicit detail in the selection of methodology and data collection must be stated with reference to the research question, providing justification for approach, study population and sample size, and collection tools. The feasibility of implementing the methodology within a given timeframe or setting should also be outlined. This may include anticipating any impact on the clinical department, and plans to mitigate disruption of the study's environment.

Where relevant, the presentation of proposed methodology must describe how consent will be obtained from the participants (*see* Chapter 4: Research Ethics Applications).

HOT TIP

HOT TIP:

The researchers should be able to defend their methodology. It can be helpful to ask the following questions to ensure the feasibility and appropriateness of a selected approach:

Why choose these methods and why are they suitable for this study?

Will my methodology answer my research question?

Are there tools available that I can use to get my data?

Are these tools tested for reliability and validity?

How will the data be analyzed?

Can I do this with the time, funds, populations, expertise, and other resources available to me?

3.3.7 *TIMELINES*

When making a case for research, a detailed account of the steps in the process is warranted. This should indicate each task or step to be completed, in what sequence it will be undertaken, and the objectives at each time point. The researcher must define the tasks and plan a schedule for meeting these deliverables, ensure the task list is as comprehensive as possible and that the schedule is realistic. The use of visual aids such as flowcharts, tables, or a Gantt chart (a type of horizontal bar chart to suggest duration of respective steps) can be used to document the timeline (see also Table 3.2).[4] The timeline can also suggest accountability of each task and can be referenced for determination of authorship at the time of publication. Case example 3.3 outlines a proposed timeline for a simple clinical survey study.

CASE EXAMPLE 3.3

In designing a simple study involving surveying of radiation therapy staff within a single department, the following would be a feasible timeline, from the point of submission to the Research Ethics Board (REB) to the completion of a manuscript reporting the study's findings.

TABLE 3.1 Survey Study Timeline.

Date	Deliverable	Lead (Team Member)
January 5, 2013	Submission to Research Ethics Board (REB)	PI
February, 2013	Introduction to managers	Team
February, 2013	REB revisions	Team
March 1, 2013	Projected approval by REB	
March 15, 2013 (two week open)	Survey distribution	CI
March 22, 2013	1 week reminder	CI
March 29, 2013	2 week reminder (close of survey next day)	CI
Spring/Summer, 2013	Analysis of data	Team
Fall, 2013	Abstract submission for Spring conferences	Team
Fall, 2013/Winter, 2014	Manuscript preparation	Team

ww is through use of a Gantt chart. While it is difficult to present as much information in this format, a Gantt chart often affords a clearer perspective of the distribution of the workload and overlapping tasks.

TABLE 3.2 Gantt Chart.

	2013												2014	
Task	**J**	**F**	**M**	**A**	**M**	**J**	**J**	**A**	**S**	**O**	**N**	**D**	**J**	**F**
Submission to REB														
Introduction to Managers														
REB Revisions														
REB Approval														
Survey Dissemination														
Survey Reminder														
Survey Close														
Data Analysis														
Abstract Submission														
Manuscript														

3.3.8 BUDGET

Most research requires funding. This may be minimal in many cases, with nominal costs such as photocopying, peer-reviewed journal access, and research time being absorbed by a host department. In other cases, costs might be significant or even prohibitive. Funding can be attained via internal (from one's own institution) or external (drug company, charity, sponsorship) sources, and a detailed budget is thus critical to the success of any research proposal. A good budget will itemize all the funds that are necessary to complete the study and provide justification for each expense.[5] The budget should ensure that all estimates are clear and reasonable, and elaborate how each budget line was estimated. The basic budgetary considerations for most research, without consideration of costs for elements unique to a given intervention, are included as Table 3.3.

The cost of research can be divided into direct and indirect costs.

3.3.8.1 DIRECT COSTS

Direct costs are what the PI considers necessary to do the work. Direct costs may include staffing (including benefits), consultants, technical or support staff, equipment, supplies, patient care costs, services, computer hardware and software, postage, photocopying, travel, and other miscellaneous items.[6,7]

3.3.8.2 INDIRECT COSTS

Indirect costs are what the institution pays to support the research.[7] Indirect costs are not always obvious and may include research space, electricity, telephone expenses, and janitorial and security services, if any of these are required beyond the standard demands of the environment in which the study is being conducted. Every project has associated indirect costs. These are real costs and while they may be absorbed by a department, the researcher should nonetheless identify them in the proposal.[5] Indirect costs also include in-kind funding, not calculated in dollars, but in dedicated (protected) time of the researcher or team members.

TABLE 3.3 Cost considerations that may be associated with research.

Cost	Examples and Considerations
Personnel	
Staffing	includes base salary plus benefits (e.g., medical benefits). Staff may include radiation therapists, medical physicists, registered nurses, physicians, or others. In many cases, these items are considered in-kind contributions, and the salaries of investigators are generally not considered here.
Consultants	experts who have specialised knowledge but have a limited role in the study, or are engaged in an isolated element of the conduct of the study. For example, a consultant may be an expert in survey development, and assist in building and validating an online survey tool.[6] This budget line might also include a biostatistician.
Technical/Support staff	research assistants who collect or enter data

TABLE 3.3 *(Continued)*

Cost	Examples and Considerations
Services	costs of paying for a task rather than hiring a person to do the task. For example, paying a data entry company to enter the responses to a survey, or a transcription service to prepare data from focus groups or interviews.[6]
Infrastructure	
Equipment	hire or purchase of equipment specific to the research, such as experimental immobilization devices, ionization chambers,
Computer Hardware/ Software	the hire or purchase of a dedicated computer or laptop for a research assistant. Specialized software for survey development, dosimetry, or statistical analysis must also be considered.
Business Supplies/Services	
Postage	cost of mailing surveys or invitations to participate to study population if done in hard copy.
Photocopying	cost of photocopying consent forms, data collection forms and other necessary documentation (estimate built from cost per page and the number of pages per form[6])
Other Supplies	folders, clipboards, highlighters, and any other supplies necessary for data collection or analysis, especially if required in bulk
Telephone/Conferencing	teleconferencing fees for meetings of the study team if not all at the same site, long distance charges for calling participants, etc.
Travel	
Travel	travel for site visits or training for researchers, and also travel and parking costs for participants if the research requires dedicated travel or appointments).
Dissemination	
Conference Presentation	submission, registration, and presentation at conference to present findings (consider airfare, car rental, fuel, parking, lodging, per diem)[5]
Manuscript Preparation	costs associated with manuscript preparation and publication (especially in open-access journals)

The budget should be as clear and precise as possible. The objective is to convince the reviewers that each item of the budget is absolutely essential to the successful completion of the project.[7] The justification need not be complicated or long, but it should be accurate and as representative of the real costs as possible.[6] In drafting a budget, it is advisable to have the head of department, business administrator, or experienced researcher reviews the figures (projected costs) to ensure that the salaries, employee benefits, and other items are correct. If resources from other departments are involved, those departments may also want to review the budget to ensure the details for the use of their resources are accurate.[7]

If the proposal is successful and the project is funded, the PI has the ultimate responsibility of overseeing the progress of how the funds are being allocated. If the PI decides that money needs to be reallocated from one budget item to another, it may be possible to do so. The PI must be familiar with guidelines for expenditures and communicate with the funding agency and justify his or her decision to reallocate funds. The funding agency will then respond by either accepting or refusing the request.[5,7]

3.3.9 RESEARCHER AND INSTITUTION QUALIFICATIONS

Some research proposals may require validation of the experience and qualifications of the researchers involved. In these cases, the curricula vitae (CVs) of the proposed team members or letter of support from a department head may be attached as appendices. These documents will provide evidence that the researchers have the necessary experience and expertise to conduct their research project safely, effectively, and ethically. It may be necessary to include the qualifications of the investigators' organization as a further means to indicate that adequate facilities and resources will be available for the completion of the study.

3.4 ADDITIONAL CONSIDERATIONS FOR RESEARCH GRANT/ FUNDING PROPOSALS

To support a research project, it may be necessary to apply for financial aid from a research grant or funding organization. This requires considerations in addition to those for a simple research proposal to accompany REB, or a business case to garner departmental support for a project. In medical radiation sciences, funding may be available from a variety of sources including employers, regional or national professional organizations, tertiary academic institutions, product vendors, and other government research funding agencies with a focus in a particular field of research. The successful funding of research is highly dependent on the research team being able to prepare a thorough research proposal that will ultimately convince the selection committee of the necessity of the work being proposed and its overall merit. Applying for funding is a competitive process, and a well-written research proposal will maximize the likelihood of success.

3.4.1 FOLLOW SUBMISSION GUIDELINES

In writing a proposal that will be submitted for a competitive call for funding, the guidelines detailed in the call should be followed. A novice researcher might mistakenly take the instructions to be simply a recommendation, but they are stringent and will be different for each submission. Some example instructions that may be specified include: the number of pages or word count, number of copies to be submitted, and formatting (font style, font size, spacing, and referencing).

3.4.2 LINK TO STRATEGIC DIRECTION

Successful proposals will be closely aligned with the priorities and goals of the organization funding the research. If a research activity is disconnected from the funding organization's mission, vision, values, and goals, or stated purpose of available funds, it will not be considered a priority by reviewers, regardless of the general merit of the proposed work. Focusing on the priorities of the organization providing the funding may increase the likelihood of a proposal receiving funding and support.[2]

3.4.3 LONG-TERM IMPACT

The proposal must revolve around a solid research question, that when answered, will make a significant contribution (big or small) to the base of knowledge on the topic.[8] Researchers must be sure the proposal clearly addresses a problem, while also demonstrating how the proposed research will contribute to improving clinical practice, education, or whatever other end goal is under consideration.[9] Applicants must convince the reviewers that their project will make a real contribution to the state of current knowledge and ultimately to patient care, as there are many worthy research questions and limited resources[8].

3.4.5 *WRITE FOR THE LAY READER*

Research grant applications are typically reviewed by a panel or board. The group of people reviewing the application may include experts in the field of study, but may also include nonexperts or laypeople. The research proposal must be written in clear language that describes the research in a manner that does not require foundational knowledge in the subject area.[1]

HOT TIP

Each funding call receives many applications that the selection committee must review and score. Make sure your proposal is the one that they want to read. The proposal must make a strong and succinct initial argument to sum up the proposal and capture the reviewers' attention, so ensure that your abstract acts as a stand-alone summary of the entire proposal.[10]

The preparation of a successful research proposal may, at first, appear to be an overwhelming task. An effective strategy is to divide the proposal into smaller, more manageable components that once completed, will constitute the proposal in its entirety. This will make the overall task appear more achievable.[11] It is also important to identify available resources that may assist in writing a grant proposal. For example, many hospitals have research departments with personnel who can offer support.[12] Similarly, the involvement of colleagues with experience in research is valuable, as they can reflect on their own experiences and provide coaching and mentorship, critical appraisal, and moral support.[11] Given the amount of work (and often rework) involved, and the number of people who may need to be consulted or engaged in the project, it is also important to start preparing the proposal as far in advance as possible. While great work is often done in the 11th hour, one may run into a roadblock that cannot be addressed hours before the proposal is due. Care taken in preparing a proposal can increase the likelihood that the project will be supported by the necessary stakeholders, such as funders, ethics boards, administration, and those in a position to provide the necessary time to investigators to complete the research. A well-researched and organized proposal will also provide a solid foundation for the research process. Consider it an "upfront investment for downstream return."

HOT TIP

Top five things to avoid while writing your research proposal:

1. Technical language and jargon: This will make your proposal difficult to review, so avoid it as much as possible. If technical words are used, define them clearly.
2. A question that is hard to understand: The research question should not be overly complicated.
3. Too broad a scope: Do not promise too much with a single research study. Future efforts can always build on past research.
4. Methodology or tools that do not answer your research question: Ensure that you consult with experienced researchers to ensure that your methodology will measure the outcome of your work. Be prepared to defend your methodology.
5. Too few (or too many) references: Demonstrate familiarity with the work being done. Present what is already evident in the literature and how it rationalizes your work. Focus on the gaps in the literature and outline how your proposed work will speak to the gap.

KEYWORDS

- Investigators
- Rationale
- Objectives
- Timelines
- Research budget

REFERENCES

1. Barbieri, R. L.; Ladd, K. M.; Hill, J. A. Ten steps to writing a research proposal. *Fertil. Steril.* **1996**, *66(5)*, 690–692.
2. Bliss, D. Z. Writing a grant proposal: part 6: the budget, budget justification, and resource environment. *J. Wound Ostomy Continence Nurs.* **2005,** *32(6)*, 365–367.
3. Ellett, M. L. Budget for a research proposal. *Gastroenterol Nurs.* **1993**, *15(5)*, 205–207.
4. Clark, W.; Polakow, W. N. The Gantt Chart. London, 1952.
5. Merrill, K. C. Developing an effective quantitative research proposal. *J. Infus. Nurs.* **2011**, *34(3)*, 181–186.
6. Paterson, B. Writing a successful research proposal. *The Canadian Nurse*. **2002**, *98(7)*, 16–17.
7. Parahoo, K. Nursing research: principles, process and issues; Palgrave Macmillan: New York NY, 2006.
8. Shortell, S. M., The emergence of qualitative methods in health services research. Health. Serv. Res. **1999**, *34(5 Pt 2)*, 1083–1090.
9. Smajdor, A.; Sydes, M. R.; Gelling, L.; Wilkinson, M. Applying for ethical approval for research in the United Kingdom. *BMJ* **2009**, *339*, b4013.
10. American Psychological Association. Publication Practices and Responsible Authorship. http://www.apa.org/research/responsible/publication/index.aspx (accessed August 4, 2013).
11. Vivar, C. G.; McQueen, A.; Whyte, D. A.; Armayor, N. C. Getting started with qualitative research: developing a research proposal. *Nurse Res.* **2007**, *14(3)*, 60–73.
12. Bowling, A. Health care research methods. Part 2. *Nurs. Stand.* **1991,** *5(49)*, 33–35.

CHAPTER 4

RESEARCH ETHICS APPLICATION

LAURA D'ALIMONTE MRT(T) BSc MHSc

Clinical Specialist Radiation Therapist, Odette Cancer Centre, Sunnybrook Health Sciences Centre, Toronto Canada
Lecturer, Department of Radiation Oncology, University of Toronto, Toronto Canada

BONNIE BRISTOW MRT(T) BSc
Research Radiation Therapist, Odette Cancer Centre, Sunnybrook Health Sciences Centre, Toronto Canada

ROSANNA MACRI MRT(T) BSc MHSc
Ethicist, Ontario Shores Centre for Mental Health Sciences, Whitby Canada
Lecturer, Department of Radiation Oncology, University of Toronto, Toronto Canada

CONTENTS

An important component of conducting any research study is the ethical considerations that should be addressed before embarking on the research journey. For research involving human subjects, ethical considerations must ensure that research is conducted in a manner that respects the inherent worth of all human beings including their right to information, safety and wellbeing.

4.1 HISTORICAL PERSPECTIVE

4.1.1 BACKGROUND

Research has enriched and improved the lives of millions of patients receiving radiation therapy. There have been significant advances that have been made possible as a result of this research. For example, in a recent and relatable context, novel research conducted by the University of Toronto on Stereotactic Body Radiotherapy (SBRT) for the treatment of spinal metastases has led to the increased knowledge of the efficacy and safety of this highly precise treatment. Published work describes the experiences of the institution, from theory to practical details of the technique as a guide for other interested institutions.[1] An essential principle of ethics is that although research can benefit society, it can also cause harm. There is therefore an inherent responsibility to ensure that research meets high scientific and ethical standards that respect and protect participants. This necessitates a thorough assessment of the entire study protocol, including the purpose and hypothesis, study design, study populations, interventions or procedures, as well as data analysis and dissemination of the information learned during the course of a research study.

People participate in research for various reasons, either because they can benefit directly from the study, as in clinical trials (*see* Chapter 8: Clinical Trials), or because their participation will contribute to the expansion of knowledge and may benefit others in the future. Research, therefore, must be conducted in an ethical manner to ensure public confidence.[2]

The purpose of all research is to search for an answer to something that is poorly understood or is unknown. In many instances, this exploration may expose both participants and researchers to inherent risks.[2] Patients may be exposed to unexpected side effects or toxicities of novel treatment modalities. Novice researchers may be vulnerable to coercion from supervisors to conduct research in unsafe conditions. These risks may range from insignificant to consequential. Before the routine implementation of Research Ethics Boards (REBs) in academic healthcare centres, several research studies were conducted that resulted in participants being harmed, at times resulting in death. Case Example 4.1 reflects on one such study, the Tuskegee Syphilis Experiments in the United States.

CASE EXAMPLE 4.1

Tuskegee Syphilis Experiments

Between 1932 and1972, the United States Public Health Service conducted the infamous Tuskegee syphilis experiment.[3] The purpose of this clinical trial was to study the natural progression of untreated syphilis in rural African American men. Approximately 600 impoverished labourers (399 with syphilis + 201 control group without syphilis) were recruited and told that by participating in this study they would receive free medical care, meals, and free burial insurance. The participants were informed that they were being treated for "bad blood," however the men were never told of their syphilis diagnosis or that their doctors had no intention of treating their disease. Instead the researcher waited for the participants to die to collect their data.[4]

While this is an extreme example, ethical principles and guidelines are important to protect and respect participants and to prevent a repeat of such injustices. Canada's Tri-Council Policy Statement (TCPS, and TCPS-2) is a joint policy of three federal research agencies, which promotes the ethical conduct of research involving humans, and is considered the national standard. The three federal agencies represented by the TCPS-2 are; the Canadian Institutes of Health Research (CIHR), the Natural Sciences and Engineering Research Council of Canada (NSERC), and the Social Sciences and Humanities Research Council of Canada (SSHRC).[2] The policy is based on the underlying value of respect for human dignity, which is expressed through the three core principles: respect for persons, concern for welfare, and justice. Respect for human dignity incorporates the moral obligation to respect autonomy and the inherent worth of all human beings while protecting those with developing, impaired or diminished autonomy.

4.1.2 HISTORICAL CONTEXT

Experimentation on human subjects has a tragic history. One of the most memorable and arguably extreme example of experimentation without restrictions occurred in Nazi Germany during World War II.[5] During this time, selected prisoners were subjected to various experiments which were designed to help German military personnel in combat situations to aid in the recovery of military personnel who had been injured, and to advance the racial ideology backed by the Third Reich.[6] For example, there were studies to learn how to treat hypothermia. In one experiment, subjects were forced to endure a tank of ice water for up to three hours. In another, naked prisoners were forced to remain outside in below freezing temperatures for several hours. The researcher then assessed various methods of rewarming the survivors.

Modern research ethics came into existence as a result of these World War II atrocities. The Nuremberg Military Tribunals, held from 1945 to 1946, included the Doctors' Trial, which specifically focused on the medical doctors accused of participating in Nazi human experimentation.[7] The Nuremberg Code was drafted as a result of the Tribunals. This Code outlined standards for judging physicians and scientists who had conducted experiments on concentration camp prisoners and became the prototype of later codes intended to assure that research involving human subjects would be carried out in an ethical manner.

Unfortunately, despite the introduction of the Nuremburg Code, several unethical studies continued to take place in North America and around the world. For instance in the United States, during the Cold War years from 1944 to 1974, more than 4,000 secret and classified radiation experiments were conducted by the Atomic Energy Commission (AEC) and other government agencies, exposing thousands of unknowing and innocent American citizens to radioactive fallout. Another infamous study, conducted on more than 700 American mentally disabled children until the 1970s, purposefully infected students from Willowbrook State School in Staten Island New York with hepatitis.[8] These types of experiments were recognized internationally as inhumane and unethical and gave rise to several other codes.

The most influential ethics codes developed to guide human experimentation include:[9]

- The Nuremberg Code (1947): consists of 10 research ethics principles[10]
- Declaration of Helsinki (1964, revised in 1975, 1983, 1989, and 1996): developed by the World Medical Association to guide primarily physicians conducting medical research involving human subjects. This was the first significant attempt from the medical community to regulate research itself[11]
- Belmont Report (1979): developed by the National Commission for the Protection of Human Subjects of Biomedical and Behavioral Research, United States Government to guide American researchers; prompted in part by problems arising from the Tuskegee Syphilis Study and was meant to provide broad principles to guide ethical decision making in research[12]
- International Ethical Guidelines for Biomedical Research Involving Human Subjects (1982, revised in 1993): developed by the Council for International Organizations of Medical Sciences in collaboration with World Health Organization to apply the Declaration of Helsinki in developing countries engaging in large-scale trials of vaccines and drugs along with other research

Many others followed including the TCPS, published in 1998 and revised in 2010. This is an evolving and living document.[2] The TCPS guides Canadian researchers in the conduct of research involving humans and describes the principle standards and procedures for governing research on human subjects in Canada and abroad. Research projects must also comply with relevant federal and provincial laws. For instance, all research must be conducted under privacy legislation and adherence to confidentiality and security requirements. Any investigator in the research team must be appropriately trained to ensure confidentiality and proper ethical protocol. The Interagency Advisory Panel on Research Ethics provides an online tutorial course available online.[13] Some research institutions have made this tutorial mandatory for REB review.

4.1.3 WHY ETHICS REVIEWS ARE NECESSARY

Research studies promote evidence-based practice and should meet the highest scientific merit (social and scientific value and validity) in addition to ethical standards prior to commencement of the research. Study investigators and ethics personnel are responsible not only to advance knowledge but to also ensure that all participants are protected and not exposed to more than minimal risk. Minimal risk research, as defined by the TCPS-2, is "research in which the probability and magnitude of possible harms implied by participation in the research is no greater than those encountered by participants in those aspects of their everyday life that related to the research.[2]" There should be a suitable process for obtaining informed consent, a system for fair and equitable subject selection, and protection of participant privacy and confidentiality.

Institutions create REBs to determine the ethical acceptability of any research that involves humans, which is under the auspices of the institution or conducted by their faculty, staff or students. This is independent of where the research is conducted. Most institutions issue annual reports to summarize activities and exhibit accountability. REBs must be independent in their decision making. They are able to approve, reject, propose modifications, suspend, or terminate any proposed or ongoing research according to the institution's policies, national and international documents and pertinent laws.

The REB is an independent committee composed of medical professionals and lay members with a variety of expertise relevant to the research disciplines and methodologies covered by the REB. Membership and size of the REB varies with institutions and should ensure competent independent research ethics review. Members come from a wide range of disciplines including ethics, law and will include at least one member of the public with no affiliation with the institution to help expand the perspective and ensure accountability to the community. Knowledge of research ethics involving humans is important. To ensure independence of REB decisions, the REB should maintain an arm's length relationship with the institution, and institutional senior administrators should not serve on the REB.

4.2 PREPARING THE SUBMISSION

Most REBs have stringent guidelines, which need to be reviewed prior to submission preparation. If there are questions or uncertainties regarding the process, the REB office should be contacted for clarification. Understanding the submission process and what forms are required for submission is important to ensure timelines are met and there are no surprises that will preclude or delay approval. For some review processes, multiple sets of the entire submission package might be required.

The REB submission package generally contains the following documents:

- REB application form
- study protocol
- consent forms
- subject recruitment procedures such as posters
- any written information to be provided to subjects
- data collection tools such as interview scripts, questionnaires, and templates for recording data from chart reviews
- information about payments and compensation available to subjects
- current curriculum vitae of the investigator(s)
- any other supporting documents that the REB may request

A checklist may be provided by the REB and can help with the organization of the submission. It may be required for the checklist to be submitted with the rest of the documents. All recruitment materials including letters, posters, and advertisements must include version dates and be approved by the REB. Telephone recruitment materials in the form of a telephone script must also be approved.

Many institutions are moving towards an online submission portal to manage and track submissions. This saves on paper, but may also add a layer of complexity to the process if registration and training are required.

The researcher should investigate such requirements well in advance, and seek assistance as necessary.

4.2.1 ETHICAL CONSIDERATIONS

REB application forms vary from institution to institution. However, there are certain commonalities that can be expected. These sections may present in a different order or under various headings, but will generally include the following considerations.

4.2.1.1 IDENTIFICATION OF THE TEAM

Information regarding the research team provides insight to the responsibility and accountability of those conducting the work, as outlined in Chapter 3 (Research Proposals). The Principal Investigator (PI) is the responsible leader for the research team. The PI must ensure compliance with institutional requirements, and must be an employee or have an appointment at the institution. A current curriculum vitae and any other relevant documentation should be available upon request. The investigators should be qualified by education, training, and experience, should meet all the qualifications specified by the applicable regulatory requirements, and should provide evidence of such qualifications through up-to-date curriculum vitae and other relevant documentation requested by the REB.

It is important that researchers be completely familiar with the appropriate use of any investigational products used in the study, in the product information, and in other information sources provided. Everyone assisting with the study should also be properly informed about the protocol, the investigational products, and their respective study-related roles. The PI and coinvestigators (CI) should have received training in research ethics. The REB may require that researchers complete a form of training in research ethics or good research practice before REB approval will be granted. Many institutions now have onsite clinical research courses that can be taken by employees to acquaint them with the guidelines and policies related to the conduct of appropriate and ethical research.

For example, TCPS-2 has an online tutorial, which gives an introduction to TCPS-2 for researchers and REB members. An international standard known as Good Clinical Practice (GCP) has also been defined by the International Conference on Harmonization to guide clinical trials involving human subjects, and many institutions have developed formalized training courses to prepare researchers for the ethical conduct of research. *See* Chapter 8 (Clinical Trials) for more information on GCP.

HOT TIP

The PI is the leader of the research team and is responsible for the conduct of the research, and for the actions of any member of the research team. If the PI or other members of the team are no longer participating in this research, or if they have left for another institution, the REB must be notified in writing and a new, equally competent individual should assume the new role of PI.

4.2.1.2 DISCLOSURE OF CONFLICT OF INTEREST

Any real, potential or perceived individual or institutional conflicts of interest (COI) that may have an impact on the proposed research must be disclosed by the researchers. To preserve the independence and integrity of ethics review, it is important that members of the REB also avoid any perceived conflicts of interest. The REB should have a method to acknowledge and resolve COIs declared by investigators by obtaining full information on the COI; assessing the likelihood that their judgment may be influenced; and assessing the possibility of harm that is likely to result. The REB must act independently from the parent institution and its autonomy must be respected by the institution. The REB should assess the probability that the researcher's prudence may be influenced by private or personal interests, and assess the severity of any harm that may result.

Appearance of a conflict may be as damaging as a real conflict. The REB may require that the researcher renounce the interests in conflict. In that case the researcher may be asked to withdraw from the research or allow others to make the research-related decisions. Prospective study participants need to know about any potential COIs to make an informed decision whether to participate. COIs may also undermine the respect for participants that is basic to the principle of Justice. Dual roles of researchers and their associated obligations such as acting as both a researcher and a radiation therapist treating a given participant, may create conflicts, power imbalances, undue influences, or coercion that could affect relationships with others and decision making.

4.2.3 STUDY SUMMARY

The REB requires a clear picture of what is proposed to be done, including why the study is being conducted, the specific research question that the researcher hopes to answer, a detailed description of the design of the study, the number of participants required to conduct the study (including inclusion and exclusion criteria and sample size justification) and a detailed description of the study intervention. The latter includes the standard of care, risks, duration of study visits and extra time commitment for participants, and data analysis.

4.2.4 RECRUITMENT AND CONSENT

A detailed description of the recruitment process will be required in this section. Specific items to address include how the participants will be recruited, who will recruit, and who will obtain consent. Consideration must be given for those participants who are incapable of providing consent. If a substitute decision-maker is required, the process for identifying this individual must be outlined. In addition, if communication difficulties exist (e.g., potential participant does not speak English), any measures in place to address these barriers should also be identified.

Consent in healthcare is commonly defined as the "autonomous authorization of a medical intervention by individual patients.[2]" For the purpose of this chapter, the term consent means free, informed and ongoing autonomous authorization of participation in research by an individual.[2] There are three components to consent: disclosure, capacity and voluntariness.[2] Therefore, an individual participating in research should do so freely and without coercion, force, or manipulation. The participant should be fully informed of all relevant information including potential risks and benefits as well as be able to understand the information and appreciate the potential consequences of his or her decision. Certain factors may lessen a person's capacity to exercise autonomy, such as insufficient information or understanding. Participants may be concerned about alienating authority figures, such as caregivers, researchers, or the community to which they belong. Other limitations may include barriers to accessing resources. These factors need to be addressed prior to any research being carried out, to ensure participants are sufficiently protected.

Some people may be unable to exercise the autonomy necessary for participation in research, such as children and those who lack the necessary mental capacity due to progression of disease or other cognitive impairments. Those individuals who lack capacity to make their own decisions may still be able to participate in the decision-making process.[2] Additional measures are needed to protect these individuals and to ensure that their wishes are respected. These measures will generally include getting consent from an authorized third party who is entrusted to make decisions on behalf of the prospective participant. While considerations for these populations tend to relate more to consent to treatment, there are still instances where their inclusion in research may be valuable. A paediatric oncology nurse at the Princess Margaret Cancer Centre in Toronto reflects on considerations in consenting children for research in Case example 4.2.

CASE EXAMPLE 4.2

Needs Assessment of Paediatric Radiation Therapy Patients towards the Development of a Computer-based Educational Program.

Susan Awrey RN BScN

Paediatric Radiation Nurse Coordinator Princess Margaret Cancer Centre/The Hospital for Sick Children, Toronto, Canada

The following is an example of research involving paediatric radiation therapy patients and their parents at Princess Margaret Cancer Centre and the Hospital for Sick Children.

The paediatric population is quite challenging when it comes to research projects given the age of the child or teenager, their developmental age, and medical condition. Many times we are speaking directly to the parents or guardians and must be reminded to talk with the patient as well. In efforts to develop a computer-based educational tool as collaboration between the Princess Margaret Cancer Centre and the Hospital for Sick Children in Toronto, it was felt to be important to get the input of the target population in guiding development of the resource. The first stage of research for our educational tool was the needs assessment for a computer-based program about paediatric radiation. The questions involved computer use, games, preferences on the computer, and questions regarding their disease and treatment. The parents were also asked questions about resources, computer use, and understanding of their child's disease.

The research project relied on children ages 4–12. This is an age where the parent would need to give consent for the project but because we were interviewing the children and asking for their ideas and input, we also needed their assent. We first approached the parents about the project, the expectations, and our goals, prior to obtaining consent. If they agreed, we would then approach the child. The children were required to give assent to the project as well before we could continue. The project was explained to them in terms they could understand based on their age and development. The child and parents were told that they should feel free not to answer the questions if they felt uncomfortable and could stop at any time. All the children approached gave their assent to proceed with the project.

Although the paediatric population involves many challenges, these patients are integral to their own treatment journey and all components of it, including research initiatives. These children have been through many procedures and processes, and have a greater understanding than we often give them credit for!

Researchers must disclose all information related to free and informed consent, including sufficient opportunities to discuss and consider participation. Consent is dependent on capacity, the ability to understand the elements of the information relating to the decision, and the ability to appreciate any reasonably foreseeable consequences of participating or not participating in that specific research project. If the individual cannot give consent, a substitute decision-maker may do this. Researchers must also be aware of possible coercion due to their clinical influence over the prospective participants and must be sensitive to the power imbalance in employment; some employees may believe they have no choice when approached by their employer or manager to participate in research. In the case of educational research, this might apply to the teacher and student relationship.

Informed consent should include explanations of the following:

- that the study involves research
- purpose of the study
- study treatments or intervention that differs from the standard of care
- probability for random assignment to each treatment
- study procedures to be followed, including all invasive procedures

Additionally, the participant's responsibilities, any risks or inconveniences to the subject, and anticipated benefits should be explained. If there is no intended clinical benefit to the subject, the subject should also be informed of this.

Alternative procedures or courses of treatment that may be available, and their important potential benefits and risks must be made known to the participant. The subject must understand that participation in the study is voluntary and that they may refuse to participate or withdraw from the study at any time without suffering any repercussions.

Most REBs have strict requirements regarding the contents of the informed consent form. Some REBs provide an ICF template for researchers to use to guide them in creating a form. A separate consent form must be written for different groups within the same study, such as control groups and investigational groups.

4.2.5 RISKS, BENEFITS, AND SAFETY OF PARTICIPATION

It is the responsibility of the research team to describe any potential harms or benefits to be expected for participants in the research study. When describing these it is important to include not only the potential physical harms but also any anticipated psychological factors that may harm the participant. For example, a study asking cancer survivors how they felt when they were first diagnosed or going through treatment may evoke suppressed or unresolved emotions. In the case of providers or students as participants, it should be clear that refusal to participate would not impact employment or status in an academic program. Also, any information disclosed or collected in the course of the study cannot be provided to an employer or instructor. Risks, benefits, and reassurances relevant to the study and to the population at hand should be presented clearly in the proposal and in related participant consent forms. The members of the REB will use this information and weigh the potential risks against the potential benefits during the review process.

Participants should not be expected to incur expenses that are a direct result from participating in the research study. Therefore, participant reimbursement may be considered. This could cover such expenses as travel and parking. Participant payment should be disclosed in this section and include what is being reimbursed and in what form the reimbursement will be provided. It is important to note that reimbursement should be for expenses, time, or inconvenience only and should not be used to encourage participation in the research study. This might be seen as coercion to participate or to prompt certain responses or results from participants.

4.2.6 PRIVACY AND CONFIDENTIALITY

Personal information must be treated in a confidential manner and participant anonymity must be maintained at all times.[2] The Canadian Constitution guarantees basic rights and freedoms which include protection of privacy.[14] There are inherent risks related to the identification of participants and the potential harms they may experience. These risks may occur at any point in the research including data collection and analysis, dissemination of results, storage and retention of information, and disposal of records or information storage devices. Consent includes the right to privacy.

Researchers and institutions performing research have an ethical duty and an obligation to guard confidential information. This includes the protection of information from unauthorized access, use, disclosure, modification, loss or theft. Confidentiality is essential for trust between the researcher and research subject as well as for the integrity of the research study. Assurance of confidentiality involves several considerations:

Physical security – the safeguard information through use of locked filing cabinets, and locating computers containing research data away from public domain.

Technical safeguards – use of encryption, computer passwords, antiviral software, firewalls and other measures that protect data from unauthorized access, modification or loss.

Administrative security – development and enforcement of rules regarding who can access personal information about participants

Ethical concerns about privacy diminish as it becomes more difficult to link information to a particular individual. Researchers should consult the REB if they are unsure whether information is identifiable. The REB requires details regarding the measures for safeguarding information and for its collection, purpose, dissemination, retention and/or disposal. Researchers should determine privacy risks and threats to the security of information at all stages of the research life cycle, and ensure proper measures are in place to protect information.

4.2.7 FUNDING, CONTRACTS, AND AGREEMENTS

Full disclosure of funding sources (if applicable), the nature of the funding source (e.g., industry, funding agency) and the status of the funding is required. It may be important to consider how the study will be conducted should funding not be obtained. This can help the REB to determine if the necessary resources are in place and if the team has adequately prepared for any costs inherent in realizing the project.

The itemized budget from the proposal is required with the submission package to demonstrate that there are sufficient funds for the study and to determine whether there are related COIs. An example of a COI related to funding would be an investigator receiving a direct personal payment for the research. The itemized study budget should reflect all costs associated with the completion of the study (e.g., database extraction, student payments, participant reimbursement) (*see* Chapter 3: Research Proposals). The REB must be assured that studies have sufficient funds to complete the proposed research. Exposing research subjects to potential harms and inconveniences of research without secured funding and the prospect of project completion is unethical.

4.3 SUBMISSION PROCESS

4.3.1 TYPES OF REVIEWS

The REB adjusts the level of review to the level of risk presented by the research, a proportionate approach, and assesses the research by considering risks, benefits and ethical implications of the proposed investigation. Two types of review are possible; one is an expedited (or delegated) review and the other is a full board review. Research that has a lower level of risk involved may qualify for an delegated review, including studies involving only current standards of care or with prior approval from another REB. All other studies require a full board review.

4.3.1.1 DELEGATED (EXPEDITED) REVIEW

A delegated REB review may involve a subcommittee of the REB and is delegated to an individual or individuals from the REB. Studies that qualify for delegated review include:

- research protocols that involve minimal risk
- amendments to already approved (non Health Canada) protocols where there is no increase in risks of human research participants
- chart reviews
- database development

- annual renewals of currently approved minimal risk research or where the research does not involve new interventions to current participants
- renewal that does not involve the recruitment of new participants, and where the remaining research activities are limited to data analysis

Delegated reviewers may confer with other reviewers in the REB or refer projects back to the full REB if they decide that full board review is required. If delegates refuse ethics approval, the full REB will review the study before communicating the decision to the researcher.

4.3.1.2 FULL BOARD REVIEW

A Full Board review will be indicated for a study that qualifies as involving greater than minimal risk. It is thus assigned for review by the entire REB. Full Board review studies include:

- clinical trials of drugs, devices, natural health products or psychosocial interventions
- investigations that collect significant personal health information
- investigations where the participant population is particularly vulnerable (children, pregnant women, minority groups etc.)

4.3.2 WHEN TO SUBMIT

All documentation for any study must be submitted to the REB for approval before recruitment or data collection begins. A submitted protocol may be prescreened to provide an assessment of whether the protocol qualifies for an expedited or delegated review or if it must go through a Full Board review. Any queries are sent to the Principal Investigator.

4.3.3 TIMELINES FOR THE REVIEW PROCESS

It is important to ensure there is sufficient time allowed for REB submissions. REBs have regular meetings to review research applications that are not assigned to delegated review. Frequency and timelines will vary with institutions and the volume of research that is conducted. Some institutions have specific submission deadline dates for new submissions while others have no posted deadlines and are reviewed on a first-come, first-served basis.

The length of time to be expected for a new study to be approved by REB is dependent upon the quality and completeness of the submission as well as whether the review is delegated or Full Board. Other factors include the complexity of the study, any risks that are involved, the availability of reviewers, and the time taken by investigators to respond to the REB with any required revisions. A decision from the board can be expected approximately six to eight weeks after submission, though this may depend on the size and process of individual REBs.

4.4 RESEARCH ETHICS BOARD DECISIONS

REB decisions are based on current scientific and ethical standards to protect participants. After review, individual proposals will be referred back to the primary investigator with comments and/or suggestions for revision. The REB will provide in writing their approval of the study, or indicate their requirement for more information, clarification, or modifications. If they require any changes, the researcher is responsible for addressing them and resubmitting the amended protocol to the REB. After approval has been granted, the study may be opened and recruitment and data collection may commence. The REB will provide in writing the decision of the ethical review of the study.[2] REB decisions can take one of two forms; approval or approval pending revisions. In either scenario, the REB will provide a letter outlining terms of condition, comments from the board, requirements for more information, clarification or modifications.[15]

4.4.1 APPROVAL PENDING REVISIONS

This is the most common response to receive from the REB. In this situation, the REB requires changes, clarification, or modifications to occur before approval is granted. It is the responsibility of the researcher to address each of the comments of the review board and to resubmit all amendments. In addition it is the responsibility of the researcher to have obtained final approval from the REB before proceeding with study activation.

4.4.2 *APPROVAL*

When approval is obtained, either outright or after revisions, the REB will submit a letter outlining successful study approval. This approval letter will contain a unique study identification number, which should be quoted when any further communication occurs with the REB. In addition, the approval letter will reference all approved study sheets with the approved version date. Most REBs maintain stringent working guidelines; it is a good idea to review these guidelines before commencing any study.[2]

Generally, REB applications are approved for one year. If the study takes longer than one year to complete, the application will need to be renewed. If any significant changes or unanticipated adverse events occur during the research process, the researcher is required to report this to the REB.

4.4.3 *AMENDMENTS*

Possibly, initial implementation of methodology or preliminary results may provide insight that suggests the need for a change to the initial study protocol. Any desire to deviate from the initially approved protocol (be it a change in recruitment, intervention, or administrative changes such as the addition of a coinvestigator) must be approved by the REB prior to implementation. For minor deviations, this can often be accomplished through submission of an REB amendment. Standardized forms can guide the PI through submission of an amendment, and criteria are normally made available that can suggest the magnitude of change that requires an amendment as opposed to an entirely new REB submission. Amendments can often be approved in a shorter period of time than would be required for a full submission.

4.4.4 ANNUAL RENEWAL

If the research is not completed after one year, a study renewal form will be required after that initial year for annual study renewal. The annual renewal normally consists of the submission of a form which should contain an overview of the study to date including:

- accrual to date (recruitment or collection of necessary sample size)
- anticipated accrual
- number of participants on active treatment
- number of participants in follow up
- any minor or major deviations from protocol

When a study is complete, a study completion or closure report must be sent to the REB indicating study closure.

Research contributes to the foundational knowledge of all healthcare professions and aids in driving healthcare forward. All modern day research is driven by ethical principles, which aim to protect participants. Therefore, ethical considerations regarding the research design must be considered before the research study begins. To ensure research is conducted in an ethical manner, submission to and approval from local research ethics boards must be obtained prior to conducting any research activity.

Once REB approval is obtained, the research can then be commenced. It is important to keep ethical considerations and principles in mind throughout the process of conducting the research and executing the methodology outlined in the proposal and REB application.

HOT TIP

Tips for REB Success:

1. Carefully review the submission process prior to application.
2. Contact the REB if you are unsure of how to fill out forms, seek signatures, or address certain items.
3. Give yourself enough time!
4. Review, and ask others to review, your submission package prior to submitting.

KEYWORDS

- Nuremburg Code
- Research Ethics Board
- Informed consent
- Conflict of interest
- Confidentiality
- Research protocol

REFERENCES

1. Sangha, A.; Korol, R.; Sahgal, A. Stereotactic body radiotherapy for the treatment of spinal metastases: an overview of the University of Toronto, Sunnybrook Health Sciences Odette Cancer Centre, technique. *J. Med. Imag. Radiat. Sci.* **2013,** *44(3),* 126–133.
2. Canadian Institutes of Health Research; Natural Sciences and Engineering Research Council of Canada; and Social Sciences and Humanities Research Council of Canada. Tri-Council Policy Statement: Ethical Conduct for Research Involving Humans. Interagency Secretariat on Research Ethics: Ottawa, Canada, 2005.
3. Kenny S.C. Tuskegee Syphilis Experiment. In: Encyclopedia of Jim Crow; Brown, N., Stentiford, B., Eds. Greenwood Press: Westport, CT, 2008.
4. Jones, J. H. Bad Blood: The Tuskegee Syphilis Experiment.; Free Press: New York, 1993.
5. Katz, J.; Capron, A. M.; Glass, E. S. Experimentation with human beings–The authority of the investigator, subject, profession, and state in the human experimentation process, 1st ed.; Russell Sage Foundation: New York, 1972.
6. Advisory Committee on Human Radiation Experiments. Postwar Professional Standards and Practices for Human Experimentation. In: The Human Radiation Experiments: Final Report of the Advisory Committee; Advisory Committee on Human Radiation Experiments; Oxford University Press: New York, 1996; pp. 74–96.
7. Advisory Committee on Human Radiation Experiments. Government Standards for Human Experiments: The 1960s and 1970s. In The Human Radiation Experiments: Final Report of the Advisory Committee; Advisory Committee on Human Radiation Experiments; Oxford University Press: New York, 1996; pp. 97–109.
8. Krugman, S. The Willowbrook hepatitis studies revisited: ethical aspects. *Rev. Infect. Dis.* **1986,** *8(1)*, 157–162.
9. Emanuel, E. J.; Wendler, D.; Grady, C. What makes clinical research ethical? *JAMA*. **2000,** *283(20)*, 2701–2711.

10. US Government Printing Office. The Nuremberg Code: Trials of war criminals before the Nuremberg military tribunals under control council law No 10. US Government Printing Office: Washington DC, 1949.
11. World Medical Association. WMA Declaration of Helsinki – Ethical Principles for Medical Research Involving Human Subjects. http://www.wma.net/en/30publications/10policies/b3/index.html (accessed July 24, 2013).
12. The National Commission for the Protection of Human Subjects of Biomedical and Behavioral Research. The Belmont report: Ethical principles and guidelines for the protection of human subjects of research. ERIC Clearinghouse: Bethesda, MD, 1978.
13. Government of Canada, Panel on Research Ethics. The TCPS 2 Tutorial Course on Research Ethics (CORE). http://www.ethics.gc.ca/eng/education/tutorial-didacticiel (Accessed September 15, 2013).
14. Dodek, A., The Canadian Constitution. Dundurn: Toronto, 2013.
15. Holden, L.; Stanford, J.; Barker, R., Clinical Research Made Easy—A Guide for Research in Radiation Therapy. *J. Med. Imag. Radiat. Sci.* **2009,** *40(4)*, 160–164.

PART 2
METHODOLOGIES

CHAPTER 5

QUANTITATIVE METHODOLOGIES AND ANALYSIS

MICHAEL VELEC MRT(T) BSc PhD(c)
Radiation Therapist, Radiation Medicine Program, Princess Margaret Cancer Centre, Toronto Canada

SHAO HUI (SOPHIE) HUANG MRT(T) MSc
Radiation Therapist, Radiation Medicine Program, Princess Margaret Cancer Centre, Toronto Canada
Assistant Professor, Department of Radiation Oncology, University of Toronto, Toronto Canada

CONTENTS

Quantitative research is a process of using numerical data to systematically obtain information, and is commonly used for testing hypotheses. The characteristics of quantitative research include using numbers to summarize findings, looking for relationships between variables, and comparing differences between or among groups. Quantitative research is quite different from qualitative research. It often starts with a certain hypothesis or theory, and uses an experimental design to test it. Qualitative research, in contrast, often uses a more holistic perspective to generate a theory (*see* Chapter 6: Qualitative Methodologies and Analysis).

Although the two research approaches are quite different in many aspects, they both are systematic approaches that can be used for the same topic and can often be complimentary to each other. Consider the example of assessing pain experienced by a patient. One could phrase an open-ended question such as "describe your pain" which is a qualitative approach. Alternatively, one could request that the patient rate his or her current level of pain from a scale from 0 (not having any pain) and 10 (the most excruciating pain). This allows the respondent to numerically weigh the degree of pain, and provides the researcher with different information. The latter is the quantitative approach, and the data collected can be of greater or lesser value to the researcher, depending on the intent of the research.

This chapter focuses on the application of quantitative research methods to design a study aimed at testing a hypothesis in a rigourous and scientifically valid manner.

5.1 STUDY DESIGN: BASIC CONSIDERATIONS

5.1.1 STUDY DESIGN

5.1.1.1 RETROSPECTIVE RESEARCH

A quantitative research study can be classified as retrospective if a study is conducted using existing data, or prospective if the study data is not yet available and will be collected once started. For example, assessing setup variation using previously acquired cone-beam computed tomography

(CBCT) images on patients who have already been treated would be a retrospective study design. Given that the outcomes are likely already known, the focus of the study is on the factors that might have contributed to these outcomes.

5.1.1.2 PROSPECTIVE RESEARCH DESIGN

A prospective study is focused on the outcome. Collecting setup variation information for patients to be treated in the next three months would be prospective. Prospective studies can be further classified as being nonexperimental or observational (i.e., no intervention is given), or as being experimental in nature. Ideally, an experimental design involves a controlled intervention assignment under a controlled manner, and includes a control group where no intervention is performed. An example is a randomized control trial (*see* Chapter 8: Clinical Trials). The basic process is illustrated in Figure 5.1.

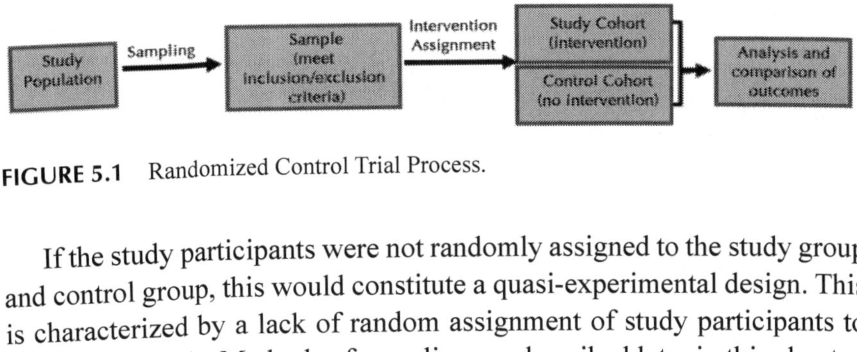

FIGURE 5.1 Randomized Control Trial Process.

If the study participants were not randomly assigned to the study group and control group, this would constitute a quasi-experimental design. This is characterized by a lack of random assignment of study participants to prospective study. Methods of sampling are described later in this chapter.

The strength and limitations of these two methods are outlined in Table 5.1.

TABLE 5.1 Strengths and limitations of prospective and retrospective research.

Type of Study Design	Strengths	Limitations
Prospective	Control of sample size and data quality Less likelihood of missing data Ability to balance confounding factors	Often requires consent of participants Less control of timeline for recruitment and data collection
Retrospective	Easy to conduct Ability to control timeline	Less control of sample size and data quality Susceptible to missing data and imbalance of confounding factors

5.1.2 CHOOSING STUDY ENDPOINTS

In an experimental design, the primary endpoint of a study is the measured outcome of interest for two or more groups. Although many outcomes are measured in clinical research, in practice one should identify the most important outcomes for designing the study, and consider others to be secondary or exploratory endpoints. Later in the chapter, it will be demonstrated how choosing the primary endpoint affects the required sample size and the statistical tests required.

5.1.2.1 VARIABLES

The term variable is often used to describe the data endpoint in a study. There are two types: independent and dependent variables. Independent variables are tested by the researcher, and have a presumed influence on the dependent variable. For example, when one investigates whether weight loss during radiation therapy may result in a change in setup accuracy, weight loss is the independent variable and setup accuracy is the dependent variable. For a retrospective study, the researcher should therefore select enough patients from each group (patients with weight and patients with no weight loss) and measure the setup accuracy of all of them to assess any differences between groups.

To make the measurement consistent, it is important to clearly define the variable in advance so others can measure the variable under the same conditions. The definition of the variable should be unambiguous, reproducible, and as specific as possible. An example concerning the evaluation of time-saving with the use of volumetric modulated arc therapy (VMAT) is presented as Case example 5.1.

HOT TIP

Selection of the study endpoint is an important element of quantitative study design. The following questions can guide the researcher in this process:

- What has been done in the literature?
- Which variables should be measured to best serve your study purpose?
- How reliable and practical is the measurement of the variable?

CASE EXAMPLE 5.1

In assessing whether VMAT intensity-modulated radiation therapy (IMRT) could save time compared to "step-and-shoot" IMRT treatment, time could be measured in many ways:

1. from the time the patient enters the room to the time he or she exits the room
2. from the time the radiation therapists (RTTs) begin to set the patient up to the time the patient is brought off the couch
3. from the start of the acquisition of the cone beam scan to initiation of the first beam
4. from the initiation of the first beam to the termination of the last beam

> These different measurements of "time" serve different purposes. In this case, the fourth definition seems to be most appropriate, as VMAT would mainly affect treatment delivery time, not the treatment process. Options 1–3 are less direct and may introduce confounding variables (i.e., more chances for patient-specific variables to be introduced into the measurement).

5.1.2.2 OBJECTIVE AND SUBJECTIVE MEASURES

Measurement methods can be classified in two ways. Objective measures are used to measure physical quantities and qualities using equipment. Subjective measures are used to rate the quantities and qualities using human judgment.

For example, to measure the effectiveness of training on the RTT's competency in performing image-guided radiation therapy (IGRT), one can choose either:

- objective measures – time and accuracy of image-matching by radiation therapists before and after training, or
- subjective measures – having therapists rate their comfort level of image-matching before and after training

5.1.2.3 TYPES OF DATA

Quantitative data can be classified according to increasingly precise levels of measurement, with more statistics being appropriate for higher levels, each scale building on characteristics of the previous, as follows:

Nominal scale: Also known as categorical data, the nominal scale is a data classification by categories that are mutually exclusive, meaning that the relationships between or among categories, meaning that something can be attributed to a single category, but that there is no ranking order or direct relationship between categories. Symbolically, A=B or A B (e.g., gender: male vs. female).

Ordinal scale: The ordinal scale addresses data that can be ranked in order such that A>B or A<B. The intervals between the groups, however,

are not always equal (e.g., age groups: child, teen, adult, senior, or cancer stages: I, II, III, IV).

Interval scale: Interval scale data can be ranked, and they also have equal divisions, or intervals, between categories, but the zero value is meaningless in that it is an arbitrary convention (e.g., temperature in Fahrenheit or Celsius).

Ratio scale: The ratio scale is similar to interval scale it as it has order and equal intervals but it does have a fixed meaningful zero, meaning that values can be assessed relative to one another (e.g., age, time, and weight).

From a statistical perspective, it is important to consider each scale as representing either discrete (nominal or ordinal) or continuous (interval or ratio) variables. The mathematical operations permissible for lower scale variables are also permissible for higher scale variables, and are summarized in Table 5.2.

TABLE 5.2 Levels of measurement and associated characteristics and statistical tests.

Level of Measurement	Put into Category	Arrange in Order	Calculate Values	Determine Ratio
Nominal	✔	✘	✘	✘
Ordinal	✔	✔	✘	✘
Interval	✔	✔	✔	✘
Ratio	✔	✔	✔	✔
Examples of Permissible Statistics	Mode, %, Chi-square test	+ median, percentile	+ mean, standard deviation, correlation, t-test	+ log

5.1.3 VALIDITY

The quality of a study is largely reflected by the validity of the study. There are two types of validity; internal validity and external validity.

5.1.3.1 INTERNAL VALIDITY

Internal validity addresses whether there is sufficient evidence to support or reject hypotheses, and on a more basic level addresses whether the researcher is measuring what they believe they are measuring. It depends on the study design and sampling method. Internal validity can be influenced by experiences, environmental factors and the study sample's characteristics. Examples are discussed in the following sub sections.

Practice effect: The practice effect is the potential impact on research outcomes of a change in behaviour or performance of participants as a result of practice or repeated exposure to the measure. For example, when conducting an image matching exercise on the same group of RTTs after training, better matching results achieved posttraining may be as a result of training, but also from familiarity of same dataset. This can represent a threat to internal validity.

Instrumentation effect: Instrumentation effect is the potential impact on research outcomes of a change or difference in the measurement device, observer, or scorer used to assess the dependent variable. For example, when asking an RTT to perform image matching on a newer version of imaging software after training, the better matching result may also come from better visualization of image on the new software. This represents a threat to internal validity.

5.1.3.2 EXTERNAL VALIDITY

External validity determines if the finding is generalizable to a larger population. Factors that could impact the external validity, include:

The Rosenthal effect: Also known as the expectation effect, the Rosenthal effect occurs when the researcher expects certain effects and thus unconsciously biases subjects to perform better towards the desired effect. For example, if a researcher gives antianxiety medication to patients, and the observer knows who gets the medication, he or she may tend to observe greater effects on the study group and ignore the changes on the control group.

The Hawthorne effect: The Hawthorne effect refers to changes in behaviour resulting from attention participants believe they are getting from researchers. For example, RTTs may wash their hands more often when the public health officer visits and observes the hand hygiene practice. To avoid this bias, observation without the knowledge of the participants is preferred, though an argument cannot always be made for the ethics of this

5.1.4 BIAS

Experimental study should be undertaken with the minimization of bias in mind. Bias is any force that could cause overall deviations from the "truth," known or unknown, and comes in many forms. For quantitative research, the potential for bias should be reflected on often and reported as a study limitation if unavoidable.

Bias can appear in many forms and stages in the research process. It can happen before the study is conducted if the researcher is particularly set on proving what they believe to be true rather than designing a valid experiment to gather proof. This skew can carry through to the reporting of results and publication and a reason why rigourous peer-review is required for publication. During an experiment it can take the forms of preferentially selecting certain groups while excluding others, (i.e., sampling bias), or if a particular measurement tool is inaccurate (i.e., systematic measurement bias).

5.1.5 IDENTIFYING THE STUDY HYPOTHESIS

In considering the study's primary endpoint, measurement scale, and overall design, it is worthwhile to frame the research question for an experimental design in the form of a hypothesis or a logical estimate of the outcome of the study, which should be supported by previous research, existing literature, or a plausible theory. A hypothesis can be classified as nondirectional, in that it specifies only the existence of a difference, and not the nature of this difference. A directional hypothesis, however, would propose the type of relationship to be expected, using such terms as "worse," "stronger," "less toxic," etc. Case example 5.2 suggests a directional and nondirectional hypothesis in the investigation of aloe vera in skin reaction management.

At this point it is necessary to introduce the following two naming conventions as they will be referred to in the discussion of inferential statistics. From a statistics standpoint, the hypothesis chosen by the researcher is actually termed as the alternative hypothesis, or H_A. The counterpart to this is the default position, which simply states there is no difference between the groups, and is termed the null hypothesis, or H_0. The researcher does not explicitly need to state the null hypothesis. The task of the researcher in conducting research is not to prove the H_A to be true, but rather to reject the H_0 if the evidence allows. Case example 5.2 provides an example of the hypotheses assigned to a research question regarding the use of aloe vera during radiation therapy treatment.

CASE EXAMPLE 5.2

Consider the research question "Does aloe vera use during radiotherapy affect the intensity of acute skin reactions?"

Alternate (H_A) hypothesis:
Non-directional hypothesis: "Aloe vera use during radiotherapy affects the intensity of acute skin reactions"
predicts there will be a difference, but not whether the reaction is expected to be better or worse
Directional hypothesis: "Aloe vera use during radiotherapy reduces the intensity of acute skin reactions"
specifies how the groups will differ
should be supported by proper evidence or theory

Null hypothesis (H_0):
"Aloe vera use during radiotherapy does not affect the intensity of acute skin reactions."

5.2 STUDY DESIGN II: ERRORS AND SAMPLING

As a researcher the first step in designing a study is to determine the goal of the study and outline the basic design. The next steps are to determine how study subjects are to be chosen and then how the outcome of the study will be measured. If care is not taken at the outset in selecting the most appropriate sampling method, the researcher may run into difficulties drawing any valid conclusions from the study.

5.2.1 CRITERIA AND SAMPLING METHODS

Sampling refers to the process of selecting study subjects from a defined population, such as a population of patients, of RTTs, or of interprofessional staff in a department. A sample is needed because it is generally impossible or costly to study an entire given population. The key requirement of proper sampling is that the sample should be representative of the study population so the finding from the sample can be generalized to the study population in question. For example, can the results from patients studied at one cancer centre be applied to the patients treated at other cancer centres?

Minimizing bias is essential in sample selection. For example, sifting through a pool of subjects and hand picking each one for study can skew the results in a certain direction while ignoring the complex, and likely large, variability in the patient population as a whole.

5.2.1.1 INCLUSION CRITERIA

A transparent and objective way to determine the subjects studied is to establish an upfront set of inclusion criteria. Inclusion criteria are conditions, which must be met before the subject can be potentially included. Whether they are or are not included will also depend on the sampling methods and in the case of prospective studies, whether or not they actually consent to participate. These lists of criteria are often mandatory for prospective studies and clinical trials in identifying who will be eligible to be approached, but they are also useful for retrospective studies. They can be employed by other researchers studying the same topic by trying to reproduce a prior study, or for explaining possible differences in outcomes of similar studies. Common criteria in the radiation therapy setting may include:

- disease type, disease stage, and treatment modality

- dose and fractionation schedules
- age, race and sex

The researcher should aim for the inclusion criteria to be as comprehensive and yet broad as possible, to avoid any bias, and yet to be clear about the nature of the population under investigation and the potential generalizability of results.

5.2.1.2 EXCLUSION CRITERIA

Some subjects will meet the defined inclusion criteria but might not be appropriate for study, as the specific cases might be difficult to handle logistically, or may confound the results. Accompanying exclusion criteria thus list the conditions under which subjects who do meet the inclusion criteria will still be rendered ineligible for study. Examples could include:

- non-English speaking subjects
- patients with specific major preexisting comorbidities
- prior history of radiation therapy treatment

Language could be justified if it is prohibitively costly for the researcher to provide translated materials or services, and comorbidities if the patient's baseline status could confound the independent variable being studied (e.g., radiation induced toxicity). A prior history of treatment could complicate dosimetric analysis, or, in the case of an educational intervention, suggest that the subject would have a higher baseline understanding of the treatment modality. The researcher should be cognizant that having too many exclusion criteria could affect the external validity of the study, particularly if excluded for criteria that are prevalent in the target population.

It is still likely after applying relevant criteria that the pool of eligible subjects will be large. It would be unnecessary to study them all. However, if a representative sample of a larger defined population is studied it can be assumed that any outcome observed in the sample could be reasonably also observed in the larger population. Therefore sampling methods are needed to select subjects from the eligible population to narrow the sample to a cost-effective, ethical, and scientifically useful number. Sampling can generally be classified into two types:

5.2.1.3 PROBABILITY SAMPLING

Probability sampling involves the selection of a sample from a population, based on the principle of randomization or chance. The researcher chooses and applies the probability mechanism by which the sample is selected. Individual subjects have no control over who would be selected. Random sampling is one of the probability methods. It gives each individual an equal chance to be selected using randomization methods (e.g., tossing dice, flipping a coins, etc.). It is generally more representative than nonrandom samples and easier to estimate sampling error. However, it requires accessibility of entire targeted population and needs to ensure that refusal of participants did not bias towards one group. Due to limited resources and the challenge in sampling using truly random approaches, sometimes it is impossible to randomly sample the entire population. Probability sampling is considered to have less selection bias than nonprobability sampling because selection is based on chance and the subjects nor the researcher decide if that specific subject will be included in the study.

5.2.1.4 NON-PROBABILITY SAMPLING

Non-probability sampling is a technique where the samples are gathered in a systematic process that does not give all the individuals in the population equal chances of being selected. For nonprobability samples, subjects consent whether to participate in the study or not.

Convenience sampling: Convenience sampling is an example of the nonprobability methods. It capitalizes on the most easily accessible members of the target population. It is easy to conduct but may not be representative. An example would be sending out an online questionnaire to survey patient's radiotherapy experience. It is easy to conduct as the sample consists of whoever responds. However, the sample could be considered biased towards those having computers access, understanding English, and perhaps even those with a higher socioeconomic status.

Quota sampling: Quota sampling is another nonprobability method that is considered more representative than convenience sampling. It requires that the researcher identify a priori (before the investigation) that important subgroups exist in the population who need to be included in the sample. Identification of the subgroups in advance could be a challenge. Similar quotas should be maintained between subgroups. For example, suppose an experiment regarding comfort level of using cone-beam CT for image guidance for head and neck cancer radiotherapy is administered. The researcher believes RTT experience is an important independent variable. If the ratio of the RTTs with 3 versus >3 year experience was 4:3 in the population, then the sample should maintain a similar quota of experienced RTTs to be considered representative (i.e., un-biased).

For prospective studies involving patients, the researcher should document how many subjects were approached and consented, and how many refused participation.

5.2.2 *SAMPLE SIZE DETERMINATION*

One of the most common difficulties the novice researcher encounters is the determination of the number of subjects needed for a study. A representative sample depends on not only sampling methods but also sample size. Using too few samples may be a wasted effort, as it prevents the researcher from drawing meaningful conclusions. Using too many samples is inefficient and may be unnecessarily costly or time-consuming. There is an ethical consideration as well. Individuals should not needlessly be exposed to potential risks if their participation would not contribute additional value to the research. Conversely, too few subjects might also make the risk assumed by some to be futile. An optimum sample size is one, which is adequate for making useful inferences from a sample to a population.

Ideally, the researcher will make an informed choice in choosing the sample size. The process can be complex and consultation with a biostatistician may be helpful. However even the biostatistician will require certain information from the researcher to provide a useful estimate of sample size to allow for a proper statistically meaningful comparison between two groups.

From a statistical point of view, it is ultimately desirable to assess if the null hypothesis (H_0, no effect) can be rejected, and the H_A accepted.

Because only a sample of the entire population is going to be studied, two important errors can emerge. These are known as Type I and Type II errors and efforts to minimize them form the basis of sample size determination.

5.2.2.1 TYPE I ERROR

Incorrectly rejecting the null hypothesis when it is actually true is known as a Type I error. In essence, it is a false positive error because the researcher falsely accepts the H_A when it is not true. For example, statistically concluding that aloe vera use during radiotherapy reduces the intensity of acute skin reactions (rejecting H_0), when it in fact does not reduce the reactions, is a Type I error. By the statistical nature of taking a sample from a population, Type I errors occur unbeknownst to the researcher, as it is possible, with too small a sample, that chance leads to inclusion of a group that tended to have less acute reactions than the broader population, completely unrelated to the interventional use of aloe vera.

Therefore one ideally wants to select a sample size that minimizes the Type I error rate, also called the level of significance, denoted as α. This is the first piece of information the biostatistician would need and is typically set at 0.05 for the vast majority of studies. This can be interpreted that the researcher will accept a 5% (5/100 or 0.05) chance of committing a Type I error.

5.2.2.2 TYPE II ERROR

Failing to reject the null hypothesis (H_0) when it is actually false is known as a Type II error. It is a false negative, because the researcher erroneously fails to reject H_0. In the example of aloe vera use, it would be the equivalent of statistically concluding that aloe vera use during radiotherapy does not reduce the intensity of acute skin reactions (failing to reject H_0), when it in fact does reduce toxicity.

The type II error rate is denoted as β. When determining the required sample size one more often refers to the concept of maximizing the statistical power ($1-\beta$). Power is the chance of correctly rejecting H_0 when H_0

is false. As power increases, the type II error rate decreases. The desired statistical power is the second portion of information the biostatistician would require in determining the required sample size. The desired power level varies more widely than α, ranging from 70–90% depending on the study question.

In some situations, minimizing one type of error may be more important than minimizing the other type. In a clinical scenario for example, a false positive (i.e., type I error) may be considered dangerous if it leads to unnecessary and potentially harmful treatment. For example, concluding that drug X is a superior antiemetic than the current standard of care, and implementing drug X in general practice, could lead to substandard nausea control amongst future patients.

5.2.2.3 *EFFECT SIZE*

The third component that needs to be given thought when determining sample size in the effect size. This is the minimum difference between two groups the researcher would like to detect after executing the experiment to make an inference about effect. For example, a researcher may wish to compare the two means between two groups. Case example 5.3 examines this concept in the context of rectal dose with IMRT.

CASE EXAMPLE 5.3

A researcher studying whether IMRT for prostate cancer reduces the maximum rectal dose at planning. He or she might identify an effect size corresponding to a mean reduction in the maximum rectal dose of at least 1Gy. This is not to say that IMRT will cause a difference of 1Gy, but rather powering the study to detect this magnitude. The actual difference may be bigger, which would strongly support H_A. Or, the actual difference may be less than 1 Gy and the researcher may decide that a difference of that magnitude is not clinically important enough to be worthy of a change in practice. Detecting a smaller effect, if desirable, requires a larger sample size

The most appropriate effect size could be estimated from existing literature and published scientific papers. Alternatively one could conduct a small pilot study or even a single case study help determine the potential effect size. Consider the Figure 5.2 of two pairs of normal distributions. Figure 2a demonstrates a very small effect size, which is this case is the difference in means (i.e., peaks) of distributions. Note that not all data points in the dashed group are larger, but on average the group is larger. Figure 2b demonstrates a larger difference between the groups as the means are further apart.

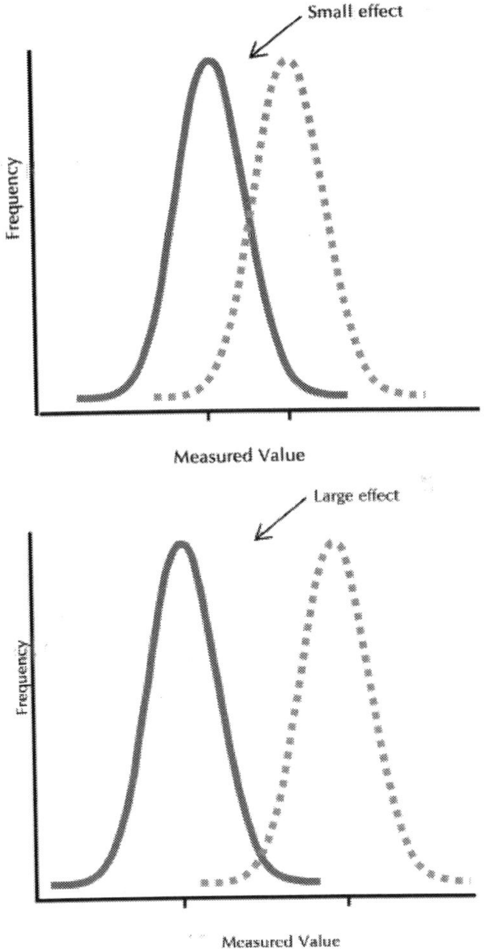

FIGURE 5.2 (a) Normal Distribution (Small Effect Size). (b) Normal Distribution (Large Effect Size).

In addition to the difference in means, one also needs to similarly estimate the standard deviation of the groups. Note that in this figure the curves all have the same standard deviations, visualized as the spread of data around the mean (curve peak). Having larger variations in the data is akin to trying to detect a signal (i.e., difference in means) when there is more noise (i.e., larger standard deviations, or more spread). This is due to the larger amount of overlap between the distributions.

After gathering the previously described information, α, β (or 1–β), and appropriate effect size, one can then undertake a power analysis with the help of a biostatistician or simple online tools. This would identify the minimum sample required to detect, with a reasonable likelihood, a given effect size. During this stage, it is often useful to vary the different parameters to see their effect on the required sample. See the Hot Tips for general rules of thumb. In practice, adjusting α or β requires a trade-off.

HOT TIP

When establishing a manageable but worthwhile sample size, consider the following:

- Higher power requires larger sample sizes
- The larger the effect size the more likely the experiment will find a significant effect
- The larger the standard deviation of the population, the lower the statistical power
- The smaller the significance level, the lower the power
- More accurate the measurement methods (i.e., the smaller the standard deviation of repeat measurements), the smaller the required sample

After settling on the inclusion and exclusion criteria and determining the required sample size, the researcher needs to step back for a moment. Consideration must be given to whether the study environment has enough subjects (e.g., patients) that will meet the established criteria, and that can reasonably be accrued to complete the study within a reasonable time frame. Many researchers may be disheartened to find that very large samples are often required yet their research is bounded by cost, resources, access to subjects, and time. Insight about recruitment rates could be gleaned from departmental statistics on new patient volumes, daily treatment appointment numbers, average incidental rates, or staff numbers, depending on the target population.

HOT TIP

There are a few historically generated "magic" sample sizes the researcher could potentially use (n = number of subjects):

- n = 5: minimum for a dosimetric comparison when the data is paired (e.g., comparing two planning techniques on the same patients)
- n = 10: minimum for a dosimetric comparison when the data is un-paired
- n = 20–30: minimum per cohort or study arm for cohort study; this is also considered as the boundary between small and large samples

In summary, when choosing sampling methods and sample sizes one needs to consider the available study population and if the proposed study methods can reach them all. Using a suitable sample size is essential if the researcher wishes to test a hypothesis. And finally, the practicality in recruiting the intended subjects in a reasonable time period should be considered.

5.2.2.4 ERRORS IN MEASUREMENT AND SAMPLING

As previously acknowledged, quantitative research is based in the detection of true differences that exist and, in the case of a two-group comparison, whether or not the difference is due to chance. Therefore is it useful to consider whether or not the variables are being measured with accuracy and precision. This will inform prestudy planning (including sample size determination) and eventual data analysis.

Accuracy: Accuracy refers to the degree with which the variable being measured actually reflects what the researcher thinks it reflects. An average deviation from the "true" value can be considered a systematic error. As accuracy increases, the systematic error decreases. Accuracy can reflect both the internal and external validity of a study. As defined earlier in this chapter, internal validity represents how well the variable being measured actually reflects what the researcher intends to measure, while external validity suggests how well the study sample reflects the larger intended population

It is worth noting that it is much easier to characterize the accuracy of certain variables (e.g., height, dose, objective measures of toxicity, etc.) than others (e.g., patient opinions, subjective measure of toxicity etc.). In many instances it may be prohibitive to determine accuracy; therefore the researcher should strive to reduce sources of bias wherever possible. The researcher should consider instruments, including surveys and questionnaires, that have previously been validated and reported in the existing literature (*see* Chapter 7: Survey Methodologies and Analysis).

Precision: Precision is the degree with which the measurement of the same value varies after repeated measurements. Variation (i.e., standard deviation) around the average measurement can be considered random error. As precision increases, the random error decreases. These errors will never be eliminated completely, but it is important to be aware of them and how they impact the experiment.

Precision is often easier to characterize by repeating measurements on the same subject after a period of time has passed. For example, this could be accomplished by recalculating a measurement with the same tool (e.g., skin-surface distances at each treatment, or recalculating dose in the treatment planning system), or getting the same or different people to perform the measurement and characterize the intra and interobserver variation, respectively. Using measurement tools that are precise can also improve the power of a study. Consider again Figure 5.1. More precise tools can reduce the noise (standard deviation or spread of the curve) so that the signal (difference in means or peaks) can be detected. Case example 5.4 reflects on a practical example of validity in research measures.

CASE EXAMPLE 5.4

Consider the uncertainties in the following scenario. An RTT wishes to compare the dose to the patient's rectum between IMRT and newer VMAT techniques in the treatment planning system for patients receiving prostate radiotherapy. It is reasonable to assume the dose calculation is an accurate measurement of the dose received by the patient because the treatment planning system has been commissioned and tested properly, and we know the radiation being delivered by the linear accelerator agrees with the treatment planning system calculation within 1–2%. Therefore, it is internally valid. The accuracy of how well the sampled patients reflect the prostate cancer patient population as a whole (i.e., external validity) will be determined by the inclusion and exclusion criteria, and the sampling methods used. The dose calculation itself is likely also very precise because modern treatment planning systems are very robust, in that you will get the same rectum dose (within a few cGy) after recalculating the planned dose. Over the entire sample however the investigator also replanned a subset of patients a second time with both IMRT and VMAT and compared it to the initial IMRT and VMAT plans. This was done to quantify the variation introduced by intraobserver plan optimization.

5.3 DATA ANALYSIS: EXPLORING THE DATA

Quantitative data analysis is the process of applying statistical methods to understand data and derive conclusions. Statistics are mathematical procedures to describe, synthesize, analyze and interpret quantitative data. More simply, they allow the researcher to condense many data points into a few key values.

5.3.1 *CHECKING DATA QUALITY*

Before any actual analysis the researcher is encouraged to check the data quality and scan for obvious errors. Possible causes could be that the incorrect unit or method of measurement was used, the incorrect measurement or formula for calculation was applied, or simply a typographical or transcription error (e.g., data entry errors). Some data may also be missing.

Next, any outliers in the data should be scrutinized. There is no exact definition of an outlier, but it can be thought of as any data point whose value is extreme in relation to the rest of the data, or which exceeds the typical variation of the data. An outlier could be an error, or a valid data point caused by a confounding factor the researcher had not yet considered.

Missing or erroneous data will not only reduce the study power, but also introduce bias. For explainable erroneous data, one should either correct them if possible or disregard them from the analysis if not.

HOT TIP

A simple method to catch outliers that is also an essential initial step for exploring the data is to plot the data in a graph. This allows for two things:

- Visualization of data trends and variable associations, specific distributions (e.g., data follows a bell curve for certain statistical tests)
- Visualization of data points that fall outside the trends (e.g., potential outliers or errors); note that these could potentially be missed with some of the descriptive statistics described below

5.3.2 DESCRIPTIVE STATISTICS

There are two types of statistics: descriptive statistics and inferential statistics. Descriptive statistics says what the data looks like, and it involves organizing, summarizing and displaying data. In contrast, inferential statistics are aiming at finding whether there is a relationship, which involves estimation, establishing relationships, and hypothesis testing.

Descriptive statistics allow the researcher to condense a set of numbers into a few simple values, including measuring central tendency and dispersion, which helps to understand and identify trends as well as describe and summarize the data.

5.3.2.1 MEASURES OF CENTRAL TENDENCY

Measures of central tendency describe how the data is clustered together, and include:

- the mean, or average of the total
- the median, or middle value
- the mode, or most frequently occurring value

5.3.2.2 MEASURES OF DISPERSION

Measures of dispersion describe how the data is spread out, and include:

- the range, or minimal and maximal values
- the standard deviation, or the average of the squared difference from the mean

Graphing allows visualization of the data and is complementary to calculating measures of central tendency and dispersion. Barker provides a series of examples of the various types of graphs.[1]

The histogram is a particularly useful form of graph. It represents a plot of frequency on the Y axis, for defined intervals (or bins) of continuous data. Below, as Figure 5.3, are three different stylized histograms (the bins have been replaced by a smooth curve). The spatial relationship between mean, median and mode can depict whether the distribution is normal or skewed. The normal distribution is of particular importance in quantitative research as most biological data, after enough measurements, will follow this bell-shaped distribution. Some statistical tests used for hypothesis testing require the data to be normally distributed.

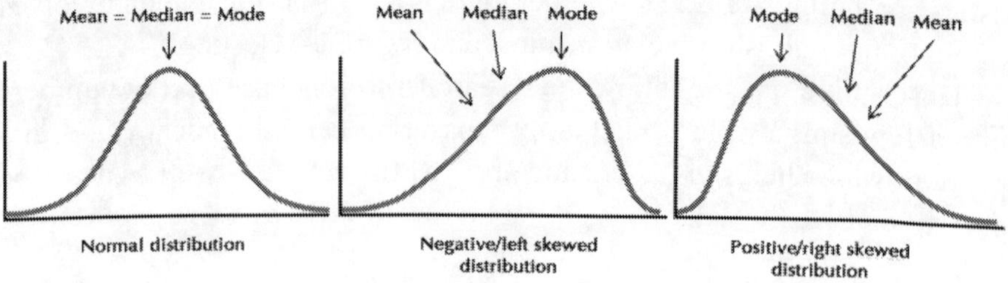

FIGURE 5.3 Mean, median, and mode in varying distributions.

Think of a skew as a normal distribution with the tails pulled in one direction. For highly skewed distributions, the preference is to report the median value. For normal distributions, the mean is preferred which is the peak of the left figure. The standard deviations represent how wide the curve is on either side of the peak.

5.3.3 PEARSON'S COEFFICIENT: RELATIONSHIPS BETWEEN VARIABLES

It is often useful to explore if there is a relationship between two variables. Correlation, for example, suggests how much one variable tends to change when the other variable changes. The strength of association is a measure of the linearity of the relationship and reported as the correlation coefficient (also called Pearson's coefficient), r.

Significance of Pearson's coefficient, r:

- when r is 0 there is no linear relationship
- when r is positive there is a trend where the variables change in the same direction (i.e., when one increases, the other increases)
- When r is negative, there is a trend where one variable increases while the other deceases

The larger the absolute value of r and closer to 1, the stronger the association is between these two variables. The common convention is that an r value less than 0.4 represents a poor agreement between the variables, 0.4 to 0.75 a fair or good agreement, and greater than 0.75 an excellent agreement. It is important to know that strong correlation does not imply causation, but rather it only means there may be an association between two variables. Consider the following pair of correlation plots in Figure 5.4 with varying degrees of noise, and r values. Fitting a trend line to the data, called linear regression, allows one to create a model (i.e., equation) that may be used to predict one variable when only the other is known.

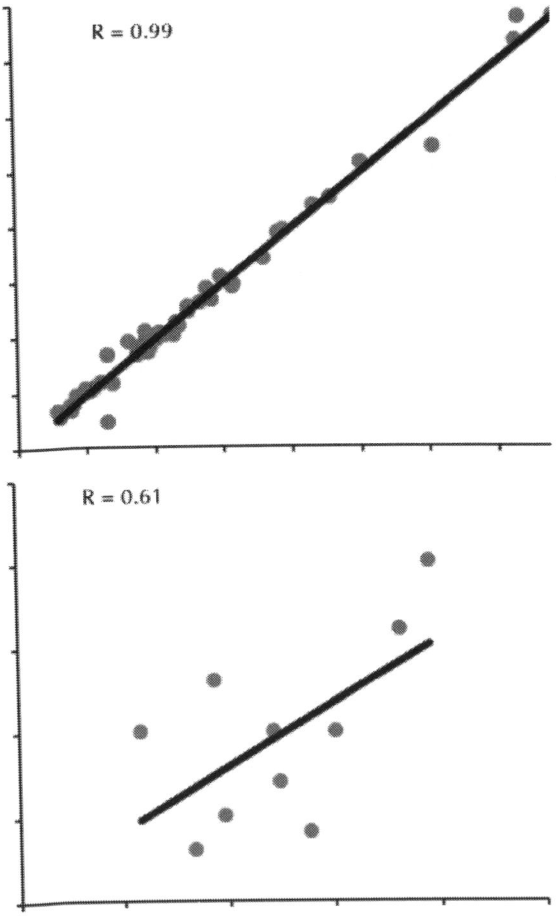

FIGURE 5.4 (a) Highly Correlated Correlation Plot. (b) Moderately Correlated Correlation Plot.

The correlation in Figure 5.4a is high, while in Figure 5.4b it is moderate. The ability to accurately predict the Y value, if the X value were known, would thus be better with the left plot, given the smaller amount of variation away from the trend line. Essentially r describes how well the data fits the trend line (i.e., when $r=1$, all data points are exactly on the line). The equation of the trend, provided by many statistics programs, can be used to model values of X and Y that the researcher does not have in the data.

HOT TIP

A few notes of caution with analyses using correlations:

- They can be sensitive to outliers especially when fewer data points are used (Figure 5.4b); therefore checking the data is essential for errors
- It is important not to attempt to predict variables outside the range for which the model was made or plotted
- The relationship may actually be nonlinear, so the researcher should plot the data and confirm if a straight line is appropriate; sometimes data transformations (e.g., logarithmic scale) are required

5.4 DATA ANALYSIS II: HYPOTHESIS TESTING (INFERENTIAL STATISTICS)

The second most frequently employed type of statistics used in quantitative research is inferential statistics. Inferential statistics allow the researcher to make inferences, or draw conclusions, about the characteristics of a population based on the sample data that has been collected. The researcher can then make confident decisions to reject or accept the null hypothesis with acceptable uncertainty. One should be aware of the following concepts when selecting and applying statistical tests.

5.4.1 PARAMETRICS

It is important to determine whether or not the data collected follows a normal distribution, in that it follows the bell-shaped curve expected of most biological data, where the majority of samples tend toward a central mean, with some data demonstrating higher or lower values on either side of this mean, or whether it is skewed in some way.

5.4.1.1 PARAMETRIC TESTS

Parametric tests are those statistical tests that can be employed when the researcher is confident that data follows a normal distribution (*see* Figure 5.3a), as the tests rely on assumptions about the probability distributions of the data. Normally distributed data can be described or modeled well using descriptive statistics (e.g., mean, standard deviation). When using parametric tests, the data needs therefore to fit the assumptions or else the result could be misleading.

5.4.1.2 NON-PARAMETRIC TESTS

Non-parametric tests make no assumptions about data distribution. Most parametric tests have a nonparametric counterpart, and it may be tempting to just apply a nonparametric test in all instances, to avoid consideration of the distribution of data. However, it should be noted that nonparametric tests are often somewhat less statistically powerful than parametric tests, and it is thus preferable to use a parametric test if the researcher is confident of the distribution. If not normally distributed (*see* Figures 5.3b and 5.3c), it is more appropriate to employ a nonparametric test.

5.4.2 PAIRING OF DATA

Different tests must be used when the samples are un-paired, or independent, as opposed to when they are paired, or dependent.

5.4.2.1 PAIRED TESTS

Paired tests are also considered repeated measures tests, and can be employed to test two measurements obtained for the same group of subjects, usually at different time points, such as before or after an intervention. Paired tests have greater statistical power, as each subject acts as its own control and individual differences can be partially accounted for. This approach can also be used for specially designed studies called case-control or matched pair studies.

5.4.2.2 UN-PAIRED TESTS

Un-paired tests should be employed when the measurements come from two different samples or cohorts. The cohorts were likely originally assigned to ensure relative comparability of characteristics between groups, but the comparison of measurements taken from a control versus someone who has not received the intervention cannot not be as strong as taking a repeated measurement from a single subject.

5.4.3 SIDEDNESS

For certain tests, the researcher may need to specify whether or not the hypothesis being tested is directional, meaning that the difference in values can be confidently known to be either positive or negative. The alternative would be that data is nondirectional, meaning that the researcher is looking solely at whether there exists any difference. These situations require one-sided or two-sided tests, respectively.

5.4.3.1 ONE-SIDED TESTS

A one-sided test is only warranted if the researcher can be certain that any measured difference would only be observed in one direction. For example, in an investigation comparing skin surface dose with and without

0.5 cm of bolus, it would be acceptable to employ a one-sided test (i.e., assuming that skin surface dose could only increase with bolus) because it is not possible for the surface dose to decrease with the presence of bolus.

5.4.3.2 TWO-SIDED TESTS

In all other cases, a two-sided test should be employed, and this is often considered the default choice. A two-sided tests would allow the acknowledgement of an effect in either direction, and would avoid the potential for an effect to go undetected in the un-tested direction (i.e., committing a type II error in the opposite direction).

5.4.4 P-VALUE

Often misunderstood, the *p*-value is the probability of obtaining a result as or more extreme than what was observed, assuming there is no real effect (i.e., H_0 is true). When the *p*-value is less than the specified level of significance (α), the researcher can reject H_0. This is commonly called a statistically significant result. When the p-value is larger than α, the H_0 is fails to be rejected. It is reported as a fraction (e.g., 0.05) but is better interpreted as a percent chance (e.g., 5%).

5.4.5 DEGREES OF FREEDOM

The concept of "degrees of freedom" is not particularly intuitive, and is determined differently for various statistical tests. Hendee described the number of degrees of freedom as "the number of observations that are free to vary without restriction" and offers the following simple example: a box with *n* chocolates has *n*-1 degrees of freedom, because after *n*-1 chocolates have been eaten there is no freedom in choosing that last one in the box.[2] Fortunately, most statistical software packages automatically identify the appropriate degrees of freedom for the researcher. In practice, the degrees of freedom relates to what critical value the test's statistics (examples in the following section) will be compared to, and ultimately whether or not H_0 will be rejected.

HOT TIP

Consider the following question when choosing and applying a statistical test:

- What type of data and difference (e.g., means, proportions etc.) are you comparing?
- How many groups are you comparing (1, 2, or >2)?
- Is it parametric or nonparametric? If parametric, does the data fit the assumptions of the test?
- Does the test require a minimum sample size or frequency count, and does your data meet this threshold?
- What is the null hypothesis for that test?

5.4.6 STATISTICAL TESTS

It is not feasible to describe all the possible tests within the scope of this chapter, but a few key examples are presented here. The researcher is referred to more comprehensive statistics resources for further insight about specific tests or applications.

5.4.6.1 THE T-TEST: COMPARING MEANS BETWEEN TWO SAMPLES

One of the most commonly used inferential statistics used is the *t*-test, which compares the mean difference of continuous variables (e.g., interval or ratio-type data) between two groups. The *t*-test is a parametric test that assumes the data is normally distributed. Statistical software packages can be used to apply tests of normality to see how well the data fit a normal distribution. Alternatively, the researcher can simply plot the data in histograms. This is where exploring the data before "blindly" applying statistical tests becomes essential! In the example, the data of each group appears to follow a normal distribution therefore applying the *t*-test should be valid. Note that with small sample sizes (e.g., <30) the data is less likely to be modeled well by a normal distribution, and may appear skewed.

To calculate this test, the *t* statistic needs to be calculated by the following equation using the mean, variance, and sample size (n) for each study group.

$$t = \frac{mean_1 - mean_2}{\sqrt{\frac{variance_1^{\,2}}{n_1} + \frac{variance_2^{\,2}}{n_2}}}$$

This takes into account the possible effect (e.g., difference in means), and the different sample sizes and variance in each group. In essence, one is calculating the ratio of the difference to the data variability, or the signal to noise ratio.[3] Calculation of the *t* statistic varies somewhat depending on whether the variances and sample sizes are the same or different between the groups.

The *p*-value associated with the *t* statistic must then be calculated, which can be done automatically by many statistical software packages. Alternatively, one can look up the *p*-value in tables included in most statistic textbooks. The p-value actually comes from the distribution of possible *t* statistics. Figure 5.5 reflects two probability distributions of the *t* statistic and their relationships to the level of significance (α). The significance level, and whether the H_A is directional or nondirectional determines what critical value the *t* statistic must exceed in magnitude for the result to be considered statistically significant.

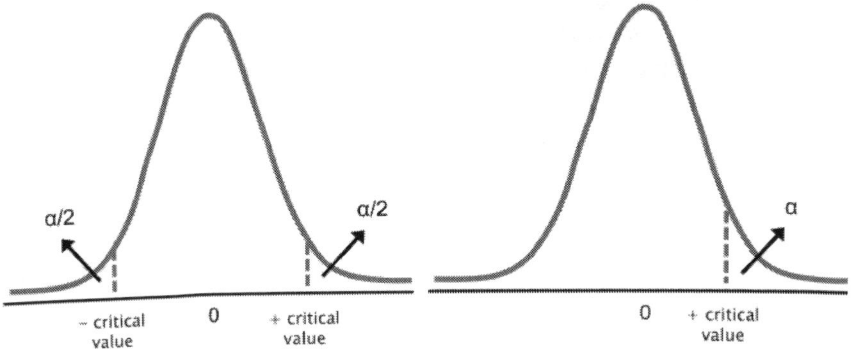

FIGURE 5.5 (a) Two-Sided Probability Distribution. (b) One-Sided Probability Distribution.

The *t* distributions look similar to a normal distribution when the sample size is large, and have long tails. It is important to note that the *t* distribution is a theoretical distribution, centreed around zero that does not come directly from the specific data. It is selected rather from a family of curves that is chosen by the degrees of freedom for the test. The degrees of freedom for the *t*-test is related to the sample size (degrees of freedom $= n_1 + n_2 - 2$).

In the above distributions, α represents the areas under the curves between a critical value and the tail(s). For a nondirectional H_A (Figure 5.4, left curve) α is divided in half for each side of the *t* distribution and hence a two-sided test is being applied. For a directional H_A (Figure 5.4, right curve), α is fully applied to one side of the t distribution and hence a one-sided test is being applied. A one-tailed test is therefore more powerful to detect an effect in one-direction because it does not divide α. That is, the critical value is lower for a one-sided test. The H_0, is that the mean difference is zero (i.e., there is no difference between groups). Case example 5.5 presents a practical application of the t-test.

CASE EXAMPLE 5.5

Suppose a researcher wants to compare the mean age of head and neck cancer patients receiving radiation therapy between those that are positive for human papilloma virus (HPV), and those that are negative. The data is graphed below as a histogram (Figure 5.6), and it is obvious there is some difference in the means between the groups. However, before drawing any conclusions about a correlation between age and HPV status at diagnosis, it must be determined whether this could be attributable solely to chance. The hypotheses are as follows:

- H_0: There is no difference in the mean age at diagnosis between HPV (+) and HPV (–) patients
- H_A: There is a difference in mean age at diagnosis between HPV (+) and HPV (–) patients

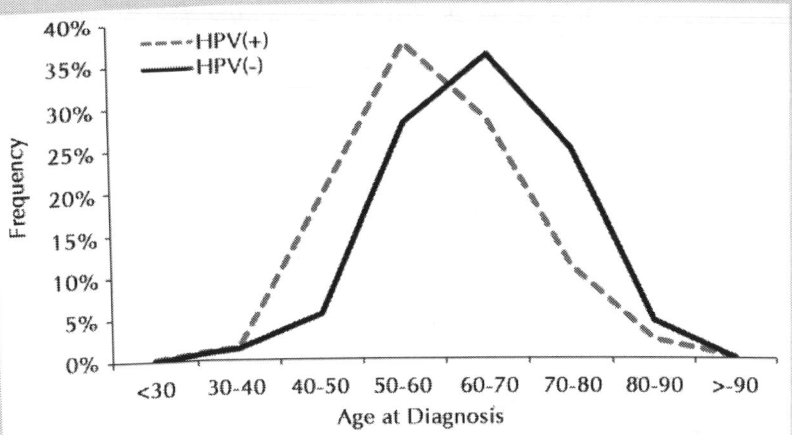

FIGURE 5.6 Histogram of age at diagnosis for patients receiving radiation therapy for head and neck cancer, based on HPV status.

For a difference in means to be considered statistically different from 0 (nondirectional or two-sided test where $\alpha=0.05$) the calculated t-statistic has to be greater in magnitude than either the positive or negative critical values. Because this is nondirectional, this application of the test checks both whether the mean difference is significantly greater or significantly smaller.

If the researcher got a *p*-value of 0.01, it could be concluded that the mean diagnosis age of 65 for HPV(–) patients is significantly higher than the mean diagnosis age of 55 for HPV(+) head and neck cancer patients. Statistically there is therefore a 1% chance of observing a mean difference of at least 10 years assuming there is actually no true difference. If the critical value was set at 5%, this probability of 1% is encompassed here, therefore H_0 is rejected, and it can be assumed that the alternative hypothesis (H_A) is likely true, although it does not actually prove the H_A true.

5.4.6.2 CHI SQUARE TEST – COMPARING FREQUENCY DISTRIBUTIONS OR PROPORTIONS BETWEEN TWO CATEGORIES

The chi-square test for independence is a nonparametric test designed to determine whether the frequencies of two outcomes, or difference in proportions, for two defined groups are statistically significant. This test can be applied to nominal data, and does not require that the data follow a specified distribution.

To understand how this test works it is helpful to organize the actual *observed data* in what is called a contingency table. Table 5.3 presents the frequencies for two binary outcomes, counted for two mutually exclusive groups. This would be called a 2x2 contingency table (plus marginal cells with the row and column totals):

TABLE 5.3 2 × 2 Contingency Table.

Observed Count	Outcome 1	Outcome 2	Total
Group 1	n = a	n = b	Row total = a+b
Group 2	n = c	n = d	Row total = c+d
Total	Column total = a+c	Column total = b+d	Grand total, n = a+b+c+d

The null hypothesis (H_0) for this test and table is that the groups and outcomes are independent of each other or have no relationship. In other words, any possible differences in the distribution of outcomes (a/b vs. c/d) between the groups are due to chance. The alternative hypothesis (H_A) is that the groups and outcomes are dependent, and the distribution differences between the groups are not due to chance (i.e., there is a real difference in the proportions). In addition to the actual observed counts above we need to calculate the *expected count*, or the frequency we should expect to see if H_0 is true:

Expected count = (row total X column total)/n

The chi-squared statistic, χ^2, is calculated by summing the difference in the frequency between the observed and expected frequencies in each of the cells of the contingency table:

$$\chi^2 = \sum \frac{(observed\ count - expected\ count)^2}{expected\ count}$$

As with the *t*-test statistic, the χ^2 statistic is then used to look up the associated *p*-value on the chi-squared distribution. Because χ^2 is always positive due to the summing of squares, its distribution (not shown) is quite different than the t-statistic. This distribution also varies greatly depending on the degrees of freedom, which for chi-square is given by the number of Groups or categories – 1.

If the observed and expected proportions counts were nearly equal, χ^2 would be very small, *p* would be large. There may not be enough evidence to reject H_0. If χ^2 is large, however, and the associated *p*-value is smaller than the specified significance level (e.g., α=0.05), then the observed and expected proportions are likely not due to chance. Therefore we can reject H_0. Case example 5.6 provides an example in the course of a patient satisfaction survey.

CASE EXAMPLE 5.6

Suppose a researcher conducted a patient satisfaction survey where patients were given the choice of being "satisfied" (outcome 1) or "not satisfied" (outcome 2) with the quality of care they received. The researcher hypothesizes that patients with different diagnoses, say prostate (group 1) and breast (group 2) cancer, would rate their satisfaction differently.

If the p-value is 0.03 after performing the Chi-Square test, the researcher would conclude that the proportion of "satisfied" patients is significantly different between prostate and breast cancer patients. Statistically, this means there is a 3% chance of finding a difference in the observed and expected counts equal to or larger than the one observed, assuming H_0 is true. Because 3% is a low probability, one concludes that there is an association between diagnosis and patient satisfaction.

HOT TIP

There are few rules that should be observed for the proper application of the Chi-Square test:

- It requires the data to be organized into categories or groups, and that actual counts are entered into the contingency table and not percentages
- The value in any cell of the table must be >5 and the total observations must be >20, otherwise a different test must be used (Fisher's exact test)
- It assumes the samples are randomly selected from the population, but it is acceptable for one random sample to be classified into two or more groups

5.4.7 POST-HOC AND MULTIPLE COMPARISONS

A common temptation for the novice researcher is to compare many more variables for statistical significance between two groups, after testing the primary endpoint (the first H_0 vs. H_A). The risk is that with each new comparison that is tested and new H_A, one will eventually detect a difference that is statistically significant though it occurred by chance alone, and not by the experimental design. Even with a p-value set at 0.05, there is still a 5% chance that an observed difference was the result of chance. Unless the study was initially powered for these multiple comparisons, the type I error rate will be inflated. It is possible to simultaneously compare more than two groups using specific tests designed to do so (e.g., analysis of variance, or ANOVA).

The simplest method to avoid this is to use a somewhat arbitrary stricter α level upfront (e.g., 0.02 instead of 0.05). However, the researcher should be cognizant of the trade-off between α and power (1-β). More formal corrections can also be used. The Bonferroni correction for example, replaces the originally desired significance level for only one comparison (e.g., 0.05) with a new one equal to the original level, divided by the number of comparisons to be made by the researcher (e.g., 0.05/5 comparisons =0.01 for five comparisons).

Perhaps most importantly, the researcher should consider carefully whether such *post-hoc* testing, making unplanned comparisons after the study has been conducted, is even clinically relevant. If the researcher deems a comparison to be relevant, these additional tests are often called exploratory analyses or hypothesis-generating tests, with the presumption that future studies will be properly powered to study the addition comparisons.

5.4.8 STATISTICAL VERSUS CLINICAL SIGNIFICANCE

Although inferential statistics are used in hypothesis testing, they give no information on whether or not the result is practically meaningful or clinically important. With a large enough sample size, nearly any comparison can become statistically significant. Therefore it is important to frame the magnitude of the statistically significant value in the clinical context.

For example, a researcher may conclude that the rectal dose for prostate patients with one planning technique was on average 10 cGy lower ($p<0.02$) compared to an older technique. While this was statistically significant, the researcher notes that the uncertainty in planning was approximately the same magnitude based on recreating plans with the same technique after a period of time has passed (e.g., the precision was approximately 10cGy). Additionally, they note that the difference is less than 1% of the total prescribed dose for prostate radiation therapy and therefore might conclude the newer technique does not justify clinical implementation compared to the added expense.

5.4.9 THE BENEFIT OF A BIOSTATISTICIAN

While it is important for the researcher to understand the basic principles and considerations of statistical analysis, it is often beneficial to solicit the expertise of a biostatistician. Many academic institutions and hospitals will have a biostatistics department, thus providing the researcher ready access to biostatistics expertise. Contrary to popular belief, such expertise is not limited to data analysis stages, but can lend insight to study design, including determination of sample sizes. Case example 5.7 provides the perspective of a biostatistician at the Princess Margaret Cancer Centre, with a strong background in collaboration in radiation therapy research.

CASE EXAMPLE 5.7

The value of a collaborating biostatistician

Tony Panzarella MSc PStat
Manager, Biostatistics Department, Princess Margaret Cancer Centre, Toronto, Canada

I have been a practicing applied statistician for almost 30 years. While I have been involved in many research studies. It has been a wonderful experience to work alongside very talented cancer researchers. I have learned a lot from my research colleagues, and, in turn, I hope they have learned a lot from me. Many years ago a senior scientist within my organization was an invited speaker at a meeting of biostatisticians. During his talk he made an important distinction between a consulting biostatistician, on the one hand, and a collaborating biostatistician, on the other. He went on to say that although a biostatistician could play both roles, they should strive to be, foremost, a collaborating biostatistician.

With years of experience now behind me I could not agree more with this position. Not only is this better professionally for the practicing biostatistician, but I would argue, even more so for the researcher!

A biostatistician is, after all, not only trained to handle analyses of data, but is also well versed to deal with the often crucial issues of study design and data collection. Too often a biostatistician is approached at the end of a study to perform a data analysis, but they discover in the process shortcomings, sometimes serious, in the study design. For example, the design chosen may be inappropriate to answer the primary question, or the sample size is too small to detect a clinically important difference as statistically significant. Unfortunately, no amount of sophisticated analysis can salvage a poorly designed study.

Success in research often involves assembling a team of individuals, with complementary skills, in the planning phases of a study. This team should include a biostatistician. Failure to do so, or seeking their assistance at a late stage, can compromise the validity of a study and waste valuable resources in the process.

The responsible use of quantitative research methods requires very careful considerations at each stage of the research process. Too often, researchers follow the temptation to rush out and "just measure something" before thinking about how to obtain information that will actually be of use and how they will interpret it. It is not possible for this one chapter to be a comprehensive lesson on all aspects of quantitative research methods. Rather, it is meant to serve as a guide and to highlight the most important aspects of properly conducting a valid quantitative study, from study design to data analysis.

KEYWORDS

- Hypothesis
- Variables
- Validity
- Bias
- Error
- Sampling
- Statistics

REFERENCES

1. Barker, R. F. Deciphering Statistics in Research: A Beginners Guide to Statistics for Radiation Science Professionals. *Can. J. Med. Radiat. Technol.* **2007,** *38(3)*, 34–45.
2. Hendee, W. R.; Ritenour, E. R. Medical Imaging Physics, 4th ed.; Wiley-Liss Inc: New York, 2003.
3. Bureau, Y. Inferential Statistics for Radiation Scientists: A Brief Guide to Better Statistical Interpretations. *J. Med. Imag. Radiat. Sci.* **2012,** *43(2)*, 121–131.

CHAPTER 6

QUALITATIVE METHODOLOGIES AND ANALYSIS

CAITLIN GILLAN MRT(T) BSc MEd FCAMRT

Radiation Therapist, Radiation Medicine Program, Princess Margaret Cancer Centre, Toronto Canada
Assistant Professor, Department of Radiation Oncology, University of Toronto, Toronto Canada

CATHRYNE PALMER MRT(T) MSc

Director, Medical Radiation Sciences Program & Assistant Professor, Department of Radiation Oncology, Unversity of Toronto, Toronto Canada

AMANDA BOLDERSTON RTT MSc FCAMRT

Provincial Professional Practice and Academic Leader, British Columbia Cancer Agency, Fraser Valley Cancer Centre, Surrey Canada

CONTENTS

This chapter builds on a peer-reviewed article by Palmer and Bolderston entitled "A brief introduction to qualitative research," published in the Canadian Journal of Medical Radiation Technology *(2006).*[1] *Excerpts are incorporated with permission.*

6.1 THE NATURE OF QUALITATIVE RESEARCH

Qualitative research is an interpretative approach, which attempts to gain insight into the specific meanings and behaviours experienced in a certain social phenomenon through the subjective experiences of the participants.[2] The researcher builds abstracts, concepts, hypotheses, or theories by asking such questions as "why," "how" and "in what way[3,4]?" Qualitative research has an alternate view of reality than quantitative research. It is a view that stresses the importance of social processes and subjective experience, and the meaning attributed to social situations from the subject's perspective. It lends itself to an exploration of processes and meanings rather than the "quantity, amount, intensity, or frequency" of quantitative research.[5] It is often an iterative process whereby the theory and hypotheses emerge from the data as it is collected, making the researcher key to the data collection and analysis processes. The study design is emergent and flexible, responsive to the changing conditions as the study progresses. The goal is to understand the phenomenon from the viewpoint of the participants; with its particular institutional and social context intact; this data and context is lost if attempts to quantify the data are made.[6]

Qualitative research differs from quantitative research in more ways than simply the methodological approach to data collection and analysis. It is based on different principles and philosophies, where the researcher examines the data for patterns, concepts, and relationships between variables, often returning to the setting to collect more data or test emerging hypotheses. Thus, qualitative research builds theory inductively over a period of time.

Key elements and rationale for qualitative research include:

- Use for problems where little is known about the topic
- Application in a natural setting where it is important to account for social, cultural, and historical aspects of the setting

- Smaller samples (fewer participants or subjects)
- Flexibility, with permission for modifications of the research and/or techniques
- Simultaneous collection and analysis of data

6.1.1 *RATIONALE AND CHALLENGES*

The value of qualitative methods is reliant on the choice and rigour of the study design. Qualitative methodologies are often seen as the "poor cousin" of the more quantitative approaches, but a lack of numbers and p values does not negate their value.[7] In fact, in many areas and depending on the nature of the research question, the state of knowledge on the subject, and the rigour with which the work is undertaken and analyzed, a qualitative methodology may be more appropriate and contribute more insight to the topic at hand. Qualitative research is thus not a "soft science," but rather one that is more appropriate in certain contexts and requires as structured an approach as quantitative research. Qualitative research can also be strengthened by using a combination of data collection methods (a process known as triangulation or mixed methodology) and by analysis of the data by more than one person. Denzin and Lincoln refer to the role of the qualitative researcher as "bricoleur," or someone who incorporates several approaches or methods of interpretation to create a "pieced-together set of representations that are fitted to the specifics of a complex situation.[5]" It is also often a good preliminary approach to provide insight necessary to inform a future quantitative study.

6.2 QUALITATIVE FRAMEWORKS

The amount of lingo and terminology that seems to accompany qualitative research is often a distractor to those wishing to experiment with these methodologies. Understanding of the many background theoretical constructs, such as positivism, postpositivism, and constructivism, while relevant and interesting, is not essential to valuable forays into qualitative research (though the constructs are explored in an accessible manner by

Bunniss and Kelly in the context of medical education research).[8] There are a few concepts, however, with which the researcher should be familiar. A basic understanding of these approaches to building knowledge in the qualitative world can inform the collection and analysis of data made possible through the individual methodologies discussed in the next section.

6.2.1 GROUNDED THEORY

Grounded theory seeks through research to generate theory rather than to prove or disprove it.[9,10] For this reason, research begins with a study situation and investigators then aim to understand the situation and develop a theory based on what is understood. As its name implies, grounded theory is "theory that is grounded in the words and actions of those individuals under study.[11]" Previous understandings of relationships or theoretical underpinnings are put aside as investigators are encouraged to enter a research situation with an inductive and open-minded approach to interpreting data. This is in contrast with most approaches to research, which are hypothesis-testing as opposed to hypothesis-generating.[9] Data collection and analysis serve the purpose of allowing for the emergence of a theory, thus suggesting an iterative process whereby data collection, coding or categorization of data, and note-taking occur simultaneously, with literature being consulted as relationships and themes are identified.[9]

6.2.2 ETHNOGRAPHY

Historically, ethnography is a term that originated in the 19th century in reference to a descriptive account of a community or culture, under the umbrella of anthropology.[12] Over time, it came to represent both the first-hand experience of a researcher in such a community, and also the comparative interpretation of different contexts. Ethnography is based in the direct immersion of the researcher into the environment under study, with a focus on the broader culture, including the relationships between study subjects.[9,11] It is inherently unstructured, in that the environment studied by the researcher is natural rather than an artificial condition created by the researcher.[12] For this reason, formal interviews, focus groups, or even observational studies would not be considered ethnographical. To maximize the likelihood that subjects in the study environment do not alter their behaviour (known as the Hawthorne Effect, see Chapter 5: Quantitative Methodologies & Analysis), ethnography often requires the investigator to be immersed in the environment for a significant amount of time. An alternative is not to disclose to study participants that they are being observed, but this may be difficult to warrant. The concept of deception is discussed later in this chapter. Data collection is equally unstructured, usually with more than one methodology or source of information, including observation, informal conversation or interview, and collection of documentary evidence.

Ethnography is often confused with grounded theory, but Morse clarifies the distinction in noting that an ethnographic approach can be applied to a grounded theory study, and the two are thus not mutually exclusive.[13,14]

6.2.3 *PHENOMENOLOGY*

Phenomenology is the objective study of subjective experience. It concerns a description and understanding of the "lived experience" of individuals, including their perceptions, judgments, and emotions.[15] Meaning is attributed to phenomena or events and creates experience, which can differ between subjects for the same event.[16] Phenomenology seeks to find the common thread, or essence, between individual experiences.[4] Woodgate describes the use of a phenomenological approach to understand children's experience with cancer, recognizing the importance of reporting the children's perspective of reality rather than the researcher's perspective.[17]

6.3 METHODOLOGIES

Qualitative research is predominantly an emergent process, whereby the designs and outcomes are formed as the research takes place. It is perhaps for this reason that qualitative methodologies are often inextricably linked with the frameworks and theories that govern them.

Data collection methodologies that are commonly used in qualitative research are the interview, the focus group, direct observation, the document review, and the case study. Table 6.1 provides a concise view of the benefits and drawbacks of each methodology, with the broader purpose, benefits and potential drawbacks of each elaborated in this section. For each methodology, an example within the context of radiation therapy is also highlighted.

TABLE 6.1 Considerations in Qualitative Methodologies.

	Benefits	Drawbacks	Examples
Interviews	Closer rapport between researcher and subject Semi-structured less time-consuming than unstructured Allow for the same basic information to be collected from all interviews	Time, feasibility, cost Potential for interview bias Lack of structured consistency leads to question of reliability of the collected data	Gillan et al. (2010): Telephone interviews held with interprofessional past participants at a continuing education course relating to image-guided radiation therapy, to assess perceptions of interprofessional education[18] Tran et al. (2012): Interviews with patients as part of a mixed methodology to evaluate an online education tool for radiation therapy patients[19]
Focus Groups	Gather a range of information in a relatively short time span Activate forgotten details of experience Reduce apprehension and discomfort amongst subjects being singled out	Considerable preplanning and organizing Sample is not random or representative, as group is usually strategically constructed Data quality is influenced by the motivation and skills of the facilitator	Turner et al. (2013): Radiation therapy focus groups to understand perspectives on radiation therapy research culture at a single institution[20] Cashell (2010): Radiation therapy focus groups to explore the perceived value of reflective practice in the clinical environment[21]

TABLE 6.1 *(Continued)*

	Benefits	Drawbacks	Examples
	Facilitator can explore related but unanticipated topics as they come up Do not require complex sampling techniques	Use the actual words and behaviours of participants to answer research questions – cannot count or measure Power hierarchies within certain interpersonal and professional relationships can affect the information that is provided	Bolderston et al. (2008): Focus groups held with radiation therapists (RTTs) and students to explore experiences of students with English as a second language[22] Bolderston et al. (2010): Radiation therapy focus groups discussing the concept of caring[23]
Document Review	Useful adjunct to triangulate data Rich in information	Challenges in accessing and interpreting data Time demands of processing the information Potential data overload	Trad (2013): Review of course syllabi, orientation packages, hospice volunteer logs, student journal entries, and other documents as part of a case study of the use of engaged scholarship in building radiation therapy students' understanding of palliative care through hospice volunteer rotations[24]
Observation Studies	Researcher witnesses subjects "first-hand" Process, behaviours, and interactions can all be studied	Researcher bias Observation aids or tools may be difficult to use Hawthorne effect (tendency to act differently when aware of participation in a study)[25]	Rees et al. (2013): Video-recorded observations of bedside teaching to investigate power relations between students, teachers, and patients[26]

6.3.1 INTERVIEWS

An interview offers the possibility of gaining insight into the subject's world and a deeper understanding of the nature or meaning of the subject's everyday experiences. This can be done in an unstructured and informal way, as might be applied to ethnological research, or could be more semistructured or structured. In a structured interview, the subjects are asked the same questions in exactly the same way using an interview script.

A structured interview is somewhat similar to a survey as there is no room for deviation or exploration of issues outside of the set questions, but being qualitative it gains different insight and requires a qualitative approach to analysis. A structured interview may also be used to test a hypothesis.[6]

A semistructured interview might allow for the use of prompts beyond the scripted questions, to encourage elaboration of a given idea or topic of conversation. The questions are formatted but the interviewer may deviate from the scheduled questions if an unforeseen discussion point is proving fruitful, using either prescribed prompts or a more informal conversation approach.[27] A study by Hsien et al. used semistructured interviews to investigate follow-up care after palliative radiation therapy.[28] Four prepared questions were used (*see* case example 6.1) and participant responses guided further questions, prompts for elaboration, and validation of responses.

CASE EXAMPLE 6.1

In Their Own Words: A Qualitative Descriptive Study of Patient and Caregiver Perspectives on Follow-Up Care after Palliative Radiotherapy

Hsien et al. used the following questions and prompts to guide semistructured interviews of patients and caregivers to evaluate perspectives on follow-up care after palliative radiation therapy.[28]

1. Please briefly share your cancer history or experience with me.
2. What happens at these follow-up appointments?
3. Who is the main person/team looking after your (the patient's) cancer care?
4. How should follow-up care be done after palliative radiotherapy?

> Five patients and four caregivers were interviewed, and while these Initial questions were all asked, no two interviews followed the same course, as the semistructured design allowed the interviewer to engage in conversation with participants. It was found that participants had a strong belief that follow up care after palliative treatment should encompass treatment outcomes, side effects, and psychosocial support. The medical oncologist was seen as the key professional in their follow-up care, and that personalized follow-up plans were necessary given individual needs.

In contrast, unstructured interviews are free flowing discussions, which can take the interviewer and interviewee in a direction that deviates from the intended subject. The data that can be generated from unstructured and semistructured interviews can be rich and provide more in-depth appreciation of a subject matter than a survey.[27] It is this type of approach that is often used as part of an ethnography study, to supplement observation and integration into the community under investigation.

HOT TIP

> Interview questions should rarely be posed as questions that could be answered with simply a "yes" or a "no" (closed-ended questions), as they will not likely yield data that is as rich. Rather than asking "Do you feel comfortable reporting radiation therapy incidents in which you are involved?" reframe it as "Describe your level of comfort in reporting radiation therapy incidents in which you are involved."

6.3.2 *FOCUS GROUPS*

A focus group is a carefully planned interview of five to 10 persons designed to obtain perceptions on a defined area of interest in a nonthreatening environment. It is a moderated discussion about a particular subject that aims to identify and understand the participants' views.[2,6,27] Traditionally, focus groups are a valued methodology for their tendency to allow for the emergence and discussion of themes that might not otherwise have been touched on or raised by the investigator, or many participants themselves, individually.

Group dynamics can lead to a richer discussion through emergence of forgotten or repressed information, thus enhancing the data collected.[2] If one participant were to make a certain point or give an opinion, others might become engaged in a discussion of that point in a way they would not have been had they been in a one-on-one setting. Successful focus groups are reliant in the make-up of the group: its size, timing, format, and composition.

It is usual practice to have the focus group facilitated by an experienced moderator, external to the social context being investigated but familiar with the subject matter. This reduces the interviewer bias (or power differential). An experienced moderator can also ensure all participants are able to convey their views, build on the thoughts of others, and offer contradictory opinions where desired, within a nonthreatening environment. Since there is a vast amount of data generated it is also helpful to have a separate note taker or audiotape of the session.

The drawback to the participatory nature of the focus group, such as in an interprofessional or practitioner-patient setting where the power relations might come into play, is the potential for the methodology to influence negatively the quality of the data generated. Conscious of who else might be present in the focus group environment, a participant might hesitate to make certain points or disagree with others in a way they would not if their views and perceptions were voiced only to an investigator.[29] There is also the potential, however, that these differing perspectives, expressed in a well-moderated focus group, contribute to a richer understanding of a topic. An example of this, highlighting the insight into imaging literacy in radiation oncology provided by interprofessional focus groups, is discussed in case example 6.2.

CASE EXAMPLE 6.2

Defining Imaging Literacy in Radiation Oncology Interprofessionally: Toward a Competency Profile for Canadian Residency Programs.

A series of four interprofessional focus groups was held between two academically affiliated radiation medicine departments in a study by Gillan et al. (2013).[30] The aim was to investigate elements or competencies that professionals believed should be included in an imaging competency profile for radiation oncology residents. Medical physicists, RTTs, and radiation oncology staff and trainees were represented in each group to stimulate conversation and debate. This dynamic helped to highlight areas of consensus and differences of opinion. For example, oncologists tended to feel more strongly than their physics and therapy counterparts regarding the importance of being physically able to perform certain imaging-related tasks, such as cone-beam computed tomography image registrations, rather than simply understand the principles and be able to identify areas of concern. All agreed that there was a lack of structure in Canadian radiation oncology residency programs, and the focus groups in this investigation sparked a dialogue between trainees and staff regarding how imaging competencies might be better achieved.

6.3.3 *OBSERVATION*

The main purpose of using observation studies in healthcare research is for the researcher to witness first-hand what people say and do in "real life," rather than relying on the subject's interpretation or recollection of the situation.[2]

There are two main types of observation studies: participant observation and nonparticipant observation. Participant observation is employed in ethnography studies, with a reliance on the researcher becoming immersed in the social situation that is being investigated, to the point that they are accepted as an integral member of the community. This method is ideal when the researcher is investigating areas of his or her own practice, as the researcher is already an insider.[6,27] The researcher enters the situation with no clear intentions or objectives and as the events or behaviour unfolds, the researcher records the observations after the event has occurred. This is also known as unstructured observation.[2,6,27]

Whereas participant observation is complete participation, Cohen et al. describe nonparticipant observation as complete detachment.[6] This method often relies on charts or checklists to allow the researcher to catalogue events as they occur. The nature of the interaction, the process undertaken, or the behaviours of the subjects are all themes that could be observed.

6.3.4 DOCUMENT REVIEW

Many projects, especially those undertaken by novice and student researchers with limited time or resources, involve the review of documents or charts. There is often a misconception that a chart or document review is a fairly straightforward research methodology. However, as with all methodologies, there are challenges to generating rigourous and valuable data. Sources of primary documents that a researcher may consider reviewing for data include minutes from meetings, departmental policies, publications from national and provincial associations, and newspaper articles. The first thing a researcher must ensure is the accessibility of the documents in question: this can be a significant issue if certain documents are considered confidential.[27] If accessible and available, management of the selection of the documents is essential, as this method could result in vast amounts of documentation that must be sifted through for valuable data. Similarly, an analysis of the content of the documents could result in data irrelevant to the initial research question.[6,27] Trad made use of course syllabi, orientation handouts, student journal entries, volunteer logs, and numerous other documents in an assessment of the value of student hospice placement in undergraduate radiation therapy education.[24] While not all information would have pertained to the research question, a thorough researcher was able to identify and organize information to provide a rich dataset to shed light on the topic.

Reflection on the content, and the document itself, forms the crux of the analysis. This evaluation is divided into two processes: external and internal criticism. External criticism questions the authenticity of the documents (i.e., that it truthfully reports on the subject), and ensuring the document is genuine. Internal criticism is the rigourous analysis of the content of the document, seeking answers to questions such as:

"What kind of document is it; policy, government statute, meeting minutes?"
"What does it actually say?"
"Who produced it and what is known about the author?"
"When was it produced?"
"Is it complete[26]?"

While the evidence or data generated can be both thorough and worthwhile, the researcher should be aware that data overload and the time demands of processing and coding are considerable.[6,27]

6.3.5 CASE STUDY

A case study is a methodology that is often applied informally as a teaching strategy, but rarely as a mode of inquiry unto itself. While the term "case study" is traditionally applied to the experience of a single patient, other units of analysis can be considered here. Implemented at the level of an individual patient case, it can guide decision making, and at the level of an organization it can be a form of health services research to guide program evaluation.[31] At any level, it is a valuable means to triangulate other sources of data or methods of investigation. Yin suggests that case studies might be considered when the investigation seeks to answer the "how" or "why" of a situation, when the behaviour and context of the subject cannot be manipulated, or when the boundaries and relationships between the subject and the context are unclear.[32] Cases can be explanatory (complex causal links), exploratory (no single, clear set of outcomes), or descriptive (contextual description).[32]

To avoid the common pitfall of having a case study become a simple narrative, it is important to keep it manageable in scope through a process known as "binding," where boundaries relating to time, place, and context are applied.[31] For example, as reported by Baxter and Jack, an investigation of decision making in reconstructive surgery after mastectomy might employ case studies to gain insight on decisions made by women in their thirties within six months of mastectomy receiving care at a tertiary care centre in a specific hospital.[31]

6.4 DATA COLLECTION

6.4.1 *SAMPLING*

Unlike in quantitative investigations, where the aim is usually to maximize the ability to generalize results to a broader population, qualitative studies generally strive to gain insight into a particular population or phenomenon. For this reason, the approach to sampling is quite different.

Qualitative study samples tend to be smaller, and investigators should be concerned with harnessing the "richest" sources of data.[33] A necessary sample size cannot be calculated based on a required power of the investigation. It is often not determined at the outset of the study at all, instead only finalized at the point of data saturation through an iterative process, when new themes, insight, and categories stop emerging with further sampling.[33]

There are four traditional approaches to sampling in qualitative research.

6.4.1.1 *CONVENIENCE SAMPLE*

Convenience sampling is the use of the most accessible subjects or environment. While most qualitative sampling includes a degree of convenience, it is the least rigourous approach to selecting subjects.[33] A researcher investigating patient perspectives on sexual health after gynecological treatment might choose to attend a radiation follow-up clinic and approach any patients who had a history of gynaecological radiation treatment. This might not ensure a representative sample, but it would be a fast and simple method to accrue subjects.

6.4.1.2 PURPOSEFUL SAMPLE

Based on the researcher's understanding of the richest sources of information and the variety of samples required, purposeful sampling involves selection of subjects that will likely provide the most valuable insight to the investigation.[33] This may involve a stratification of necessary variables such as age, gender, experience, professional group etc. The value of opposing views should also be considered. In many cases, key informants or content experts are sought to provide the most information on a given topic.

6.4.1.3 CRITICAL CASE SAMPLE

Especially in the use of case studies, where it might be that a single or very few "subjects" or cases are included, it is important to articulate the objective of the study, and select cases that will help to meet that objective. Selection of a typical case can highlight a common set of values or provide a general understanding of a phenomenon. Through exploring a typical case, potential causal relationships might be explored, and could be considered representative.[34]

An extreme or intense case sample is, as the name suggests, the selection of a case that lies far from the average or "typical," and in its intensity can be prototypical or paradigmatic.[34] For example, in investigating radiation therapy incident analysis, there is value in exploring the Therac-25 cases, which involved patient deaths, to highlight systematic issues that might inform analysis of incidents on a much smaller scale.[35]

A diverse or deviant case sample would include a minimum of two cases, representing what are believed to be the extremes or range of values or relationships.[34] The researcher might select these based on a set of variables for which cases can be identified that differ with respect to a variable. It is this variation that can be highlighted through deviant case sampling.

6.4.1.4 THEORETICAL SAMPLING

Theoretical sampling is the most iterative in its approach. It is based on the desire to build a story or framework out of the data collected, and thus relies on ongoing data analysis to inform the inclusion of future samples.[33] As themes emerge, new samples are selected to elaborate on identified ideas or concepts. Theoretical sampling is the key approach to grounded theory methodologies, as the researcher works to build a theory out of collected data.

6.4.2 ETHICAL CONSIDERATIONS IN CONSENT AND ACCESS

When determining and approaching a sample population, it is important to consider the unique ethical issues inherent in qualitative research. While ethics in research has been covered earlier in this book, the unique issues here warrant special consideration. For additional reference on this topic, Wright et al. explore several practical and ethical considerations in the use of focus groups in radiation therapy, and many of the principles discussed will also apply to the broader set of qualitative methodologies.[36]

6.4.2.1 RELATIONSHIPS

The relationship between the researcher and any subjects in the investigation is important in many ways. This relationship can impact the quality of the data collected, but should also be considered in terms of the safety and interests of the subject. An interviewer, moderator, or acknowledged observer can be seen as being in a position of power in a given situation, and a conflict of interest might arise if there is also a pre-existing power differential, be it actual or perceived. Patients being interviewed by a professional who could be in a position to provide direct care might feel that refusal to participate or to "give the right answers" could lead to inferior care. A staff member being interviewed by a superior might similarly fear negative repercussions for the expression of certain opinions.

If such a dynamic is identified, it might be prudent to engage an external facilitator to conduct the data collection – someone who is deemed impartial and does not have a pre-existing relationship with the subject. The relationship of the researcher to the investigation is discussed further later in this chapter, relating to reflexivity.

6.4.2.2 CONSENT

While most qualitative investigations involving subjects requires their express consent, interviews and focus groups can trigger memories, experiences, or situations that are uncomfortable or painful to the subject, and the investigator must be well-versed in the ethical considerations in attending to such potentialities.[37] For example, in interviewing a cancer patient about end of life decisions, someone who might consent at the start of the investigation could become distressed during the interview. The researcher must thus understand when to "continue with the interview and gain more insight about the topic under study or to stop the interview and give advice or refer the participant to an appropriate treatment or counseling service.[37]" In investigations where sensitive issues are likely to emerge, it is common practice to include in the research protocol a plan for managing this, including informing (and reinforcing) potential participants of their right to withdraw and having a process in place for referral or otherwise addressing the subject's emotional needs. In most situations, the express permission of the subject is required before a referral can be made, given concerns and stipulations regarding confidentiality in research.

6.4.2.3 CONFIDENTIALITY

While confidentiality has been addressed elsewhere in this book (*see* Chapter 3; Research Ethics Applications), it is important to note the inherent relationship in much qualitative research between the richness and completeness of the data and the identity of the subject. Confidentiality can thus be a challenge as the researcher must strike an ethically appropriate balance between reporting the data and the ethnographic context, and maintaining the anonymity of the participant. In some circumstances, the researcher might choose to code participants. For example, Gillan et al., felt it was important to acknowledge the profession of focus group participants in a study of interprofessional perspectives on imaging competency amongst radiation oncology residents (*see* Case example 6.2).[30] A coding system thus allowed for differentiation between medical physicists, RTTs, and radiation oncologists, as the researchers acknowledged that this would not provide sufficient information to identify the participant.

6.4.2.4 DECEPTION

There is a conflicting dynamic in qualitative methodologies where the formalization of a relationship between the researcher and the subject, through the process of consent, is felt to impact the situation under investigation and weaken the quality of any collected data. This comes into play primarily in ethnographic research, such as with participant observation, where the researcher is directly immersed in the environment, and might not be identifiable as a researcher. While intentional deception through nondisclosure of research intents was once common practice in sociological research, it is now more strictly regulated by governing ethics boards and principles in most jurisdictions.[38,39] Methodological and ethical considerations must be weighed and decisions justified to deceive research subjects through not disclosing that they are part of an investigation or the nature of the investigation.[38]

6.4.2.5 REFLEXIVITY

Reflexivity is the consideration of the impact of the researcher's personal background, values, and construction of meanings on the carrying out of research and the interpretation of data.[40] By describing relevant aspects of what the researcher brings to the investigation in this way, the reader is better able to "explore the ways in which a researcher's involvement with a particular study influences, acts upon, and informs such research.[40]"

The information thought to be most relevant here is the professional background of the investigators, and thus warrants consideration.

6.5 ANALYSIS AND INTERPRETATION

6.5.1 DATA SATURATION

Data collection usually continues until the researcher begins to achieve data saturation or until resources are exhausted. Data saturation is the point at which no new ideas, themes, or points of view emerge with each new opportunity for data collection, and suggests that a full appreciation of a topic can be built from the data collected. This can be considered similar to the idea of power in quantitative research, though there is no true method to assess prospectively how many subjects must be included to reach saturation. Qualitative researchers predominately use inductive data analysis, which means that critical themes emerge out of the data.[16]

6.5.2 TRANSCRIPTION

It is generally recommended that interviews or focus groups be audio recorded to ensure the completeness and accuracy of data, and such recordings must be transcribed to text prior to analysis. Transcription can often be outsourced to either an administrative assistant who regularly transcribes physician clinic notes, or to a professional transcription service. Transcribing recordings oneself, however, does build an early familiarity and intimacy with the data which might be beneficial to the analysis.

Any field notes acquired during the study, either as a primary method of data collection or to supplement audio or video recordings, should also be formally documented and organized.

It is important to treat any audio or video recordings with the same care as other forms of data when it comes to data security. Recordings may be required by institutional ethics boards to be kept in a safe and secure place for a finite amount of time.

6.5.3 CODING

The data can be sorted, broken into subunits and worked with until patterns emerge. In this way, the raw data is organised into meaningful categories for communication to others.[41] This process is often referred to as coding. Given the potential for bias, it is common practice for data to be coded independently by a researcher who was not directly involved in the collection of data, or by multiple researchers who might then meet to build consensus through refinement of categorizations.

In the latter stages of coding, it is common to distil specific quotations that might articulate key points. In cases where participants might not have been succinct, it is permissible to shorten quotations by removing text and replacing it with "…." It is sometimes also necessary to change certain words in a valuable quotation, either to maintain anonymity, clarify a reference to something, or change a tense.

For example, a quotation might initially read as follows:

> *"I've noticed that Sarah does not know how to speak to the paediatric patients at their level, and it makes them anxious. It really drives me nuts to watch her talk to them like they are adults, and expect them to understand and follow commands when they're scared! You know, it might be useful if we could have a lunch and learn. I think we need education about this. We, as radiation therapists, would benefit from it, as it would equip us to relate to different generations and populations."*

It could be more succinctly written as the following, without altering the meaning intended by the participant:

> *"I've noticed that [a colleague of mine] does not know how to speak to the paediatric patients at their level, and it makes them anxious…. We, as radiation therapists, would benefit from [education about this], as it would equip us to relate to different generations and populations."*

6.5.4 DATA MANAGEMENT

There may be hundreds of pages of raw data and sorting it can be done by hand, using a word processing system to divide text into categories, or by organizing it using one of several analytical computer software programs for qualitative data such as NVivo®, ATLAS.ti® or N6® (formerly nud*ist). Such programs can facilitate the grouping and regrouping of quotations, related field notes, and even segments of dialogue. Even those who have access to this type of resource will often choose to complete at least some aspect of the coding and analysis using paper transcripts and different-coloured marker highlighters.

As discussed earlier in this chapter, it is often desirable to highlight certain relationships, trends, commonalities and differences between subjects. Anonymization of data is important in terms of ethical conduct of research, but the process of data coding and management might involve the development of a nomenclature system for identifying certain characteristics amongst subjects.

6.5.5 RIGOUR AND TRUSTWORTHINESS

Whereas quantitative research is concerned with issues of validity, reliability and objectivity, the realities of qualitative work require these terms to be redefined, most often under the umbrella of trustworthiness.[42] The most relevant terms include:

- **C**redibility: that explanations of explored phenomena are consistent and understandable
- **T**ransferability: that there is enough information provided to allow the results to be adapted to another context or population
- **C**onformability: that there is a distinction between the researchers and the subject's ideas
- **D**ependability: that the process used to obtain the results can be replicated

Methods to ensure trustworthiness include the following steps:

1. Audit Trail: Detailed documentation of all decisions made during data collection and analysis to ensure a transparent process

2. Peer Review: This can include an independent review of the themes by research team members or a review of themes by peer(s) not involved in the research
3. Member Checking: Interpretations of the data are shared with participants to ensure that meaning has been preserved
4. Triangulation: Compare data with those from other sources (e.g., focus groups with surveys).
5. Negative Case Analysis: Deliberately look for contrasting experiences or examples to disprove emerging theories
6. Data saturation: Gather data until all themes are exhausted

6.5.6 REPORTING QUALITATIVE RESEARCH

The sound reporting of qualitative research is a difficult skill to master, and depends greatly on the specific qualitative approach, the richness of the data collected, and the method and audience of dissemination. In many cases, quotations and direct observations constitute the data points, and it is important to know how to include them in writing.

While the considerations in reporting qualitative research are beyond the scope of this chapter, it is often beneficial for someone embarking on a qualitative study to read other published work that made use of a similar methodology. The inclusion of specific quotations from focus groups, interviews, or observation studies, or passages from document reviews, will provide weight to arguments. These should be balanced, however with summative narrative and paraphrasing to highlight certain points.

HOT TIP

The reporting of response rates and descriptive statistics do not tend to be appropriate in qualitative research, as the focus is instead on relationships, experiences, and concepts.

The strength of qualitative research is in its ability to capture the details, practice, and experience of the subjects as it occurs. The types and qualities of interactions are described, thereby providing meaning to subjective experiences. This chapter provides a brief introductory overview of the value of qualitative research methodologies. A running example relates the theoretical underpinning of qualitative research to the radiation sciences. To conclude, the qualitative approach can be a useful and enlightening way to research issues in many areas of our daily practice. As Hoepfl notes, "the decision to use qualitative methodologies should be considered carefully; by its very nature qualitative research can be emotionally taxing and extraordinarily time consuming. At the same time, it can yield rich information not obtainable through statistical sampling techniques.[41]"

KEYWORDS

- Subjective
- Interviews
- Focus groups
- Reflexivity
- Saturation
- Iteration

REFERENCES

1. Palmer, C.; Bolderston, A. A brief introduction to qualitative research. *Can. J. Med. Radiat.* Technol. **2006,** *37(1)*, 16–19.
2. Polgar, S. Thomas, S. A. Introduction to Research in the Health Sciences, 2nd ed.; Churchill Livingstone: Edinburgh, 1991.
3. Mertens, D. M. Research and evaluation in education and psychology: integrating diversity within quantitative, qualitative and mixed methods. Sage Publications Inc: Thousand Oaks, CA, 2005.
4. Cresswell, J. W. Qualitative inquiry and research design. Sage Publications Inc: Thousand Oaks, CA, 1998.

5. Denzin, N. K.; Lincoln, Y. S. Introduction: the discipline and practice of qualitative research. In: Handbook of Qualitative Research; Denzin, N. K.; Lincoln, Y. S., Eds.; Sage Publications Inc: Thousand Oaks, CA, 1994.
6. Cohen, L.; Manion, L.; Morrison, K. Research methods in education. 6th ed.; Routledge: New York, 2001.
7. Neergaard, M. A.; Olesen, F.; Andersen, R. S.; Sondergaard, J. Qualitative description – the poor cousin of health research? *BMC Med. Res. Methodol.* **2009,** *9*, 52.
8. Bunniss, S.; Kelly, D. R. Research paradigms in medical education research. *Med. Educ*. **2010,** *44(4)*, 358–366.
9. Glaser, B. G.; Strauss, A. L. The discovery of grounded theory; strategies for qualitative research. Aldine Publishing Co.: Chicago, 1967.
10. Kennedy, T. J.; Lingard, L. A. Making sense of grounded theory in medical education. *Med. Educ.* **2006,** *40(2)*, 101–8.
11. Goulding, C. Grounded theory, ethnography and phenomenology: A comparative analysis of three qualitative strategies for marketing research. *Eur. J. Mark.* **2005,** *39(3/4)*, 294–308.
12. Hammersley, M.; Atkinson, P. Ethnography: Principles in practice. Routledge: New York, 2007.
13. Pettigrew, S. F., Ethnography and grounded theory: a happy marriage? *Adv. Consum. Res*. **2000,** *27*.
14. Morse, J. M. The cultural sensitivity of grounded theory. *Qual. Health Res.* **2001,** *11(6)*, 721–2.
15. Ng, C. K.; White, P. Qualitative research design and approaches in radiography. *Radiography* **2005,** *11(3)*, 217–225.
16. Patton, M. Q. Qualitative evaluation and research methods. Sage Publications Inc: Thousand Oaks, CA, 1990.
17. Woodgate, R. Part I: an introduction to conducting qualitative research in children with cancer. *J. Paediatr. Oncol. Nurs.* **2000,** *17(4)*, 192–206.
18. Gillan, C.; Wiljer, D.; Harnett, N.; Briggs, K.; Catton, P. Changing stress while stressing change: the role of interprofessional education in mediating stress in the introduction of a transformative technology. *J. Interprof. Care.* **2010,** *24(6)*, 710–21.
19. Tran, C.; Szumacher, E.; Di Prospero, L., A pilot study evaluating the usability and usefulness of a multilanguage online patient education tool for patients undergoing radiation treatment: findings from a student project. *J. Med. Imag. Radiat. Sci.* **2012,** *43(3)*, 181–196.
20. Turner, A.; D'Alimonte, L.; Fitch, M. Promoting radiation therapy research: understanding perspectives, transforming culture. *J. Radiat. Pract.* **2013,** *12(2)*, 92–99.
21. Cashell, A., Radiation therapists' perspectives of the role of reflection in clinical practice. *J. Radiat. Pract.* **2010,** *9(3)*, 131–141.
22. Bolderston, A.; Palmer, C.; Flanagan, W.; McParland, N. The experiences of English as second language radiation therapy students in the undergraduate clinical program: Perceptions of staff and students. *Radiography* **2008,** *14(3)*, 216–225.
23. Bolderston, A.; Lewis, D.; Chai, M. J. The concept of caring: Perceptions of radiation therapists. *Radiography* **2010,** *16(3)*, 198–208.

24. Trad, M. Engaged Scholarship in Partnership with a Local Hospice: A Qualitative Case Study in a Radiation Therapy Classroom. PhD Dissertation, Texas State University, San Marcos, TX, 2013.
25. Eckmanns, T.; Bessert, J.; Behne, M.; Gastmeier, P.; Ruden, H. Compliance with antiseptic hand rub use in intensive care units: the Hawthorne effect. *Infect. Control Hosp. Epidemiol.* **2006,** *27(9)*, 931–934.
26. Rees, C. E.; Ajjawi, R.; Monrouxe, L. V. The construction of power in family medicine bedside teaching: a video observation study. *Med. Educ.* **2013,** *47(2)*, 154–65.
27. Bell, J. Doing your research project: a guide for first-time researchers in education, health and social science. 5th ed.; Open University Press: Berkshire, England, 2010.
28. Hsien, J. W.; Rosewall, T.; Wong, R. K. In Their Own Words: A Qualitative Descriptive Study of Patient and Caregiver Perspectives on Follow-Up Care after Palliative Radiotherapy. *J. Med. Imag. Radiat. Sci.* (Online early access). doi:10.1016/j.jmir.2013.01.001. Published online: March 7, 2013. www.jmirs.org (accessed July 2nd, **2013**).
29. Krueger, R. Moderating focus groups, Vol. 4. Sage: Thousand Oaks, CA, 1997.
30. Gillan, C.; Uchino, M.; Giuliani, M.; Millar, B. A.; Catton, P. Defining imaging literacy in radiation oncology interprofessionally: toward a competency profile for Canadian residency programs.. *Med. Imag. Radiat. Sci.* **2013,** *44(3)*, 150–156.
31. Baxter, P.; Jack, S. Qualitative case study methodology: Study design and implementation for novice researchers. *Qual. Rep.* **2008,** *13(4)*, 544–559.
32. Yin, R. K. Case study research: Design and methods, Vol 5. Sage: Thousand Oaks, CA, 2007.
33. Marshall, M. N. Sampling for qualitative research. *Family Practice* **1996,** *13(6)*, 522–5.
34. Gerring, J. Case study research. Cambridge University Press: Cambridge, 2007.
35. Leveson, N. G.; Turner, C. S. An investigation of the Therac-25 accidents. *Computer,* **1993,** *26(7)*, 18–41.
36. Wright, C. A.; Schneider-Kolsky, M. E.; Jolly, B.; Baird, M. A. Using focus groups in radiation therapy research: Ethical and practical considerations. *J. Radiother. Pract.* **2011,** *11(4)*, 217.
37. Orb, A.; Eisenhauer, L.; Wynaden, D. Ethics in qualitative research. J. Nurs. Scholarsh. **2001,** *33(1)*, 93–6.
38. Kimmel, A. J.; Smith, N. C.; Klein, J. G. Ethical decision making and research deception in the behavioural sciences: An application of social contract theory. *Ethics Behav.* **2011,** *21(3)*, 222–251;
39. Marzano, M., Informed consent, deception, and research freedom in qualitative research. *Qual. Inq.* **2007,** *13(3)*, 417–436.
40. Nightingale, D. J.; Cromby, J. Social constructivist psychology: a critical analysis of theory and practice. Open University Press: Buckingham, 1999.
41. Hoepfl, M. C. Choosing qualitative research: A primer for technology education researchers. *J. Tech. Edu.* **1997,** *9(1)*, 47–63.
42. Corbin, J.; Strauss, A. Basics of qualitative research: Grounded theory procedures and techniques. Sage: Thousand Oaks, CA, 1990.

CHAPTER 7

SURVEY METHODOLOGIES AND ANALYSIS

RUTH BARKER MRT(T) BSc MEd

Instructor, Department of Radiation Oncology, University of Toronto, Toronto Canada

CONTENTS

Survey research is a method of inquiry that has widespread use over a diverse number of research settings. It is not encompassed well in either the quantitative or qualitative domains, but rather incorporates elements of both and requires several additional, unique considerations. Market research is a form of survey research, as is random telephone polling of an electorate to determine candidate preference. When an entire population is surveyed, this is known as a census or status survey, whereas when a subset of a known population participates it is known as a survey sample.[1,2]

7.1 THE NATURE OF SURVEY METHODOLOGY

Survey research is a systematic way to capture the beliefs, attitudes, or outcomes, the results of which can often be generalized to the larger population from which the sample was selected.[1–4] This type of research is the most common form used in social science and health service research.[5] The method has gained considerable credibility through its widespread use and acceptance in the academic environment.[4]

In health professional and medical research, surveys allow the researcher the ability to capture data that will provide insight into individuals' perspectives and experiences. It does so by self-reported data collection.[4] There are three main types of surveys that are used to collect data about individual perspectives.[4] These are:

- Epidemiological surveys
- Surveys assessing attitudes about a health service or intervention
- Questionnaires assessing knowledge of a particular issue or topic

Some examples of surveys commonly used in healthcare research are patient reported quality of life surveys, (known as HRQoL) and patient satisfaction survey scales; for example, the widely used NRC Picker Patient Experience Survey,[5] which allows comparison between hospitals on specific dimensions of the patient's experience. Results from both of these types of measures can assist in institutional planning and decision making to inform approaches to care delivery.

Radiation therapists (RTTs) have published papers in peer reviewed journals using this type of research methodology, with the subjects of the research being colleagues, patients or students.[1,3,6] There are many valid reasons to employ a survey research design to investigate a research question. This method, like any research method has advantages and disadvantages. Some advantages are:

- Ability to generalize about a large population from data collected from a small portion of that population[4,5]
- Convenience and timeliness of data collection[4]
- Ability to make planned comparisons between groups at one time or over time[4]
- Administration from and to remote locations across wide geographical locations[3,5]
- Comparison of well-developed standardized tool results across settings[1,3,4]
- Initiation of inquiry into a new area of research (exploratory), and subsequent ability to inform larger scale research design and instruments[3]
- Allows for real world data collection[5]
- Offers multiple ways to collect data (*see* Table 7.1)
- Allows for both qualitative and quantitative data collection[7], with combinations of the two giving rise to richer data[5]
- Conveys to respondents that their opinion is important[7]
- Cost efficiency (depending on data collection method)

While there are many advantages of survey research, there are also disadvantages that need to be considered before proceeding with a project using this method of inquiry. Some disadvantages of survey research are:

- Inaccuracy of subject recall and self-reporting of events compared to objective measures[3]
- If unable to obtain an adequate sample size the research project may be considered to be invalid
- Non response
- Training required for verbal formats[5]
- Cost (depending on data collection method) and time
- Possible impact of the quality of the survey instrument or the skills of the person administering the survey[5,8]
- Sampling errors
- Representativeness of the data being completely dependent on the sampling frame and method
- Quality of the data being limited by the questions on the data collection tool

7.2 STEPS INVOLVED IN SURVEY RESEARCH

Survey research follows the same basic steps as any kind of research project, with some method specific considerations. Rea and Parker outline 11 stages of the survey research process (listed below) in *Designing and Conducting Survey Research: A Comprehensive Guide* (p. 23).[4] The focus of the discussion in this chapter will be on those topics that are salient to survey research and have not been covered elsewhere in this book.

7.2.1 *STAGES OF THE SURVEY RESEARCH PROCESS*

Conducting a survey to answer a research question requires a systematic and rigourous approach to developing and implementing the instrument, and analyzing the resulting data. The following are steps that can guide the researcher in this process:[4]

1. Identify the focus of the study and method of research
2. Determine the research schedule and budget
3. Establish an information base
4. Determine the sampling frame
5. Determine the sample size and sample selection procedures
6. Design the survey instrument
7. Pretest the survey instrument
8. Select and train the interviewers
9. Implement the survey
10. Code and computerize the data
11. Analyze the data and prepare the final report

7.3 GETTING STARTED WITH SURVEY RESEARCH

Any research project begins with an idea; a conceptualization of the problem, which leads to a review of the literature to determine what is already known. Often these ideas come from observations in clinical practice or through professional experience that has made a clinician curious to know if the observations or anecdotal events are random in nature, or if there is some underlying reason that waits to be discovered. As stated in earlier chapters, starting with a literature review allows the researcher to determine if this phenomena or idea has already been investigated. If it has and there is a clear, well-researched answer, then there is no point in redoing the same study, since the work is not creating new knowledge in the area of interest. However, if there is good reason to believe that the answer may be different for the population in question, then it is appropriate to proceed.

A literature review can also be helpful to determine existing tools and how and with whom they have been used. This serves to refine and formulate the research question, determines that survey research is appropriate and enables a clear definition of the population to be surveyed. An expansion of this concept will be provided in the section on survey instruments, later in the chapter.

7.4 DATA COLLECTION

7.4.1 TEMPORAL CONSIDERATIONS

Once it has been determined that the research question is feasible and warrants further investigation using survey methods, decisions regarding when and how to collect survey data must be made. The time span of the data collection is an important aspect of survey study design. Survey methodology can take two different forms with respect to temporal considerations: cross-sectional or longitudinal design.

Cross-sectional surveys take place across a population at a specific point in time.

Longitudinal surveys use the same tool to study a particular issue over time. If the same individuals are surveyed over time, it is known as a longitudinal cohort survey. If the same population, but different subjects are surveyed over time it is known as a longitudinal trend survey.[5] The schedule of survey administration depends on the research question(s) that are at the heart of the study.

7.4.2 BUDGET CONSIDERATIONS

Survey research projects can be large and complex, and require a significant budget to complete (such as a national survey of the opinions of all breast cancer survivors). Alternatively, they can be a small, inexpensive in-house project or online survey. The research design and subsequent budget required depends on the goal of the research. If decisions will be made on the basis of the results, then a larger budget may be required to develop a more rigourous research protocol. There are granting agencies available to fund these types of projects. A detailed discussion of how to develop a research budget can be found in Chapter 3 (Research Proposals). Specific unique costs that need to be accounted for in a survey budget will depend on the data collection method, but might include:

- Online survey tool site registration or membership
- Postage for mailed surveys (often including postage-paid return envelopes)
- Cost of access to and permission to use a standardized tool
- Data analysis software
- Training of interviewers
- Questionnaire Development

7.4.3 APPROACHES

Survey research can use a variety of data collection methods. The method of data collection will depend on whether the focus of the research question is descriptive, explanatory or exploratory (*see* Chapter 1: Evidence-Based Medicine and the Scientific Method).[3] Standard data collection methods are face to face, by mail, over the telephone, by electronic means or by some combination of these. Table 7.1 is adapted from Jones, Baxter and Khan with additional references added. It provides an overview of the advantages and disadvantages of each collection method.[6]

TABLE 7.1 Advantages and Disadvantage of Survey Research Data Collection Methods.

Method of Data Collection	Advantages	Disadvantages
Face to Face (Personal)	Personal connection Able to ask more complex questions, clarify and probe[1,4] Visual aids can be used Higher response rates Subjects can be illiterate, young, frail, less fluent (i.e., less selection bias)[1,5] Quantitative and open ended questions used[2,9]	Expensive[2,4,6] Training required Time inefficient[4,6] Interviewer effects[4,6,9] Greater stress for interviewer and subject[4] Less anonymity[4] Sensitive questions[10] Scheduling[9] Subject or researcher may need to travel
Telephone	Allows clarification/probing[4] Less personal (sensitive questions)[4,10] Larger area of sampling Less expensive than face to face Higher response rates Ability to increase sample X 5 for same cost as interview[1] Technology assists[11] Rapid data collection[4]	No visual aids/cues[4] Training required Difficult to develop rapport[4] New technology impedes response rates[9,11] More expensive than other methods[4] Time consuming for interviewer
Mail	Larger target Limited visual aids[4] Impersonal-sensitive questions[10] Reduced interviewer bias[4] Anonymous[4] Standardized[1] all questions are the same Training not required[4] Less costly[4] Convenient for subjects with no time constraints[4]	Non response[6] especially for open ended question[4] Time for data compilation Lower response rates[3,4] Impersonal[4] Non response bias[12] Follow up required can lengthen the data collection period[4]

TABLE 7.1 *(Continued)*

Method of Data Collection	Advantages	Disadvantages
Electronic (Web Based Surveys)	Larger target	Non response
	Visual aids[4,13]	Not all subjects accessible[3]
	Quick response	Lower response rates
	Quick data compilation[4]	Design effects[16]
	Convenient[4]	Overuse[13]
	Cost effective[4]	Operating system requirements[13]
	Easy follow up[4]	

7.5 ENHANCEMENT AND BARRIERS TO SURVEY DATA COLLECTION

Technological advances have had both positive and negative effects on survey research data collection in recent years. The ability to take advantage of these advances is entirely dependent upon the budget for the project. For telephone surveys some of the advancements have included random digit dialing (to offset the increasing number of households with an unlisted number), interactive voice response (to reduce costs and computerize responses received over the telephone) and computer assisted telephone interviews.[11]

Some technological advances that have impeded telephone survey data collection and led to declining response rates are answering machines, caller identification, block call phone functions and the increasing use of cell phones.[11] In the latest data available from Statistics Canada, 91% of households had a home phone, but the numbers of Canadians who exclusively use a cellular phone is on the rise, especially with the younger demographics.[15] These trends should be kept in mind for telephone survey research. It is unlikely that clinical researchers will have access to these highly technical tools outside of government-led health services research (*see* Chapter 9: Health Services Research and Program Evaluation). For smaller scale projects, if using telephone data collection methods, it is important to ensure that subjects who have consented know the specific time they will be contacted, and are aware of the number that will display on a call display system. These steps will increase the likelihood of reaching the subjects and having them completes the telephone survey.

Combination methods can be beneficial in offsetting some of the collection method disadvantages noted above. There is less research available on the efficacy of combination methods; however, they can likely offset some of the noted disadvantages of individual methods. For example, a survey can be sent by mail with an option to complete and return a hard copy version, or the recipient can be directed to a web version of the survey.[13]

Two thirds of Canadians have a home computer and access to the internet, and this is expected to increase.[16] Electronic surveys are likely to dominate survey research data collection in the future, but as with all sampling techniques, the demographic characteristic of the population needs to be carefully considered if the results are to be generalized widely.[11] For clinical researchers the ability to use online surveys as part of a research project is becoming increasingly simple. There are free online survey providers that can be adequately used for data collection for small scale studies, and while these can facilitate broad dissemination and subsequent data analysis, they can be time-consuming to prepare and the researcher must be wary of considerations relating to confidentiality and security of data in an online forum. For an in-depth discussion of issues and considerations when using web-based surveys, refer to Couper and Mahon-Haft.[13,14]

A final example of a technological advancement that can make things simpler for survey research participants and researchers alike is the availability of video interviews. This modality has the advantage of the personal connection between the researcher and the subject, without the need for either party to travel. This cuts down the cost of interviewing significantly and can be particularly useful where subjects (such as radiation therapy patients) may not be willing to return to the clinic or hospital to participate in a face-to-face survey interview.

7.6 SAMPLING

7.6.1 DETERMINING THE SAMPLING FRAME, SAMPLE SIZE AND SAMPLE SELECTION PROCEDURES

It is rare that a researcher based in clinical practice will have the financial means, or support to sample an entire population to find answers to a practical research question. As acknowledged in Chapter 5 (Quantitative

Methodologies and Analysis), this is also inappropriate. This dictates the systematic use of a rigourous and well-defined sampling strategy. Most authors strongly encourage the use of random (probability) sampling of subjects from the population in question, to allow for generalization of the results. Most of the statistical tests used to analyze data are based on the assumption that the data has been drawn from a random sampling of subjects. The basis for survey research is grounded in statistics and the linkages between the sampling process and the application in this method of research are often overlooked.[4] There are also nonprobability methods of sampling, but there are limitations to their use. The research results from this type of sampling are considered to be less rigourous and not generalizable beyond the subjects themselves. Each will be described briefly from the perspective of survey research, though many of these approaches have been touched on in the previous two chapters.[2,4,5,9,17,18]

The starting point for a sampling process is to determine the sampling frame defined as "a complete and accurate list of the population to be sampled.[1]" This is the pool from which a selection of subjects to participate in the survey is drawn. It does not mean all subjects will have all the requirement characteristics for the final study sample, but will be eligible to be included in the sampling unit. Note that when one refers to sample subjects, the unit of analysis is often individual people (e.g., patients), but it could also be individual institutions or groups of people or institutions, depending on the focus of the research question[4]. Often novice researchers think that a large sample size can make up for any number of methodological weaknesses, but statisticians caution that "when a selection procedure is biased, taking a large sample does not help. This just repeats the basic mistake on a larger scale.[17]"

7.6.2 RANDOM OR PROBABILITY SAMPLING

Random or probability sampling requires an accurate sampling frame, where all potential subjects are assigned a unique number.[1] Random sampling can be done manually using random number tables, or computer generated random assignment to the sample.[1] One of the greatest advantages of random sampling is that it controls for many sources of variation, even those that may not have been considered. If the sample is large enough, the varied characteristics of the population will even out.[1] The main types of probability sampling techniques are; simple, systematic, stratified and cluster or multistage.

7.6.2.1 SIMPLE RANDOM SAMPLING

Simple random sampling is analogous to putting all of the unique participant numbers into a hat and pulling out the required number of participants at random.[1,18] To be truly considered random sampling, the process is actually quite complex, as the entire sample population cannot often be established and "put in a hat." True random sampling would require specialized randomization functions within a software program.

7.6.2.2 SYSTEMATIC RANDOM SAMPLING

Systematic random sampling is when the potential subjects are listed by some order that is unrelated to what is being measured; e.g., alphabetically[18]. The researcher then chooses every nth subject from a randomly selected starting point of all "N" subjects. The value of n is determined by the sampling fraction, which is equal to N/required sample size. For example for a required sample size of 100 from a population of 1000 individuals, 1000/100=10, therefore n=10 and every 10th individual on the list will be chosen from a random starting point.

7.6.2.3 STRATIFIED RANDOM SAMPLING

Stratified random sampling is similar to simple random sampling, but the researcher decides ahead of time, based on known information, that the survey sample requires predetermined proportions of participants with a specific characteristic.[18] To do this the population is sorted into groups by the critical characteristic (stratified) and then random samples are chosen proportionally from each group or strata. An example would be sorting by ethnic group or gender to ensure appropriate representation in the final survey sample that reflects the population proportion.[4]

7.6.2.4 CLUSTER OR MULTISTAGE RANDOM SAMPLING

Cluster or Multistage random sampling is a method that clusters sample units together. There is then consecutive random choice of clusters at increasingly smaller units. This method is used because it is often not possible or feasible to take a simple random sample, or if the sampling frame is not known.[4,17] For example, to survey all RTTs in Canada, each cancer centre is considered to be a cluster, then many cancer centres would be chosen at random and all the RTTs at those centres would be asked to complete the survey.

7.6.2.5 NON-RANDOM OR NON-PROBABILITY SAMPLING

Non-random or nonprobability sampling methods are often used in small, local projects due to limitations on resources, time and expertise. If there is no random selection of participants, researchers have to be careful of the statistical tests used to analyze the data (nonparametric tests are likely more appropriate) and be aware that there is no certainty that the probability of subject selection is equal among participants.[4,9] There are four main nonprobability sampling techniques: convenience, quota, snowball and purposeful.

Convenience or opportunistic is sampling based on readily available and accessible subjects (e.g., all RTTs at the researcher's cancer centre)

Quota sampling is a sample that is hand-picked by the interviewer based on some key characteristic (e.g., male African-America patients at any cancer centre in Alberta).[17]

Snowball sampling uses the opinions of nonrandomly chosen qualified participants to identify others who may also qualify as respondents.[4]

Purposeful sampling is when the researcher uses professional judgment to identify and select respondents with known expertise in a certain subject area (e.g., interview of all the Clinical Specialist Radiation Therapists in Ontario).[4]

Due to the potential complexity of sample selection, when determining the appropriate sample size and plan for the final data analysis it is highly recommended to consult a statistician early in the process.[6,12] A statistician can also advise on database development, whether the data collected will be useful to answer the research question, and how to develop a data analysis framework.[12] Wise words of advice for any researcher are "don't collect data until you know what you are going to do with them.[6]" Schmidt found that a deviation from a simple random sampling of the target population protocol led to an over estimation of results in a large scale health survey.[19] The sampling process is critical in large-scale projects. This is another good reason to consult a statistician, especially if the design is complex. This is true for smaller clinical projects also, as the goal is still to create new knowledge and contribute to the radiation therapy literature. A statistical consultation can ensure that even small, local projects will be based on sound methodology and can answer the research question. Several studies have been unpublishable due to methodological errors that were discovered too late or remain incomplete because the data collected was not appropriate to answer the research question.

7.7 THE SURVEY INSTRUMENT

7.7.1 *USE OF EXISTING INSTRUMENTS – LOCATION AND ASSESSMENT*

To find existing survey instruments (also known as tools or scales) that may be appropriate to collect data for a research project, a thorough literature search is required (*see* Chapter 2: Literature Reviews). For health research, Streiner and Norman recommend *Measuring health: a guide to rating scales and questionnaires.*[9,20] It gives a critical review of many scales that are of interest to researchers in the health sciences fields.

"Most researchers tend to magnify the deficiencies of existing measures and underestimate the effort required to develop an adequate new measure… dismiss scales too easily and embark on the development of a new instrument with an unjustifiably optimistic and naive expectation that they can do better.[9]" If possible, it is a good idea and will save the research team a lot of time to use an existing tool. Another advantage of using an existing standardized tool is that it allows for comparison across different studies. The process of properly evaluating a newly developed tool is extremely lengthy and involved. Full research projects are devoted to assessing the psychometric properties of a new tool.[21] The decision to develop an entirely new survey instrument should be based on strong evidence that there is no relevant standard survey available.[12]

Once an appropriate survey instrument is located, the researcher or team must review the background literature regarding how the tool was developed and administered, how the tool was evaluated, the sample population that was used to for testing, and the psychometric properties of the tested tool. This critical analysis will allow the researcher to confidently determine if the tool is indeed applicable and feasible for use in the proposed study population; if it can help to answer a specific research question, and if the quality of the tool will allow the results to lead to valid and reliable conclusions. Survey tools are only helpful if they convey information accurately and consistently.[6] Quality survey tools are said to be validated, having been extensively tested for psychometric properties on a relevant, targeted population.[6,12,21]

7.7.1.1 PSYCHOMETRIC PROPERTIES

Strictly speaking, the psychometric properties of a test relate to the data that has been collected on a psychological test to determine how well it measures the construct of interest. The terminology is also used broadly in the survey research literature. To determine the psychometric qualities of a data collection instrument the following properties are assessed or calculated.

Validity: relates to the tool's ability to measure the true value and measure what it purports to measure[1,3]

Face Validity: the tool looks reasonable and is assessing desired qualities[9]

Content Validity: the tool measures all relevant content or domains[9]

Construct Validity: an analysis of how well the construct (theoretical background) is being measured and is evaluated using factor analysis

Reliability: relates to consistency/stability of responses and is evaluated using Intraclass Correlation or Cohen's Kappa[1,3,9,21]

Internal Consistency: a measure of the correlations between different items on the instrument and is evaluated using a statistic called Cronbach's Alpha

For a more in-depth discussion, an excellent resource to consult is *Health measurement scales: a practical guide to their development and use* by Streiner and Norman.[9] Most resources and references refer to the reliability and validity of a test. From a statistical standpoint, it is the inferences that are made from the results that will be valid and reliable if the instrument is of high quality.[9] When using a preexisting tool these points should be reviewed for applicability and acceptability of the tool.

HOT TIP

Once an appropriate tool has been found, researchers must be careful to investigate whether the tool has been copyrighted and requires permission to use and/or if there is a fee to use the tool. This is generally a fairly simple process, and contacting the author is the best way to clarify any conditions for use.

7.7.2 MODIFYING EXISTING TOOLS

Sometimes, excellent tools can be found in the literature that do not quite meet the needs of the researcher to answer the question, or the tool has been tested and used in a different population than intended for current use. It may be possible to alter a previously validated tool but researchers should seek advice before doing so, as this is likely to reduce its power.[6] If the researcher opts to change the data collection tool in a substantive way, validity testing should be repeated, especially if the results will be used for decision making.[3] For smaller scale descriptive or exploratory projects, this element may not be as critical, but researchers need to be aware of the limitations of altering a tool as opposed to developing a new one. The use of in-house nonvalidated tools for assessing patient reported outcomes should be avoided because of their propensity to degrade the quality of the research. They also limit the ability to generalize the study results to other populations.[3] It is recognized that validated tools may be too general to use, particularly within the radiation therapy setting. The stringency of adhering to these statements are determined by the goal of the research.

7.7.3 DESIGNING NEW SURVEY INSTRUMENTS

If an appropriate existing tool cannot be located or modified for use, the research team must put the time and effort into designing a tool that will yield valid and reliable results. This is a lengthy process. The risk of not putting in the time is that the collection tool will not yield useful data or that inappropriate conclusions will be drawn. Administration of a poor quality instrument is a waste of time, energy, money and a potential risk to the reputation of the research team and sponsoring organization. Validating the psychometric properties of a survey instrument is a rigourous and lengthy procedure, however if time and finances allow, it is an extremely worthwhile exercise. The advantage is the creation of new valid and reliable tools for radiation therapy research, where relatively few currently exist.

Often the words "survey" and "questionnaire" are used interchangeably, but a questionnaire can be thought of as a tool or instrument to collect survey data whereas a survey is a research method.[5] Regardless of the route of administration of the data collection tool, the questions (also known as items) need to be structured in such a way that the respondents have no difficulty understanding what is being asked of them. Proper design of the individual items, the associated scales, and of the broader data collection tool is vital to the success of the project.[3,6]

High quality survey research requires that the measurement tool is based on a theory, hypothesis or conceptual framework.[3,9] There must be a clear research goal[6] that can describe the relationship between the variables, and each item must relate to that underlying knowledge. When constructing a tool, it is best practice to be able to justify each item's relevance to the research question.[12] It is tempting to ask as many questions as possible to get as much data as possible, but this can reduce the response rate and subsequently affect the power of the study.[6]

Survey tools (questionnaires) have a standard basic structure, regardless of route of administration. Each begins with an introduction for the participants. The essential information to include in the introduction is the: study purpose, research question, contact information for principal investigator, information about research ethics board, the time required to complete the survey, information regarding anonymity of responses and what will be done with the results.[4,7,12] In face-to-face survey interviews, the researcher must also introduce himself or herself by name and obtain permission to proceed.[4]

Following the introductory material, the items are presented. The questions must follow a logical order.[3,4] It is best to begin the questionnaire with easier questions and keep themed items together, separated by headings and more instructions if necessary.[3,4] The more important questions should be placed near the beginning of the instrument, in case a respondent does not finish.[3] Sensitive questions should be placed at the end of a survey to reduce the possibility of "break offs," which happens when a participant quits part way through if posed a question that is felt to be too personal.[8] Finally, there is rationale to leaving the demographic questions to the end, when participants might be experiencing survey fatigue and may not put thought into answers to more complex questions.[4] This, however, is rarely ever done in practice. Sensitive items will be discussed in further detail later in this chapter.

In general, survey tools should be clear, comprehensive and written for a reading level of the lowest educational level of the anticipated respondents.[3,4,6] This corresponds to a reading level of approximately 12 years of age (grade six) for the general public.[9,21] The principles of plain language usage in patient education material development also apply for survey item development. Layout should be clean and well-spaced, and the directions should be easy to follow, regardless of format. Generally a larger, simple, sans serif font such as Arial or Calibri is recommended. Web surveys have additional considerations.[12–14]

7.7.4 SURVEY LENGTH

There is no standard or rule about the length a survey instrument should be. There is evidence that longer tools have higher nonresponse rates, but instruments with more items generally have better psychometric properties. There is a tradeoff between the reliability of the tool and the number of items asked.[9] Brevity is not necessarily desirable, since it is achieved at a cost to the reliability of the tool. Opting to increase the response rate by use of a less reliable, but shorter tool depends entirely on the scope of the project and the intended use or decisions to be made based on the results.

HOT TIP

The following limits can be used a guideline for the maximum time to expect a respondent to participate in various modes of survey research.[4]

Face-to-Face Survey Interview – 30 min
Phone Interview – 20 min
Paper Questionnaire – 30 min
Web-Based Questionnaire – 15 min

7.7.5 QUESTION TYPES

There are two main types of items used in survey research: open-ended and closed-ended questions.

Closed-ended questions are the type used most often.[4] The possible answers are chosen from a fixed list of alternatives, thus the responses are more relevant, uniform, clearer for the subject, easily computerized and analyzed.[3,4] An "other" category can be used to broaden the response categories if necessary.

Open-ended questions are exactly as the name suggests. Respondents can answer as they choose. This provides rich data, but the responses are difficult to analyze.[3,4] In a study where there is not a lot of literature available to prepare questions, these types of questions can be helpful to explore the research question in a more qualitative way to aid in new tool item development. In general, open-ended questions should be used sparingly.[4]

Survey research can bridge quantitative and qualitative research methods, depending on the data collected and the questions asked. A research project that uses a survey to collect data is not necessarily qualitative or quantitative. Open ended questions generally lend themselves to contributing to a qualitative design, while closed questions asking for strictly numerical results (e.g., percentage selecting a given predetermined response) are more likely part of a quantitative design. Misconceptions exist that survey research is qualitative or quantitative, but it can be either or both, depending on the goal of the project.

7.7.6 STRUCTURAL CONSIDERATIONS FOR INDIVIDUAL ITEMS

Item construction is an important consideration when developing a survey tool. Each individual item must be developed carefully. The following list offers some advice for item construction, and case example 7.1 offers some common examples of poorly structured items.

Do:

- Use simple, unambiguous words (e.g., use reddened skin versus erythema).[12]
- Use clear, short statements[3,12]
- Use neutral, nonemotional wording[4]
- Ensure response categories do not overlap (mutually exclusive)[3]
- Avoid bias and judgmental language[3]
- Avoid questions that attribute causality (e.g., "How long were you a smoker before you were diagnosed with lung cancer?")[3]
- Word sensitive questions carefully[10]
- Use questions instead of statements[22]
- Ensure that the respondents are offered an item response that is applicable to their situation[7]

Do not:

- Ask a question that contains more than one idea (double barreled questions)[3, 22]
- Use jargon, acronyms, highly technical or complicated medical words.
- Pose negative questions[3,9,22]
- Use overly complex questions[4]
- Use leading or manipulative questions[4]
- Encourage proxy reporting (answering on behalf of another)[3]

CASE EXAMPLE 7.1

Poorly Structured Survey Items

(1) How many radiation treatments did you have?
  (a) 0–5
  (b) 5–10
  (c) 10–15
  (d) 15–20

In this example a patient who had five treatments can answer either a or b (category overlap). A patient who had 15 treatments or more than 20 treatments is unable to answer the question at all.

(2) Did you find the cancer centre parking lot and check-in kiosk easily?
  (a) yes
  (b) no

This is a double-barreled question. The patient is unable to answer about each separately, and they may not have the same response.

(3) How did you find your experience at the cancer centre?
  (a) Excellent
  (b) Above average
  (c) Good
  (d) Average
  (e) Fair

This is a leading question and the scale is unbalanced. If the patient had a poor experience, there is no choice to represent his or her views.

Some more practical examples of items that relate to radiation therapy can be found in French's 2012 article, *Designing and Using Surveys as Research and Evaluation Tools.*[7]

7.7.7 OPTIONS FOR SCALES AND ANCHORS

For closed ended items, the "answers" are provided for the respondents. When it is a multiple choice type question, the possible answers are the options. When the respondent is ranking on a scale based on his ot her belief or perception, the answers are called anchors. Scales can be nominal (named categories), ordinal (named categories with an implied direction or rank) or interval (true numerical values).[4,12] The purpose of the question will determine the response categories and how the scale of the question is structured.

7.7.7.1 LIKERT SCALE

The most common type of respondent scale seen in survey research is the Likert Scale. Likert developed a rating scale with five possible responses, Strongly Approve, Approve, Undecided, Disapprove and Strongly Disapprove.[2] There have been many modifications to this ordinal scale over the years (e.g., "Agree" categories often replace "Approve" categories). When a researcher wants to force a respondent to make a positive or negative answer, the undecided or neutral category is removed forcing those who tend to answer neutrally to make a decision with a directional response.[3]

7.7.7.2 SEMANTIC DIFFERENTIAL SCALE

Another type of ordinal scale is a semantic differential scale. This type of scale provides gradations between two opposite words (antonyms), separated by boxes or lines.[2] The responses can be coded numerically for data analysis according to which line or box is chosen. An example is shown below:

Today I feel:

SAD ——|——|——|——|——|—— HAPPY

Artino et al. outline five common pitfalls for survey design.[22] Two of the five relate to the type and number of anchors. The authors suggest that agreement response anchors (scales using degrees of agreement with a given item) can lead to acquiescence bias, where respondents have the tendency to be agreeable, and answer positively, regardless of the question.[9,23] Tool developers should use at least five response anchors to achieve stable participant responses. Too many or few anchors is ineffective.

7.7.8 SENSITIVE QUESTIONS

Researchers in health professional fields are often gathering information from the subjects that are felt to be personal or private in nature. This type of item is called a sensitive question and these require special consideration when included in survey research. Sensitive questions are those that inquire about issues that are considered to be intrusive, have a threat of disclosure to a third party, are socially desirable or undesirable (violation of a social norm), or could be a cause for embarrassment.[10]

Questions that ask about income, drug use, sexual behaviour, voting practices, religious practice, health status or even weight can be considered sensitive.[9,10] For the purposes of radiation therapy research, this could include questions that ask about smoking or alcohol consumption. At issue with these types of questions is that respondents tend to skip these questions, misreport (e.g., responses are not accurate), or decline to participate.[9,10] This can lead to a data collection problem known as social desirability bias.[9,10,13] Survey participants may misreport in either direction, for example over report for socially desirable traits and underreport for socially undesirable traits. For some issues, social desirability bias can be compounded by other factors such as education levels.[10]

These type of questions have been found to affect response rates.[4,9,10] The effect is greatest in face to face interviews, and lessened with the use of web surveys.[10,24] For face-to-face survey interviews, accuracy of reporting on sensitive questions during interviews was improved by allowing the participants to respond to sensitive questions with paper and pen and put the response in an envelope.[10] Special care needs to be taken when developing these types of questions, regardless of the way in which they will be asked.

7.7.9 PRETESTING AND PILOTING THE INSTRUMENT

The previous section has provided some rules and guidelines for producing good quality items and instruments. Before the survey tool is implemented in a study population it has to be tested.

The next section gives some practical suggestions for evaluating a new tool and justifying the use of the tool in the population of interest. This process is called pretesting the instrument.

The first step in evaluating the tool is to have the research team review all of the items carefully for spelling, wording, clarity, flow, length, reading and content and to determine whether the instrument samples all the relevant or important content or domains.[9] The purpose of this review is to look for anything in the tool that may impede its completion, and to uncover any issues with the items early on in the process.[6]

The next step is to test the tool on a limited number of people who match the study population.[6] This is known as piloting the tool. Testing should be done on a representative sample that can allow revisions based on missing data, response variation, and information from the respondents about clarity, flow and format.[3] An evaluation of the tool can be added to the end and respondents can be given instructions to mark any questions that are unclear or difficult to answer. Jones and Baxter suggest completing this tool review in a focus group setting, to encourage discussion and maximize the use of the pilot-testing volunteers' time.[6] If this is done however, this author suggests it would be prudent to make sure all of the individuals have a chance to review the items independently, before a group discussion begins. This item review process generally leads to a reduction in items from the original number that were developed and a revised version of the instrument.[3]

Pretesting and piloting are important aspects of the survey research method. Although it increases the time and cost of instrument development, the advantage is that it enables the research team to gain valuable information. This will improve the quality of the research.[3] Case example 7.2 highlights the process of developing and validating a new survey instrument.

CASE EXAMPLE 7.2

Psychometric properties of cancer survivors' unmet needs survey

In the article *Psychometric properties of cancer survivors' unmet needs survey* by Campbell et al., the authors provide an excellent example of the process an oncology research team underwent to develop and validate a tool to assess cancer survivors' unmet needs.[21] Their project was to ensure that the new tool was psychometrically rigourous; that it had acceptable reliability and validity, multidimensional measurements, collected data directly from subjects, was acceptable to subjects, and was feasible to administer in the setting in which it will be used. This article is a good illustration of the stringent processes required to develop a tool that will generate results that are generalizable and can be used for decision making. Researchers who plan to develop a new tool should review articles such as the one described to get a better idea of the practicalities of the endeavor.

Reliability was assessed using the Intra-class Correlation Co-efficient (Kappa), which measures reproducibility over time. The internal consistency was evaluated using Cronbach's Alpha. Face and content validity were determined by having subject matter experts and target group participants review the instrument. The tool was evaluated for plain language and reading level by an external source. The construct validity was evaluated using factor analysis to determine quantitatively if the instrument was measuring what was intended. The lengthy initial item development process produced 200 items, measuring 9 different domains. The final psychometrically tested tool consisted of 89 items measuring 6 domains and was tested on a population of more than 500 cancer patients.

7.8 SURVEY ADMINISTRATION

7.8.1 MAXIMIZING RESPONSE RATES

As mentioned previously, sample size is very important. Thus, it is imperative to take all possible steps to ensure the administration method produces a good response rate.[6] Researchers will lose participants from the original sample due to lost questionnaires, nonresponders, missing data and improper answers. Once this is accounted for, the sample size still needs to be large enough to be representative of the population in question, and have adequate power to give meaningful results. One of the best ways to do this is to ensure that the potential participant list is as accurate as possible.[4]

A systematic review of the literature found several factors that have a statistically significant impact on improved response rates for mailed surveys.[25] These were:

- Use of incentives
- Short surveys (as opposed to lengthy ones)
- More personalized recruitment information
- Prepaid mailings
- Precontact of participants
- Follow up mailing including another copy of the survey
- University sponsorship of the study

It is often thought valuable for the researcher to assign a unique identification number to be able to match respondents to returned surveys, send three targeted reminders to nonresponders over a two-week period and include the survey with the reminders.[3]

For other modes of survey administration, the same principles apply and should be considered for recruitment and implementation. Large scale studies aim for very high response rates (more than 70%), but often in smaller clinical studies, the response rates are more in the order of 30–40% due to study limitations.[23,26] Physicians pose unique challenges as a survey study population. Jones and Baxter note that physicians have the lowest response rates to survey research.[6] A study by Bhandari et al., with the amusing title *Does flattery work? A comparison of two different cover letters for an international survey of orthopaedic surgeons* found increased response rates when a personalized cover letter was used versus a standard cover letter.[27] The personalized approach is also supported by a related systematic review, and is likely generalizable to any health professional group.[28]

7.9 DATA ANALYSIS

Once all of the data have been collected, the next major stage is data analysis. This step will be much easier if a statistician was consulted early on in the process to guide the researchers to the correct data collection, data base preparation and data analysis plan.

The first step is to create a statistical log. This is a book or electronic file where everything that is done with respect to the data analysis is entered. Any decisions that were made or actions taken should be entered into this log. For example, the researcher would note how variable names were decided, how missing data was dealt with or how decisions were made about coding. After a few months, the researcher may not remember exactly why certain decisions were made, but the logbook will always serve as a reminder. Next, all the data from the closed-ended questions will be manually entered into a database (for face to face, telephone or mailed responses), or exported into a database for electronically collected methods.

This complete, clean dataset should be saved in an untouched form, so that there is always a backup file of the true raw data. The next step is to look carefully at the data to determine if any questions were problematic. For example:

- Is there a higher proportion of nonresponses, duplicates, or unexpected response patterns?
- Are there any break points where survey participants stopped answering?
- Is there any observed trend that may indicate a problem with the collection tool items such as social desirability bias or response bias?

Before any statistical tests are performed, the researcher must ensure that the data collection method, sampling process, and sample size obtained are congruent with the assumptions required to run the analysis. Many statistical tests are based on the assumption that the subjects have been chosen at random and that the sample size is large enough that the responses to the items should be normally distributed. The type of scale used also affects the type of statistical testing that can be done on the collected data. Chapter 5 (Quantitative Methodologies and Analysis) will provide some insight to statistical approaches to looking at data. For a detailed review of the data analysis processes as they apply to survey research, see *Health measurement scales: a practical guide to their development and use* by Streiner and Norman or *Applied Survey Data Analysis* by Heeringa et al.[9,29]

The data obtained from the open-ended questions should be prepared, coded and analyzed following the processes that are used in qualitative research methods. *See* Chapter 6 (Qualitative Methodologies and Analysis) for a review of the methods of coding, theming and analyzing this type of data.

7.10 REPORTING SURVEY DATA

Reporting the results of survey research is similar to any scientific report, and gives the complete specification of the project; for example, what was collected, from whom, and why the project was undertaken.[1] The final written manuscript follows the standard research headings of Introduction, Methods, Results, Discussion, and Conclusion. The report should allow another researcher to replicate the survey based on the description provided.[1,3] Specifics for survey research include source of data, sampling techniques (inclusion and exclusion, population and sampling frame, information about the psychometric properties of the tool if previously validated, or how the tool was tested (if researcher developed), the administration process (e.g., method and incentives), sample collection schedule and procedures, including the response rates and descriptors of responders versus nonresponders.[3]

Published standards, guidance and consensus on survey method reporting are lacking.[30] Poor reporting compromises transparency and reliability, which are both crucial components of good research. There is a need for standardized reporting, but in the absence of these standards, the suggestions above should be covered when writing up and submitting a survey research manuscript to a journal for consideration of publication.[26,30]

Survey research is a method of inquiry that has widespread use over a diverse number of research settings. The purpose of this chapter was to provide the researcher with some tools, resources and advice for embarking on survey research.

The information provided in this chapter can help to ensure that smaller practice based projects are well designed, and larger scale projects are rigourous enough to allow for generalization of the results to a larger population and decisions to be made as a result of the conclusions. As more and more RTTs become experienced researchers, the projects will become more complex and far reaching. Whether a small in-house project, or a large multicentre survey, attention needs to be paid to the rigour of the research design. High quality radiation therapy research projects, regardless of scale, contribute to our body of literature and enhance our professional profile, resulting in radiation therapists becoming important contributors to the body of knowledge in the field of radiation medicine.

KEYWORDS

- Survey instrument
- Psychometrics
- Administration
- Validity
- Pilot testing
- Likert scale

REFERENCES

1. Sapsford, R. Survey Research. Sage: London, 2006.
2. Leaver, D. Survey research techniques. *Radiologic Tech.* **2000**,*71(4)*, 364–378.
3. Alderman, A. K.; Salem, B., Survey research. *Plast. Reconstr. Surg.* **2010,** *126(4)*, 1381–1389.
4. Rea, L. M.; Parker, R. A. Designing and Conducting Survey Research: A Comprehensive Guide. Jossey-Bass: San Francisco, CA, 2012.
5. National Research Corporation: About us. www.nrxpicker.com (accessed June 29, 2013).
6. Jones, T. L.; Baxter, M. A.; Khanduja, V. A quick guide to survey research. *Ann. R. Coll. Surg. Engl.* **2013,** *95(1)*, 5–7.
7. French, J. Designing and Using Surveys as Research and Evaluation Tools. *J. Med. Imag. Radiat. Sci.* **2012,** *43(3)*, 187–192.

8. Jäckle, A.; Lynn, P.; Sinibaldi, J.; Tipping, S. The Effect of Interviewer Experience, Attitudes, Personality and Skills on Respondent Co-operation with Face-to-Face Surveys. *Surv. Res. Methods.* **2013**, *7(1)*, 1–15.
9. Streiner, D. L.; Norman, G. R. Health measurement Scales: A Practical Guide to Their Development and Use. Oxford University Press: Oxford, UK, 2008.
10. Tourangeau, R.; Yan, T. Sensitive questions in surveys. Psychol. Bull. **2007,** *133(5)*, 859–883.
11. Kempf, A. M.; Remington, P. L. New challenges for telephone survey research in the twenty-first century. *Annu. Rev. Public Health.* **2007**, *28*, 113–126.
12. Grimmer, K.; Bialocerkowski, A. Surveys. *Aust. J. Physiother.* **2005**, *51(3)*, 185–187.
13. Couper, M. Web surveys: a review of issues and approaches. *Public Opin. Q.* **2000,** *64(4),* 464–494.
14. Mahon-Haft, T. A.; Dillman, D. A. Does visual appeal matter? Effects of web survey esthetics on survey quality, *Surv. Res. Methods,* **2010,** *4(1),* 43–59.
15. Statistics Canada. Residential Telephone Use. http://www.statcan.gc.ca/daily quotidien/110405/dq110405a-eng.htm (accessed June 26, 2013).
16. Statistics Canada. Individual Internet Use. http://www.statcan.gc.ca/daily quotidien/070504/dq070504a-eng.htm (accessed June 26, 2013).
17. Freedman, D.; Pisani, R.; Purves, R. Statistics. Norton and Company: New York, 1980.
18. Crocker, L.; Algina, J. Introduction to classical and modern test theory. *ERIC*, 1986.
19. Schmidt, C. O.; Alte, D.; Volzke, H.; Sauer, S.; Friedrich, N.; Valliant, R. Partial misspecification of survey design features sufficed to severely bias estimates of health-related outcomes. *J. Clin. Epidemiol.* **2011,** *64(4),* 416–423.
20. McDowell, I.; Newell, C.; McDowell, I. Measuring Health: A Guide to Rating Scales and Questionnaires Vol 268. Oxford University Press: New York, 2006.
21. Campbell, H. S.; Sanson-Fisher, R.; Turner, D.; Hayward, L.; Wang, X. S.; Taylor-Brown, J. Psychometric properties of cancer survivors' unmet needs survey. *Support Care Cancer*. **2010,** *19(2),* 221–230.
22. Artino, A. R., Jr.; Gehlbach, H.; Durning, S. J. AM Last Page: Avoiding five common pitfalls of survey design. *Acad. Med.* **2011,** *86(10)*, 1327.
23. Krosnick, J. A., Survey research. Annu. Rev. Psychol. **1999,** *50*, 537–567.
24. Couper, M. P. Web surveys: The Questionnaire Design Challenge, Proceedings of the 53rd Session of the ISI, Cite seer: 2001.
25. Edwards, P.; Roberts, I.; Clarke, M.; DiGuiseppi, C.; Pratap, S.; Wentz, R.; Kwan, I. Increasing response rates to postal questionnaires: systematic review. *BMJ* **2002,** *324(7347),* 1183.
26. Fincham, J. E.; Draugalis, J. R. The importance of survey research standards. *Am. J. Pharm. Educ*. **2013,** *77(1),* 4.
27. Bhandari, M.; Leece, P.; Sprague, S.; Swiontkowski, M. F.; Schemitsch, E. H.; Tornetta, P. Does flattery work? A comparison of two different cover letters for an international survey of orthopedic surgeons. *Can. J. Surg.* **2006,** *49(2)*, 90.
28. Evans, J. R.; Mathur, A. The value of online surveys. *Internet Res*. **2005,** *15(2),* 195–219.
29. Heeringa, S. G.; West, B. T.; Berglund, P. A. Applied Survey Data Analysis. CRC Press: Boca Raton, FL, 2010.

30. Bennett, C.; Khangura, S.; Brehaut, J. C.; Graham, I. D.; Moher, D.; Potter, B. K.; Grimshaw, J. M. Reporting guidelines for survey research: an analysis of published guidance and reporting practices. *PLoS Med.* **2010,** *8(8)*, e1001069.

PART 3

UNIQUE CONSIDERATIONS IN RESEARCH

CHAPTER 8

CLINICAL TRIALS

LORI HOLDEN MRT(T) BSc CCRP

Clinical Specialist Radiation Therapist & Vice Chair, Rapid Response Radiotherapy Program / Bone Metastases Clinic, Odette Cancer Centre, Sunnybrook Health Sciences Centre, Toronto Canada
Assistant Professor, Department of Radiation Oncology, University of Toronto, Toronto Canada

CONTENTS

A clinical trial can be defined as a research study involving human subjects (or participants) to evaluate the effect of interventions or exposures on biomedical or health-related outcomes.[1] Clinical trials are important for establishing new treatment modalities and improving upon current standards of practice in the healthcare environment.

In radiation therapy, with the continued evolution of treatment modalities, techniques and technologies, radiation therapists (RTTs) are on the forefront of transforming this type of new knowledge into practice[2]. In the past, RTTs conducting clinical trials was not commonplace, but in the last 10–15 years, the importance of providing and practicing evidence based medicine has become increasingly recognized and reported in the healthcare disciplines.[2–5] Patients have access to a vast abundance of information from on-line sources and it is incumbent on RTTs to be as up-to-date as possible in the recent advances of scientific research.

RTTs have the opportunity to assume a variety of important roles during the research process. Initially, they may be involved with the conception or refining of a clinical question, or may directly partake in the protocol development itself, thus leading to being a coinvestigator, or primary investigator. They often play the very important role of study coordinator. This is a very encompassing role, incorporating the responsibilities of document development (e.g., the case report and data collection forms) and submission (e.g., to the Research Ethics Board (REB)), organizing data collection, or data entry. RTTs may also be the Certified Research Assistant (CRA) for a particular study, with the additional responsibility for screening patients for eligibility, trial enrollment and form completion. These are just a few of the many roles and responsibilities that an RTT can adopt during the research process.

In the literature, some authors consider it a requirement, and not just a choice, for RTTs to partake in evidence-based medicine.[3] Gambling et al. recognized the importance of research in radiotherapy and challenged readers to become more involved in the academic side of delivering treatment.[6] Even as far back as 1996, authors have recognized the importance of conducting research, however they also identified the barriers and challenges encountered by RTTs when embarking on their own trial work.[7] Subsequent articles have published on the barriers and supports of research, and interestingly, they have not changed much.[8–10] Common challenges were identified, with the most cited being: time, support, education, knowledge, or mentorship.[8–10] Certain articles have provided suggestions to deal with the financial and time barriers, and some centres are now in a position to employ "research radiation therapists" to conduct research on a full-time basis.[9] However, education can still remain a challenge.[6,10,11] Apart from the training an RTT would receive in the course of their education, there can be a lack of formalized advanced research training to guide interested RTTs in conducting research. Often, they are left to discover available courses or educational materials on their own. This can be frustrating if one does not know where to begin. Certain organizations such as the Society of Clinical Research Associates (SoCRA) do offer formalized certificate programs, but this may not be a viable option for some.[5]

This chapter will serve to help tackle the barrier of education by providing a primer for those RTTs interested in initiating their own, or collaborating on, clinical trials in their departments. It will describe the different phases of clinical trials and outline various aspects of clinical trial design and management. Hopefully, by confirming or broadening one's knowledge base, RTTs can continue to overcome the potential barrier of education and become more involved in clinical trials.

8.1 TYPES OF CLINICAL TRIAL

The term clinical trial, by definition, specifically applies to trials involving therapeutic drugs, however, it is now commonplace to hear it relate to device trials, radiation therapy technique related trials, and quality of life trials. RTTs often partake in, or assume the lead role in radiation therapy related trials, often investigating effects of treatment prescription doses, immobilization devices, or treatment planning on patient outcomes, just to name a few examples.

Although there are many different types of clinical trials (e.g., quality of life, prevention, treatment), one way of classifying clinical trials is by the role played by the investigator. By this definition, there are two types of clinical studies; interventional trials and observational trials.[1]

8.1.1 INTERVENTIONAL TRIALS

Interventional trials are conducted under controlled settings, whereby the safety and efficacy of a certain experimental treatment or novel idea is tested.[1] These are what are most commonly referred to as clinical trials. The investigators assign an intervention to participants, based on a certain protocol, and an outcome is measured. For example, one might study the impact of a new drug on controlling radiation-induced emesis. Interventional trials have a range of primary endpoints depending on the phase in which a certain intervention or treatment is being tested. Phases of clinical trial development are vital to understand in a research-based environment and therefore will be discussed in depth later in this chapter.

8.1.2 OBSERVATIONAL TRIALS

Observational trials are studies in which an outcome is observed in a group of participants; however, the investigators do not assign any intervention to them.[1] For example, a researcher could observe a specific group of adults to see the effect of different lifestyle choices on cancer incidence. In observational trials, one sees the cohort, case control or cross-sectional studies. There are differences in how these different studies are conducted, and the nuances between them have been discussed in previous chapters for the researcher's reference.

The United States National Institutes of Health (NIH) further classifies trials into five categories based on their purpose, those being:

- Quality of Life Trials
- Screening Trials
- Diagnostic Trials
- Treatment Trials
- Compassionate Use Trials

Regardless of what type or class of trial being conducted, there are criteria that must be met, and protocols that must be followed, to properly conduct the trial.

8.2 RANDOMIZATION AND BLINDING

In terms of trial design, there is a fundamental distinction in the design of trials between the above-mentioned groups. In the interventional trials, one typically sees the randomized (double-blind, single-blind, or no-blind) or the nonrandomized designs. The term randomized, when employed with respect to a trial, refers to the process whereby participants are randomly allocated to receive one or the other treatment arm. It is similar to tossing a coin. After randomization, the two cohorts are studied in the same way, with the differences in outcome being intrinsic to the treatments being compared.[11]

By using randomization in a trial, it minimizes bias in treatment assignment, and allows for "blinding." The various approaches to blinding refer to who in the study actually knows to which intervention a subject was randomized.

Double-blind: neither the subject nor the healthcare provider is aware of the treatment arm that particular to which a particular subject was assigned.

Single-blind: infers that only one side (either the patient or the healthcare provider) is aware of the assigned intervention.

No-blind: the absence of blinding.

8.2.1 PLACEBOS

Typically used in blinded studies is a strategy called a placebo, or sham treatment. In this type of study, the patient is assigned either an intervention or a placebo, however, they are blinded to which they are actually receiving.[12] Placebos are made to look and be administered in exactly the same way as the intervention. The purpose of using a placebo is to account for something known as the placebo effect. The placebo effect refers to the phenomenon that treatment effects may be due to other factors not related to the intervention itself, such as the perception that one is receiving a treatment, or extra attention and expectation by the healthcare providers. Utilizing a placebo overcomes this effect.

Double-blind, randomized, placebo-controlled trials are what are often referred to as the gold standard of research, and usually provide the most compelling evidence. It is important to keep in mind, however, that there are ethical concerns surrounding placebo-controlled trials. In circumstances where a standard of care actually exists for a patient with a condition, it may be unethical to accrue them to a trial whereby someone may receive a placebo to test a new intervention. This highlights the importance of full and informed consent and the important role that the research ethics board has in approving these studies. Chapter 3 (Research Ethics Applications) goes into greater detail on each of these subjects.

8.3 PHASES OF CLINICAL TRIAL DEVELOPMENT

Clinical trials are usually conducted in sequential order, or phase. Once sufficient data from a phase is available, trials of subsequent phases can be conducted either by the original study group or a different group of investigators. The different phases of clinical trial development are described below. Typically, one would perform a phase I trial first, followed by phases II-IV, depending on the results from the previous phase studies. It is common, though, to have some investigators begin their study in the phase II or III setting if previous work has been conducted by other investigators. By the definitions below, it becomes clear as to why this may be the case.[13]

Before the commencement of a clinical trial, new drugs often undergo preclinical studies. In this initial phase, tests are performed with the ultimate goal of testing the safety and feasibility of the drug. Based on the success of these trials, the drug can then move into the next phases of drug development (*see* Figure 8.1).

8.3.1 PHASE I CLINICAL TRIAL

A Phase I clinical trial is usually conducted with healthy volunteers. It is designed mainly to determine the pharmacological actions of the drug, and the safety and side effects, all associated with dose escalation.

Pharmacokinetic studies as well as drug interaction studies are usually considered as Phase I trials regardless of when they are conducted during drug development. Typically, phase I trials incorporates sample sizes of 20–100 individuals.

8.3.2 PHASE II CLINICAL TRIAL

In this phase of development, the primary outcome is efficacy and safety. Side effects and risks associated with the drug as well as short-term adverse events continue to be evaluated. In many situations, these trials are conducted in multicentre environments and typically involve sample sizes in the order of 100–300 subjects.

8.3.3 PHASE III CLINICAL TRIAL

These are intended to gather additional and confirmatory information about the clinical efficacy and safety under the proposed conditions of use for the drug. These trials can take usually between one and four years to conduct, and involve 300–3,000 subjects.

8.3.4 PHASE IV CLINICAL TRIAL

After a drug has been approved for market, phase IV trials can subsequently be performed. These studies are often important for optimizing the drug's use, gathering additional information regarding a drug's safety and efficacy. These trials do not usually require regulatory approval by Health Canada.

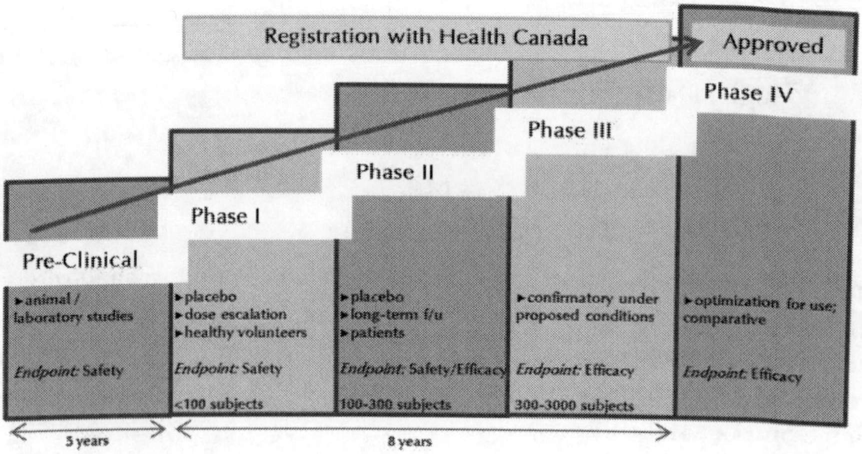

FIGURE 8.1 Phases of the Clinical Trial Process.

8.4 REGULATION OF CLINICAL TRIALS

Health Canada is the regulatory body that ensures that individuals have access to high quality, safe and efficacious products.[13] It also ensures the balance of risk versus benefit, making certain that individuals are not subject to undue risk of the therapeutic product.[14] The specific regulation that individuals conducting pharmaceutical clinical trials are governed by are Part C, Division 5 of the Food and Drug Regulations (FDR) for the Government of Canada. Division 5 is titled "Drugs for Clinical Trials Involving Human Subjects.[15]" Within this section of the FDR are numerous modules containing information and requirements on things such as: the sponsor's obligations, labeling and storing of drugs, records, and serious adverse drug reporting. There is also a subsection entitled Good Clinical Practice (GCP).

The regulations of Health Canada integrate the principles of GCP as described by the International Conference on Harmonization (ICH). The ICH makes recommendations and provides for a unified standard for the European Union, Japan, the United States, Australia, Canada, Nordic countries, and the World Health Organization. They are responsible for the development of GCP for global implementation.

Before a drug or drug product is approved for sale in Canada, it must be reviewed and approved by Health Canada. On average, Health Canada authorizes approximately 900 clinical trials per year.[13] Within Canada, the sponsor of a phase I-III clinical trial is responsible for filing that application prior to the initiation of the trial. In many situations, the sponsor is usually a private company, or the industry responsible for the manufacturing of that drug, however, when an investigator initiates a trial under his or her own sponsorship, that individual becomes the sponsor. In either case, by doing so, the sponsor agrees to be governed by the regulations of Health Canada as well as bound to comply with the GCP.

Good Clinical Practice guidelines are an international ethical and scientific quality standard for designing, conducting, performing, monitoring, auditing, recording and reporting trials involving humans.[16] By practicing GCP, one ensures the integrity of the data, as well as ensuring the rights and safety of the participants. In Canada, sponsors of clinical trials must be able to demonstrate their trial is conducted in accordance to the principles of GCP.[14] An abbreviated version of these principles includes the following:

- clinical trials must be conducted in accordance with GCP and the appropriate regulatory authorities
- before a trial is initiated, the risks versus benefits must be assessed, initiating the trial only if the anticipated benefits outweigh the risks
- the rights, safety, and well-being of the trial subjects must prevail
- the available information (both clinical and nonclinical) on an investigational drug must be adequate to support the proposed trial
- clinical trials must be scientifically sound, following a concise protocol
- the protocol must have received REB approval prior to initiation
- the medical care given and medical decisions must always be the responsibility of a qualified physician
- each individual involved in conducting a trial should be qualified by education, training, and experience to perform his or her respective task(s)
- every subject must freely give their informed consent prior to clinical trial inclusion

- all clinical trial information must be recorded, handled, and stored in a way that allows for accurate reporting, interpretation and verification
- the confidentiality of records that could identify subjects must be protected
- investigational drugs must be used as specified within the approved protocol (the fabrication, handling, and storing must be in accordance with applicable good manufacturing practices (GMP))
- procedures assuring the quality of every aspect of the trial must be implemented

The above principles ensure the rights of the subjects are protected and the data are credible, however it is important to understand that there are numerous additional criteria and mandates which are included within each respective point above, that collectively comprise GCP. Examples of these additional criteria would be record retention, audits, and the function and responsibilities of personnel working within the trial.

HOT TIP

It is good practice to always follow GCP no matter what type of research study is being conducted. As one can see, the principles of GCP encompass any and all aspects of conducting clinical trials, which are considered the most rigourously regulated research. On-line GCP courses exist, and some institutions actually provide in-house training in GCP, so it is important for the researcher to seek out the appropriate resource prior to embarking on a research project, whether a clinical trial or a patient satisfaction survey.

8.4.1 STANDARD OPERATING PROCEDURES (SOPS)

When a pharmaceutical trial is submitted to Health Canada, it is considered a "regulated" trial, and therefore, both GCP and Division 5 training must be performed and documented by all individuals prior to embarking on any tasks associated with the trial. If a trial is not regulated, for example, Phase IV trials, then the Division 5 training is only a recommendation. On top of these, regulatory authorities require that clinical research sites use standard operating procedures (SOPs).[17] Some institutions develop their own in-house SOPs, whereas others may adopt the N2 (Network of Networks) SOPs. The N2 SOPs are a national standardized set of operating procedures that are applicable to any therapeutic area in any given institution or research environment.[17]

Examples of typical SOPs are:

- database setup SOP
- protocol development SOP
- informed consent process SOP

Most institutions will provide SOP training. If they do not, however, there are external sources available from which to obtain the necessary training that complies with the requirements of individual institutions. It is important to remember that proof of training must be documented and kept with the master files of that particular trial.

8.4.2 KEY INDIVIDUALS: SPONSOR, INVESTIGATOR AND MONITOR

When conducting clinical trials, there are three key individuals responsible for the initiation, management and outcome of that trial. They are the sponsor, the investigator and the monitor. It is important to remember that each has his or her own specific role and is responsible to fulfill it accordingly. Table 8.1 outlines some of the various duties assumed by these individuals.[16] In some studies, as outlined previously, the investigator is the sponsor and therefore assumes both assigned roles.

In radiotherapy, many research endeavours are investigator-initiated. However, when the investigator is also the sponsor, as mentioned above, he or she takes on an additional list of responsibilities. It is important to list a few other very important responsibilities of the sponsor, as they relate to RTTs. The sponsor must:

- maintain accurate records and ensure that the investigator adheres to the approved protocol

- report any unexpected adverse drug reactions in an expedited manner
- keep all trial-related documents for a period of 25 years
- ensure and be able to provide proof of GCP training for all individuals involved in the trial

It is important to maintain good communication between all key individuals so as to ensure protocol compliance on all levels. One strategy in doing so is to maintain good documentation and documents themselves. All players must adhere to the same protocol, in order to ensure study compliance.

TABLE 8.1 Roles of Key Individuals in Clinical Trials Management.

Sponsor	Investigator	Monitor
Ensure protocol is being followed	Ensure all individuals active in trial, adhere to the protocol	Verify rights of participants are protected and integrity of data maintained
Ensure prompt reporting of adverse events	Personally conducts/supervises the trial	Be thoroughly familiar with the protocol, investigational drug, consent
Terminate study if drug poses significant risk to participants	Ensure prompt reporting to the Research Ethics Board (REB) of any changes or unanticipated problems	Follows SOPs for monitoring protocol
Select qualified monitors and investigators	Ensures proper training by all involved personnel	Verifies all aspects and training of individuals, for trial
Provide necessary information needed for conduct of trial	Maintains accurate and available records for inspection	Provide written reports to investigator/sponsor, after site visit
Manufacture drug, drug accountability, provide drug to participating investigators	Ensures informed consent for participants	
Maintain written Standard Operating Procedures (SOPs) for all trial activities	Drug accountability/storage/compliance	
Provide medical expertise	Annual and safety reporting	
Obtain agreement between sponsor and investigator	Obtains REB approval	
Notify all parties of new safety information		

8.4.3 IMPORTANT DOCUMENTS

Once Clinical Trials Application has been filed with Health Canada, Health Canada itself must reply with a "No Objection Letter" for drug trials or an "Investigational Testing Authorization" for medical device trails, in order for that trial to commence. Basically, this letter states that Health Canada has reviewed the submitted protocol and agrees for it to proceed.

Other required documentation that must be completed and filed prior to initiating a clinical trial includes:

- A Clinical Trials Site Information form
- A Qualified Investigator Undertaking form
- An Research Ethics Board (REB) attestation form- stating that the protocol and Clinical Trial Application form have been submitted, reviewed and approved by the REB

The first three forms can be found on the Health Canada website for reference, and all of these forms must be completed and kept with the trial's essential documents, for the required number of years.[16] The institution's research associates can provide guidance in completing these required documents. Filing a trial with Health Canada does not supercede the requirement for REB approval. This must still be obtained from each institution associated with that trial. It is unnecessary to complete the aforementioned forms for clinical trials that do not require Health Canada submission, such as trials that adhere to the licensed drug indication or are purely observational. However, this does not exclude the trial from requiring approval of a local REB. REB submissions, regardless of need for Health Canada regulation, must include a study protocol, informed consent form, case reporting forms, and appendices including all relevant reporting forms and questionnaires (*see* Chapter 4: Research Ethics Applications).

Other important and useful documents that are required by Health Canada include a Task Delegation Log, a Screening Log, a Training Log and even equipment logs. A Task Delegation Log is required, as it outlines the roles, which an investigator has delegated to individuals on his or her trial team. By doing this and signing it, the investigator is confirming that the individuals listed have the required training and education necessary to perform the listed tasks, and he or she is therefore delegating responsibility to that individual.[16] All other forms serve to ensure the integrity of the data collected and the trial itself.

8.4.4 REGISTRATION IN CLINICAL TRIALS DATABASE

Health Canada encourages sponsors to register their trial in the clinicaltrials.gov database. This is a repository of clinical trials that have been reviewed by Health Canada. It is accessible by both the general public and healthcare professionals. Patients are able to seek trials that are actively recruiting, and both are able to search it to obtain information on trial results, or current open trials as well. It is an on-line database that currently contains information on almost 150,000 cases in more than 185 countries.

Of note, as a condition of publication, the International Committee of Medical Journal Editors (ICMJE) requires a clinical trial to be registered in a clinical trials database.[18]

With a rigourous protocol developed, the process of applying to the local REB, and the steps to apply to Health Canada become less daunting and more achievable. It is the hope of the author that by giving a brief overview of clinical trials, the researcher can discover that conducting clinical research is a manageable endeavor, and one that RTTs can embark upon with the improvement in their patients care in mind. Even the smallest change in products, treatments, or technology can have a great impact on the patient, RTTs have the ability to challenge or support existing paradigms and even to create new ones.

"Not everything we count, counts.
Not everything that counts can be counted."
Let's all Count!

~ William Bruce Cameron, 1963

KEYWORDS

- Investigational trial
- Observational trial
- Randomization
- Blinding
- Placebo
- Good Clinical Practice

REFERENCES

1. ClinicalTrials.gov. Learn About Clinical Studies. http://clinicaltrials.gov/ct2/about-studies/learn (accessed April 24, 2013).
2. Harnett, N.; Palmer, C.; Bolderston, A.; Wenz, J.; Catton, P. The scholarly radiation therapist. Part one: charting the territory. *J. Radiother. Pract.* **2008,** *7(2)*, 99–104.
3. Catton, J.; Catton, P.; Davey, C. Research and the Medical Radiation Technologists: What are we waiting for? *Can. J. Med. Radiat. Technol.* **1999,** *30*, 35–44.
4. Sackett, D. L., Evidence-based medicine. *Semin. Perinatol.* **1997,** *21(1),* 3–5.
5. Gilbert, R.; Fader, K. Evidence-based decision making as a tool for continuous professional development in the medical radiation technologies. *Can. J. Med. Radiat. Technol.* **2007,** *38(1),* 39–44.
6. Gambling, T.; Brown, P.; Hogg, P. Research in our practice—a requirement not an option: discussion paper. *Radiography* **2003,** *9(1),* 71–76.
7. Challen, V.; Kaminski, S.; Harris, P. Research-mindedness in the radiography profession. *Radiography* **1996,** *2(2),* 139–151.
8. Sim, J.; Zadnik, M.; Radloff, A. University and workplace cultures: their impact on the development of lifelong learners. *Radiography* **2003,** *9(2),* 99–107;
9. Agustin, C.; Grand, M.; Gebski, V.; Turner, S. Radiation therapists' perspective on barriers to clinical trials research. *J. Med. Imaging Radiat. Oncol.* **2008,** *52(2),* 178–82;
10. Halkett, G.; Scutter, S. Research attitudes and experiences of radiation therapists. *Radiographer* **2003,** *50(2),* 69.
11. Schulz, K. F.; Altman, D. G.; Moher, D. CONSORT 2010 statement: updated guidelines for reporting parallel group randomized trials. *BMC Med.* **2010,** *8(1),* 18.
12. Chiodo, G. T.; Tolle, S. W.; Bevan, L. Placebo-controlled trials: good science or medical neglect? *West. J. Med.* **2000,** *172(4),* 271.
13. Health Canada. Drug Products. http://www.hc-sc.gc.ca/dhp-mps/prodpharma/index-eng.php (accessed May 15, 2013).
14. Health Canada. Regulations amending the food and drug regulations (1024 – clinical trials). http://www.hc-sc.gc.ca/dhp-mps/compli-conform/clini-pract-prat/reg/1024_tc-tm-eng.php (accessed September 5, 2013).

15. Government of Canada. Food and Drugs Regulations. http://laws-lois.justice.gc.ca/eng/regulations/CRC_c.870/ (accessed September 5, 2013).
16. Goldfarb, N. M. 2009 Code of Federal Regulations and ICH Guidelines GCP Reference Guide. Barnett International, 2009.
17. N2 Network of Networks. N2 SOPs. http://n2canada.ca/n2-sops/ (accessed April 26, 2013).
18. Health Canada: Applications and Submissions. http://www.hc-sc.gc.ca/dhp-mps/prodpharma/applic-demande/index-eng.php (accessed May 15, 2013).

CHAPTER 9

HEALTH SERVICES RESEARCH AND PROGRAM EVALUATION

GUNITA MITERA MRT(T) BSc MBA PhD(c)

Quality Initiatives Specialist, Canadian Partnership Against Cancer, Toronto Canada

KATE BAK MSc

Policy Research Analyst, Radiation Treatment Program, Cancer Care Ontario, Toronto Canada

ELIZABETH MURRAY MA

Project Coordinator, Radiation Treatment Program, Cancer Care Ontario, Toronto Canada

ERIC GUTIERREZ MRT(T) BSc CMD

Program Manager, Radiation Treatment Program, Cancer Care Ontario, Toronto Canada

CONTENTS

The definition of health services research (HSR) is constantly evolving; however, in general it can be defined as "a multidisciplinary field of scientific investigation that studies how social factors, financing systems, organizational structures and processes, health technologies, and personal behaviours affect access to healthcare, the quality and cost of healthcare, and ultimately our health and well-being. Its research domains are individuals, families, organizations, institutions, communities, and populations.[1]" The intent of HSR is to generate knowledge about health system performance by assessing its effectiveness, efficiency and equity.

9.1 SCOPE AND VALUE OF HEALTH SERVICES RESEARCH

In general, HSR is a broad and wide-reaching multidisciplinary field. It incorporates theoretical underpinnings from the disciplines of health care, social sciences, management science, information science, epidemiology and economics. Research topics may include the following:

- Access to care
- Quality of care
- Quality improvement
- Cost and financing of healthcare
- Population outcomes
- Clinical and program evaluation
- Health human resources
- Provider and patient behaviours
- Clinical decision making
- Knowledge translation and dissemination

Healthcare policy makers may be asked to make difficult decisions in situations where there is insufficient or contradictory information. HSR helps to synthesize and organize the available research so that decisions to improve healthcare quality and delivery are based on sound evidence. Evidence generated from HSR can and should be used to support decision making at any stage of the policy cycle. Evidence-informed policymaking is defined as "an approach to policy decisions that aims to ensure that decision making is well-informed by the best available research evidence. It is characterised by the systematic and transparent access to, and appraisal of, evidence as an input into the policymaking process.[2]"

Howlett conceptualizes the policy cycle into five distinct stages: agenda setting, policy formulation, decision making, policy implementation and policy evaluation (Figure 9.1).[3] While policy-making can occur at any stage of the cycle, conceptualizing the process in this manner can provide a clearer understanding how a policy progresses from a social and individual issue to becoming a public and formal issue on the government agenda, to how a policy may or may not eventually get implemented.[3]

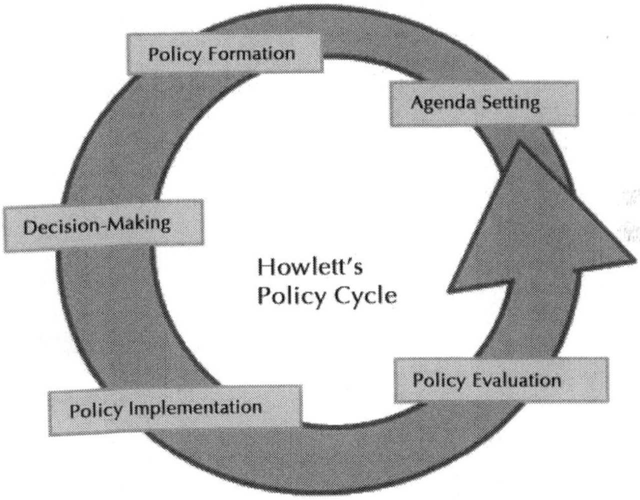

FIGURE 9.1 Howlett's Policy Cycle, demonstrating the process involved in moving a policy issue from the formal government agenda to eventual policy implementation.

9.2 FORMULATING THE HSR RESEARCH QUESTION

Developing an appropriate research question is one of the foundational elements of a successful research project. The research question should be specific and focused, and related to a timely issue for which the results may contribute to the existing body of knowledge in the health services research or policy fields.

Research projects can quickly extend beyond their intended scope, therefore the PICO format (Population, Intervention, Comparison and Outcomes) is often used to maintain research focus, as described in detail in Chapter 1 (Evidence-Based Medicine and the Scientific Method). An example of a PICO-derived HSR research question is included as Case Example 9.1. A focused research question will help the researcher pinpoint the relevant evidence or information. This should also be followed by a review of the literature to further assist the researcher in formulating and refining the research question.

CASE EXAMPLE 9.1

The formulation of a research questions using PICO can help to ensure a concise, focused, and feasible research question.

Population: prostate cancer patients
Intervention: proton therapy
Comparison: photon therapy (standard of care)
Outcome: cost-effectiveness

The HSR research question then becomes:
What is the cost-effectiveness of photon therapy versus proton therapy in patients with prostate cancer[4]?

9.2.1 *THE DONABEDIAN MODEL: STRUCTURE, PROCESS, OUTCOME*

Donabedian helps to further conceptualize HSR into a framework involving three domains: structure, process, and outcomes (Figure 9.2). This framework is often referred to as the SPO framework and is used to help situate HSR in the context of quality improvement, which can facilitate the generation of a meaningful HSR research question.[5,6] Donabedian defines the elements as follows:

Structure: relatively stable characteristics of the providers of care, including organization elements, personnel elements, and the operation of programs.

Process: the transactions associated with providing and receiving care, and may involve both providers and recipients of care.

Outcome: the change(s) resulting from healthcare, including improvements in a patient's health status, patient satisfaction, and wait times for care, and this domain ultimately validates the effectiveness and quality of medical care for patients.[6]

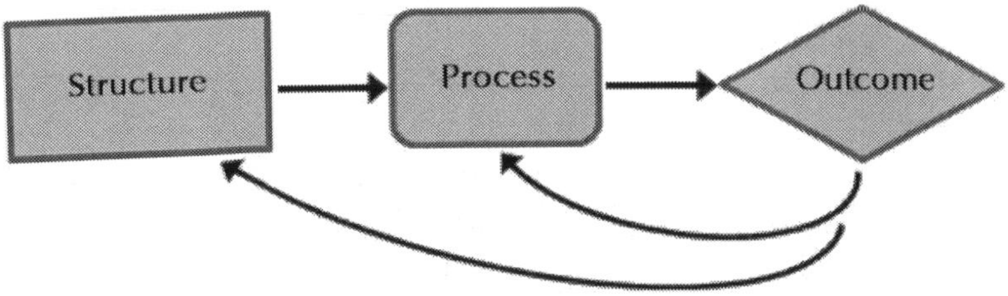

FIGURE 9.2 The Donabedian Framework.

While it is not necessary for a research question to address each domain of the SPO framework, the three components of the framework should be considered as linked together in the context of an entire systemic integration and not viewed as independent domains of quality.[5] This lens can help to better conceptualize an HSR research question to clarify the issue at hand and the various factors involved. Case example 9.2 reports on the application of the Donabedian Framework in a microlevel radiation therapy context.

CASE EXAMPLE 9.2

A radiation therapy department wished to explore a formal approach to generating efficiency in their work processes, through use of a concept known as the LEAN quality improvement strategy.[7,8]" This strategy has been tested in the healthcare industry, however, never specifically in a radiation therapy department.

A research question to address this issue was generated: "How does implementing a LEAN strategy in radiation therapy departments improve wait times for treatment?" In the context of the Donabedian Framework:

Structure: the radiotherapy department

Process: the hand-off required for each step required to move a patient from consultation to receiving a radiation treatment

Outcome: the radiotherapy treatment wait times

This investigation thus focused on how the process variables within the radiotherapy department structure of the cancer centre will influence wait time outcomes.

9.3 HEALTH SERVICES RESEARCH METHODOLOGY

Depending on the research question, qualitative, quantitative and mixed-methods approaches may be used in HSR. Other chapters review in detail how these types of methodologies are applied (see Chapters 5, Quantitative Methodologies and Analysis; 6, Qualitative Methodologies and Analysis; and 7, Survey Methodologies and Analysis).

Within HSR, qualitative methods may often be applied for health policy questions, and this is typically in the form of a case study analysis, which is an in-depth investigation of a population or a phenomenon. Increasingly, health policy makers are relying on consensus methodology, such as the Modified Delphi process.[9] As it is considered relatively unique to HSR research, the Modified Delphi Process is discussed in further detail here.

9.3.1 MODIFIED DELPHI PROCESS

The Modified Delphi process is a means of generating consensus in establishing the most appropriate healthcare approach, set of standards, or other HSR variable. It is based on the concept that a formal and structured approach to pooling expertise will lead to a more accurate or effective decision. The Process incorporates a series of iterative rounds of communication or structured debate and consensus-building amongst experts in a given area, to overcome the limitations of available evidence and eliminate bias in decision making.

The approach thus requires the participation of content experts who can provide insights on a specific topic. A preliminary compilation of statements or items is compiled from available sources, such as the published literature or an initial series of experts. This list is then circulated to all participants who then rank their agreement with each statement. The rankings are summarized, and may be discussed in a group meeting. Changes are made to the list based on insight generated in the first round, and a new list is subsequently recirculated to the group for another round of ranking. This process is repeated until an acceptable degree of consensus is reached. This approach was used successfully in a Canadian initiative that led to the development of a set of indicators for the quality of radiotherapy treatment in prostate cancer.[10]

This method usually does not require costly resources since it can be done via email or teleconference, participants can provide feedback anonymously. The use of technology also allows the research to leverage the engagement of a heterogeneous group of experts from various disciplines and geographic locations, through virtual participation in Delphi rounds. This helps reduce bias and create more reliable results. However, anonymity and multiple rounds may result in low-response rate or participant fatigue.[9]

9.3.2 *ADMINISTRATIVE DATABASES*

Another valuable source of information that can inform health services, accessed through quantitative retrospective methodology, is the use of administrative health services databases. These databases are large repositories of routinely collected information on health services transactions, the populations served, and cost, as well some outcomes such as patient deaths. Administrative health services databases offer objective and unbiased data, at the population level. Examples of these types of databases include the cancer registry databases and physician billing databases.

Administrative databases can be used for HSR to help support the development and implementation of evidence-informed policy.[2] Additionally, while administrative databases contain a wealth of information that can be used to advance HSR, it is important to acknowledge these databases are developed to support health system planning and are generally not structured for the purpose of research. Therefore, the structure of these types of databases will have limitations from a researcher's perspective. These limitations include the potential for data entry error, lack of or inconsistency in reporting, lack of access to real-time data, and often significant variability in structure and content by province and country. Databases often require special linkages between datasets through a common variable to obtain more granular detail at the level of the individual patient. This may or may not be possible depending on the capabilities of each database and the expertise and resources required to create the linkage, thus making access to such databases more challenging. Case example 9.3 reports on the implementation of a radiation therapy-specific administrative database in Ontario.

CASE EXAMPLE 9.3

Implementing a system-level database

One of the biggest barriers to policy development in radiation therapy in Canada late in the last century was the lack of available system-level databases to assess radiation therapy effectiveness on access to care policy. One of the recommendations that emerged from the Cancer Services Implementation Committee report, led by Dr. Alan Hudson and submitted to the Ontario Ministry of Health and Long-Term Care, was that a fully linked comprehensive provincial database including administrative and clinical data be developed and used for research, planning, and to strengthen the quality of and access to care.[11] Based on this report and its recommendations, a provincial database was implemented and data has been collected centrally by Cancer Care Ontario since 1997. Within this database, radiation therapy activity data is collected to produce quality, cost, and performance indicators for the cancer system. It is also used for planning and management purposes, wait times and guideline concordance, and to support funding decisions around cancer services. While the collected data is acknowledged to have limitations, it is currently the only database of its kind in Canada. Using this wealth of information should be a future consideration for HSR researcher in radiation therapy since it could be leveraged to strategically inform policy decision making around radiation treatment delivery.[11]

While the use of administrative databases for research has its limitations, there is a general acknowledgement that policies informed by imperfect information are still beneficial. This is because this process can still reduce political risk by suggesting altered courses of action if the policy does not work as expected. For example, there is a far greater political risk when policies are advocated without acknowledging the limitations of the available evidence and when policies are then adhered to regardless of the results. Accordingly, the benefits of exploiting databases designed for health services planning purposes such as those collected by Cancer Care Ontario (CCO) to inform radiation therapy delivery practices should outweigh the consequences of implementing an uninformed policy that may not produce the desired outcome. An example of this was seen during the wait times crisis for radiation therapy in Ontario in the late 1990s, which resulted in patients having to be sent to the United States for treatment at the government's expense.[12]

9.4 PROGRAM IMPLEMENTATION AND IMPROVEMENT

Health services researchers are continuously implementing and improving various programs and processes to impact access to, quality, and cost of healthcare services. There is a large body of literature that details the diffusion of innovations and the various factors that influence how knowledge, processes or products are adopted and implemented into healthcare practice.[13–15]

9.4.1 *IMPLEMENTATION RESEARCH*

Implementation research provides insights into ways of implementing innovations and identifies issues to consider when developing change strategies. No two implementation approaches will be the same, since they are often dependent on the adopters, the adoption process and the organization itself. Researchers have long established that the implementation process is often nonlinear and dynamic since adopters tend to change and adapt implementation initiatives to their own contexts and particular needs.[16] This is especially true in radiation medicine where the treatments are technically complex and dependent on a multitude of factors, including available technology and skills of the multidisciplinary team. Sophisticated software and other supplementary devices, treatment guidelines and standardized protocols are continuously being implemented to enhance the quality of radiation treatment. In case example 9.4, the implementation of a provincial patient satisfaction survey program in British Columbia is highlighted, suggesting how the data collected through this well-established initiative has led to improvements in the system.

CASE EXAMPLE 9.4

Measuring Patient Satisfaction in Radiation Therapy as a means to Quality Improvement

Cheryl McGregor RTT ACT CTIC
Resource Therapist – Planning Module, Abbotsford Cancer Centre, British Columbia Cancer Agency, Abbotsford, Canada

One aspect in measuring the quality of healthcare provided is through patient satisfaction.[17–19] The Canadian Partnership for Quality Radiotherapy reported in their 2011 Quality Assurance Guidance for Canadian Radiation Treatment Programs that the Radiation Therapy Quality Assurance Committee (RTQAC) "defines and monitors, on a continuous basis, quality indicators for the Radiation Treatment Program, and reports indicator trends to the Radiation Treatment Program Head and/or other committees or groups with responsibility for quality within the Radiation Treatment Program, Cancer Program or Organization.[20]" In 1999, as part of a quality improvement program, J. French developed a survey with both qualitative and quantitative measures of patient satisfaction within the BC Cancer Agency – Fraser Valley Centre.[21] Data from the patient satisfaction survey allows the RTQAC to evaluate the program and monitor performance. This survey has since been rolled out to all cancer centres in the province where data is collected and reported on a quarterly basis.[21]

Using a 6-point Likert scale with room for comments on each question, the survey addresses several key areas of patient care:[22]

- Information given about nature of illness and radiation therapy treatment options and side effects
- Help given to manage side effects from treatment and to address concerns regarding treatment
- Information given about support services available at the centre
- Courtesy and respectfulness of staff at the centre
- Satisfaction with appointment times, wait times, and waiting areas and services
- Comments or suggestions for improvement
- Overall satisfaction with the team, including doctors, nurses, radiation therapists (RTTs) and clerks

Included in the quarterly report are the demographic break down of male versus female, age range and the education level of the respondents as well as survey response rate. Data for each question is collected and graphed in a percentage based on the number of survey responses. The report compares results from the previous period to the current period to look for significant changes in the percentage of responses, focusing on shifts of +/– 10%. It also includes a statement of the overall patient satisfaction. There is a provincial goal to have overall satisfaction >90% at each centre. This value is reviewed at the provincial management level.

Each site reviews the Patient Satisfaction Report, looking for areas that can be improved within the program to increase patient satisfaction levels. In 2008, the Abbotsford Cancer Centre opened and within the first two periods of patient surveys there were several comments on the lack of a water supply for patients. This complaint was raised further to the Operations Committee and a water dispenser was installed in the department. Another common complaint was a lack of parking. This was raised to the host hospital management, resulting in an additional parking lot added to the property. Subsequent patient survey results showed major improvements for satisfaction in all areas that were addressed by the program. Sometimes it really is the "little things" that contribute to program improvement, and these are only possible when information is collected to guide change.

Consistent program evaluation and performance monitoring through patient satisfaction surveys is important to improve radiation therapy service delivery.[23] BC Cancer Agency has established a continuous patient satisfaction reporting system within all of their treatment centres in an attempt to maintain and improve a high quality radiation therapy program.

HOT TIP

Five key factors that influence implementation:

Leadership: involve opinion leaders early on so that they can inspire others and champion the project.

Collaboration: build strong relationships within the department, the cancer centre and the region to share updates and lessons learned.

Training, expertise and standardization: offer activities that lead to skilled behaviour and standardize processes to increase efficiency and safety.

Resources: assess the need for equipment, personnel and time.

Resistance to change: address intimidation and/or anxiety concerns and educated users about the technology/process and its benefits.[24]

9.4.2 TOTAL QUALITY MANAGEMENT: PROGRAM IMPROVEMENT STRATEGIES

The introduction of one technology or process can lead to an improvement or evolution of another technology or process. This encourages a continuous cycle of improvement. The concept of continuous quality improvement is often referred to as total quality management (TQM) in the business industry. TQM is a concept that is slowly integrating itself into healthcare, and is starting to receive attention in the field of radiation oncology. A common TQM definition is that it encompasses an organization-wide commitment to infusing quality into every activity through quantitative methods for continuous improvement. Furthermore, its aim is to improve internal and external customer satisfaction by modifying a preexisting system. Process changes in all departments are made incrementally to allow for a smooth transition within the work place. Once this transpires, changes in daily processes will follow easily.[25]

Quality gurus such as Philip Crosby, W. Edwards Deming, Armand V. Feigenbaum, Kaoru Ishikawa, and Joseph Juran have pioneered the theoretical construct of TQM. The commonality amongst them was that each was introduced as a prescriptive form, and only acknowledged the hard aspects of TQM. The soft elements are also important to consider, and are encompassed within the concept of Total Quality Culture (TQC). TQC includes several behavioural practices such as empowerment, teamwork, participative management, continuous improvement, and culture change.[26]

Huq suggests that TQM is generic enough to be considered an overall strategic plan, encompassing all business functions and employees of all industry sectors, including healthcare.[27] However, before implementing any TQM program, it is important to assess if the work culture will support TQM and TQC. Case example 9.5 illustrates a systematic literature review approach to investigating whether radiation therapy departments are supportive of a total quality culture.

CASE EXAMPLE 9.5

Total quality culture in radiotherapy departments across Ontario[28]

The purpose of this study was to investigate the prevalence of total quality culture (TQC) within radiation therapy (RT) departments within a province in Canada. A validated survey was distributed to all RT staff within RT departments. The response rate included 90% of managers (9/10) and 50% of employees (261/519). Concordance existed between managers and staff that overall RT departments exhibit a work culture that somewhat resembles a TQC. Both groups scored 55% of the categories as *somewhat agree* with TQC and 9% of categories as having no TQC. 36% of the categories were discordant between groups; managers scored a higher prevalence of TQC compared to their RTTs. Moreover, larger RT departments (>50 employees) had a higher prevalence of discrepant scores between groups. This is the first study to document the prevalence of TQC within RT departments. Strategies designed for on-going continuous improvement will benefit staff, RT managers, continuity of patient care and patient safety within RT departments.[29]

Program improvement strategies are often translated into practice through the development of knowledge translation tools, such as clinical practice guidelines, quality standards documents, reports, guides-to-practice, algorithms, various frameworks and other interactive evidence-based tools. Significant education and training is often integrated to the initiative to ensure that users have the necessary skills and knowledge to embrace the new practice. Further details on knowledge translation and dissemination of HSR are discussed later in this chapter and in Chapter 11 (Knowledge Dissemination: Value and Approaches).

9.4.2.1 MODEL FOR IMPROVEMENT: THE DEMING CYCLE

One specific framework that has become popular in healthcare to evaluate programmatic continuous quality improvement is the Deming Cycle, also known as the PDSA cycle, which consists of four phases: plan, do, study, and act. Conceptualizing quality improvement in this manner allows researchers to focus on three key system or process questions:

What is hoped to be accomplished?
How will it be known if a change leads to an improvement?
What changes can be made that will result in improvement?

The Deming Cycle is used to assess change in practice settings by planning change, trying it, observing the results and acting on what has been learned.[30]

9.4.2.2 MODEL FOR IMPROVEMENT: THE LEAN STRATEGY

Building on the Deming Cycle for continuous quality improvement, the lean strategy was developed and successfully used in the automotive industry. The healthcare industry has slowly begun to test and incorporate this strategy as well (*see* Case example 9.6). The lean strategy provides a simple step-by-step template for process improvement execution and an on-going sustainability strategy.[31] In theory, lean implementation may provide improved patient quality and safety, efficiency in throughput, continuous improvement, and improved staff morale through constant multidisciplinary staff engagement.[32–34] This may reduce the cost of healthcare and allow the medical staff to do what they do best, care for the patients.[34]

CASE EXAMPLE 9.6

A scoping literature review, which reviewed both the peer-reviewed and grey literature, was conducted to determine if the lean strategy could be implemented successfully in hospitals and specifically within radiation oncology programs. For the peer-reviewed literature, relevant databases were searched for literature published between 1950 and October 22, 2010. The grey literature was searched using two key words at a time and only the first 30 hits for each Internet search were reviewed for relevance. A total of 39 publications related to lean strategy in hospitals and cancer centres. Of these articles, one was related to a radiation oncology clinic.[5] Majority of studies have come from either Europe (43%) or the United States (43%), and the remaining were from Australia (14%). No studies were reported from Canada. All studies were published as peer-reviewed, prospective quantitative case studies. Of these cases 43% were prospective pre- and post-lean intervention studies, 35% were descriptive, 22% reported on results after implementation within a hospital program. Only one case report from the United States reported on implementing lean strategy within a bone and brain metastases clinic of a radiation oncology program.[5]

This is the first study to summarize the literature on the use of lean strategy in healthcare, and also within a radiation oncology program. The results of this scoping review have demonstrated that it is feasible to implement lean strategy within hospitals and radiation oncology clinics. However, from this review we learn that this subject area is still under-studied, with room to grow. Particularly, given the unique complexities associated with a radiation oncology program within cancer, more research is required to determine if lean strategy is the most appropriate management strategy to improve process efficiency and value for the cancer population within the Canadian healthcare system.

There are five principles that are applied to lean strategy:

1. Identification of customer value
2. Management of value stream and eliminating waste
3. Developing continuous flow production
4. Using pull techniques based on customer's consumption
5. Striving to perfection (i.e., zero waste)[6]

Value is a key concept in lean thinking, defined as the capability to deliver exactly the product or service a customer wants with minimal time between the moment the customer asks for that product or service and the actual delivery. Hence, the perspective from which value must be assessed must clearly be defined upfront. Process is divided into value-adding activities that contribute directly to creating a product or service a customer wants, and nonvalue adding activities as defined from the customer's perspective. Non-value adding activities are called waste, and in lean strategy the aim is to eliminate as much waste as possible.[7] In healthcare, lean aims to improve care by eliminating waste activities that undermine efficient treatments. Moreover, lean enhances the quality of care by reducing delays and waiting for care, and by speeding up processes related to treatment. This will lead to cost savings without sacrificing quality of care for patients.[32]

Case example 9.7 reports on the use of the lean strategy to generate efficiencies in a brachytherapy program at the Princess Margaret Cancer Centre in Toronto.

CASE EXAMPLE 9.7

Using the lean method to improve the efficiency of a MR-guided brachytherapy program

Kitty Chan MRT(T) BSc MHSc
Clinical Specialist Radiation Therapist, Radiation Medicine Program, Princess Margaret Cancer Centre, Toronto, Canada

Integrating magnetic resonance imaging (MRI) to guide brachytherapy treatment in cervical cancer has been recommended as a standard.[35,36] This increases the complexity of the treatment process and often causes inefficiency. Chan et al. conducted a study in Toronto using the lean method to evaluate the workflow and recommended changes to improve the efficiency of the process.[37]

Nine multidisciplinary staff members were interviewed and eight consecutive MR-guided brachytherapy (MRgBT) for cervical cancer procedures were observed using Lean Methods. All activities for the procedure were mapped out. Then time, description, location, number of staff involved and causes of any inefficiency were recorded. Inefficiencies of the process were categorized according to Lean value-added vs. nonvalue-added (i.e., wastes) activities. Then they were grouped using Taichi Ohno's 7 Wastes in Health Care[38].

The mean procedure time required was 8.1 h (range 6.5–9.2). The process had 17 discrete activities: 10 value-added vs. seven nonvalue-added (waste) activities were observed. The proportion of value-added versus wasted time was 79% vs. 21%. As activities were carried out on five different floors in the study hospital, all procedures wasted time on transporting the patient. Other wastes observed were waiting for the availability of the physician to review the contours and plan, and wastes on rework performing replans (*see* Table 9.1).

The Lean data suggested a long-term solution of remodeling the current process to allow dedicated radiation oncologist, radiation physicists and RTTs to work in a dedicated area; the renewed process is predicted to increase efficiency by 59% (8.1 h to 4.8 h). The short-term solution suggested was to eliminate wastes on waiting and reduce the frequency of underdeveloped talent by sharing the knowledge of replanning strategies in case review rounds.

TABLE 9.1 Wastes identified in MR-guided brachytherapy.

Ohno's 7 Lean Wastes in Health Care	**Observed Results**
Waiting	MRI availability
	MR image data transfer
	Staff member availability
Transportation	Transferring patient from operating room (OR) to MRI
Rework	Planner spends time replanning
Motion	Forgot OR equipment
	Forgot treatment quality assurance (QA) equipment
Overproduction	Lack of standard process in communication among staff between recovery to MRI scanner
Processing	Frequent communication and requests for updates regarding planning and plan QA progress
Underdeveloped Talent	Rationale for replanning not shared for subsequent procedures

9.4.2.3 MODEL FOR IMPROVEMENT: KOTTER'S CHANGE PROCESS THEORY

There are many theories detailing how to most efficiently implement programmatic changes both locally and at a system level. One of these models was developed by John Kotter and has been widely applied in the business sector[39]. However, it has also gained ground in healthcare. Kotter's theory involves eight pragmatic steps to implement change and improve programs:

Create a Sense of Urgency: For change to be successful 75% of the leaders need to "buy-in" to the change; thus, a burning platform supported by evidence and key leaders, is necessary for change management projects.

Creating the Guiding Coalition: Engage key stakeholders in the change process. Engaging strong leaders that are visible, vocal and supportive may result in more successful adoption of change.

Create a Vision for Change: A clear vision will help the project team and the various stakeholders understand what they are being asked to do and how this will be done.

Communicate the Vision: Regularly communicate the goals and vision to all involved stakeholders.

Remove Obstacles: Removing obstacles can empower people who are executing the vision, and it can help the change move forward.

Create Short-term Wins: Report on visible results by creating short-term, achievable targets and share them frequently. Each produced "win" can further motivate the entire staff and stakeholders.

Build on the Change: Kotter argues that many change projects fail because victory is declared too early. Real change runs deep. Continue looking for improvements.

Anchor the Changes in Institutional Culture: Change should be seen in every aspect of the organization and should be promoted in day-to-day work, especially by those in leadership positions.

9.5 PROGRAM EVALUATION

9.5.1 EVALUATION RESEARCH

Evaluating the effectiveness of a program by systematically gathering, analyzing and reporting data on that program, can answer important questions about a program's success and challenges, and it offers important insights for future planning. Evaluation research is thus the process of determining the effectiveness of a program.[40]

9.5.1.1 PROGRAM EVALUATION

Program evaluations can be performed at the level of an individual department or academic program or at a provincial, national or international level. Evaluations may be valuable or necessary for some of the following purposes:[40]

- assessing program changes
- identifying new avenues for improvement
- testing the success of innovative programmatic ideas
- determining if programs should be expanded or eliminated
- assessing accountability

Determining the purpose of the evaluation and who will be using the gathered data is one of the first steps a researcher needs to take. A theoretical framework must then be selected to guide the evaluation process. A commonly used framework for quality assessment in healthcare is the Institute of Medicine's six aims of quality care: safety, effectiveness, patient-centreedness, timeliness, efficiency, and equity.[41] Measures corresponding to these or similar aims can then be selected or devised. To draw sound conclusions, the measures used to gather data in the evaluation must be both valid and reliable (*see* Chapter 7: Survey Methodologies and Analysis). Next, the researcher will need to determine the most appropriate methods for collecting the necessary information.

There are three major sources of information that can be used for evaluations:[42]

1. *Existing information*: program documents and reports, minutes of meetings, related media stories, census data, etc.
2. *The people involved:* those who participated in the development and implementation of the program, the users of the program as well as nonparticipants or critics of the program
3. *Records and observations:* pictures from before and after the intervention, video records, observations of verbal and nonverbal reactions

Qualitative methods, such as document reviews, interviews, focus groups, and observation, or quantitative or mixed methods, such as surveys, may be used to gather the data (*see* Chapters 5 (Quantitative Methodologies and Analysis), 6 (Qualitative Methodologies and Analysis), and 7 (Survey Methodologies and Analysis) for more information on these methodologies). Evaluations offer an opportunity to inform future directions for programs, prove that program accreditation standards are being met, and may also provide evidence that newly implemented initiatives or improvements are successful.

9.5.1.2 PERFORMANCE MONITORING

Performance monitoring often compliments evaluations as it helps the researcher determine whether a program is meeting operating standards and predetermined targets. Indicators, which are succinct measures that serve to describe the key elements of a system, are used in performance monitoring to help compare and improve a program or system.

An evaluation of a project undertaken in Ontario known as the "IMRT Implementation Project" was conducted to highlight the innovative strategies, successes, shortcomings and lessons learned. The evaluation consisted of document analysis, interviews and electronic surveys (*see* Case example 9.8 for more details).

CASE EXAMPLE 9.8

Using Qualitative HSR Methods to Evaluate the Implementation A Province-Wide IMRT program

Bak et al. conducted a study to document a jurisdiction-wide evaluation of IMRT in one province in Canada, highlighting innovative strategies, successes, shortcomings and lessons learned.[24] To obtain an accurate provincial representation, six cancer centres were chosen (based on their IMRT utilization, geography, population, academic affiliation and size) for an in-depth evaluation. At each cancer centre semistructured, key informant interviews were conducted with senior administrators. An electronic survey, consisting of 40 questions was also developed and distributed to all cancer centres in Ontario.[24]

Twenty-one respondents participated in the interviews and a total of 266 electronic surveys were returned. Funding allocation, guidelines and utilization targets, expert coaching and educational activities were identified as effective implementation strategies. The implementation allowed for hands-on training, knowledge exchange and sharing of responsibility. Future implementation initiatives could be improved by increasing ongoing jurisdiction-wide communication, encouraging early stakeholder consultation and developing educational opportunities. IMRT utilization increased without affecting wait times or safety. From fiscal year 2008/09 to 2012/13 the absolute increased change was found as the following: Prostate 46%, Thyroid 36%, Head and Neck 29%, Sarcoma 30%, and CNS 32%. Breast IMRT from April 2011 to end of March 2013 saw an absolute increase of 26%.

This type of jurisdiction-wide implementation approach has not been previously used. The lessons learned can promote the rollout of IMRT or other complex innovations in similar jurisdictions. This evaluation offers valuable recommendations and will be of interest to those exploring ways to fund, implement and sustain complex and evolving technologies in a coordinated manner.

9.5.2 *ECONOMIC EVALUATIONS*

Health economics is the study of resource allocation decisions within the healthcare marketplace and between the marketplace and other areas of economic endeavors. Economic evaluations are methods used to identify, measure, value and compare the costs and consequences of alternative courses of action. This information can be used to support the decisions made by senior administrators. Economic evaluations can be conducted as cost minimization analyses, cost effectiveness analyses, cost utility analyses and cost benefit analyses. The method chosen depends on the number of outcomes involved within the program being considered and also if the programs differ in their effectiveness (Figure 9.3).[43]

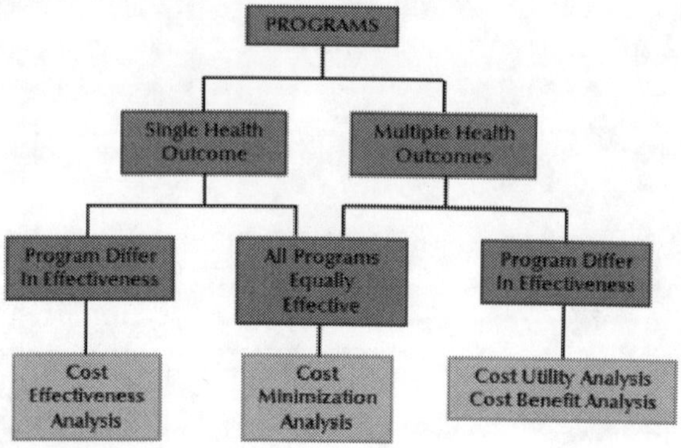

FIGURE 9.3 Selection of Economic Evaluation Models.

9.5.2.1 COST-EFFECTIVENESS ANALYSIS

Cost-effectiveness analysis (CEA) allows payers to quantify the value for money for health services under consideration. It provides a framework to focus discussion on key decision factors and uncertainties around them.[44,45] In radiation therapy, CEAs are often used to compare the relative value of different techniques. For example, two CEAs comparing IMRT to three-dimensional conformal therapy (3DCRT) were conducted to evaluate IMRT as an emerging technique. The first CEA was entitled "Cost-effectiveness of Intensity-modulated Radiotherapy in Oropharyngeal Cancer" and demonstrated that IMRT strategy for the treatment of locally advanced oropharyngeal carcinoma appears to be cost-effective when compared with 3DCRT.[46] The second CEA, "Cost-effectiveness of Intensity-modulated Radiotherapy in Prostate Cancer" compared IMRT to 3DCRT for the radical treatment of localized prostate cancer at elevated doses (>70 Gy). The results of this

CEA identified that for radical treatment courses, IMRT appears to be cost-effective when compared with an equivalent dose of 3DCRT.[47] These CEAs supported policy decision making regarding future funding for new and innovative health technology initiatives.

In radiation treatment practice, technology implementation may outpace the rate at which evidence is produced to support the use of such technologies. An example of this may be for patients with stage I nonsmall cell lung cancers (NSCLC) that are ineligible for surgery. While these patients have two curative treatment options; conventional radiotherapy (CRT) or stereotactic body radiotherapy (SBRT), no randomized trials have compared these two approaches. To determine if it is worthwhile to invest in diffusing such technologies, a CEA comparing SBRT to CRT for this patient population was conducted in a large academic centre in Ontario, from 2002–2010 (*see* case example 9.9).

CASE EXAMPLE 9.9

Cost-Effectiveness Analysis Comparing Conventional Versus Stereotactic Body Radiotherapy for Surgically Ineligible Stage I Non-Small Cell Lung Cancer[48]

Purpose: The purpose of this study was to conduct a CEA comparing SBRT to CRT for stage I NSCLC patients within a publicly funded healthcare system.

Methods: All patients with stage I nonsmall cell lung cancer treated in a single large cancer centre with CRT or SBRT from January 2002 – June 2010 were included in the analysis, with SBRT offered from 2004. Direct medical costs from the perspective of the Ontario public healthcare system were calculated, including physician billing, labour costs for RTTs, physicists, nurses, equipment maintenance staff, information technology support staff, and hospitalization due to acute adverse events. In addition, the subset of direct radiation treatment delivery costs excluding physician billings and hospitalization was calculated. Direct costs were obtained from professional groups, manufacturers and funding agencies at 2010 Canadian prices. Missing costs were derived from published literature or expert opinion. The effectiveness outcome for both analyses was life-years gained. Time-to-event data was captured using Kaplan-Meier and log-rank statistical methods. One-way and two-way sensitivity analyses were carried out to determine which factors most influenced overall costs.

Results: Of 170 patients (51 CRT; 119 SBRT) treated with a median follow-up of 24 months, the mean overall survival for the CRT group was 2.83 years (95% confidence interval (CI): 1.8–4.1 years), and 3.86 years (95% CI: 3.2 – NR) for the SBRT group (p=0.06). The mean estimated life-years gained (LYG) with SBRT compared to CRT treatment was 1.03 years. Total mean direct costs for CRT were $6,885 overall, and $5,989 for radiation treatment delivery costs. In the SBRT arm, mean costs were $8,042 and $6,962 for treatment delivery only. The mean incremental cost per patient treated with SBRT was $1,156, $972 specifically for treatment delivery. The incremental costs per LYG for SBRT over CRT were $1,120 from the public payer perspective, and $942 including treatment delivery costs only. A one-way sensitivity analysis showed that varying survival difference and direct labour costs +/– 20% led to the largest changes in incremental cost for both analyses. When simultaneously adjusting both survival difference and direct labour costs by +/– 5% to +/– 30% in a two-way sensitivity analysis to account for selection bias, potential stage migration, and efficiency of SBRT over time, the incremental cost per LYG for SBRT versus CRT was still within the threshold for accepting a new health technology.

Conclusion: In this first study of the cost-effectiveness of SBRT over CRT in a publically funded healthcare system, SBRT appears highly cost effective.

9.6 KNOWLEDGE TRANSLATION AND DISSEMINATION

The Canadian Institute of Health Research (CIHR) defines knowledge translation as "a dynamic and iterative process that includes the synthesis, dissemination, exchange and ethically sound application of knowledge to improve health, provide more effective health services and products and strengthen the healthcare system"[49] (*see* Chapter 11: Knowledge Dissemination: Value and Approaches).

While numerous conceptual frameworks have been developed, the Knowledge to Action Cycle is a conceptual framework developed by Graham (2006) to suggest how knowledge is created or produced (knowledge creation cycle) and how knowledge is applied (knowledge action cycle).[50]

This framework has also been adopted by the CIHR. Based on this framework, knowledge is first created through inquiry, and then through an iterative process, finally refined into a knowledge product. Once the evidence has matured, the knowledge may go through the action cycle for uptake into the community. Knowledge translation focuses on the use of tools and strategies to enhance research utilization by clinicians, managers and policy-makers through understanding the complex factors that can influence health professional practice and outcomes. This knowledge is relevant to guideline implementers, continuing education planners, practicing clinicians, healthcare managers, and health services researchers. Specifically, this type of research uses educational, social, organizational, incentive and embedded approaches and interventions to study the gap between best evidence and practice. Research in the area of knowledge translation can target several interventions aimed at addressing this gap.

Educational strategies include interventions targeted at work-specific, reflective, or self-directed learning to change practice instead of traditional forms of continuing education such as mailing of educational material or meetings.

Social interventions involve examining the formal and informal interactions in how information is delivered. This could include the use of opinion leaders, educational outreach and mentoring.[51,52] Patients can also be engaged to influence their access to care, the behaviour of their healthcare provider, the quality of care they receive, and their involvement decision making or management of their own health status.[53]

Organizational strategies are often used to measure the success of implementation. Specifically, this may include examining the impact before and after the implementation of institutional policies, protocols, visible and involved leadership; development of a quality culture; and support for teamwork.[14,54] The approach of the Nova Scotia Cancer Centre in Halifax to implementing and ensuring compliance with novel a novel radiation therapy incident reporting framework is highlighted in Case example 9.10.

CASE EXAMPLE 9.10

Changing the Incident Reporting Structure in the Department of Radiation Oncology: A Multidisciplinary Experience

Kathryn Moran RTT BSc CTIC
Radiation Therapist, Radiation Therapy Services, Nova Scotia Cancer Centre, Queen Elizabeth II Health Sciences Centre, Halifax, Canada

Following preliminary discussions at the national level regarding the need for a national incident reporting and learning database, and the dissemination of a preliminary radiotherapy incident taxonomy proposed by the American Association of Physicists in Medicine, we began to look at our own in-house incident reporting structure and culture, and determined existing gaps and potential for improvement.

The department had a long-standing culture of incident reporting among the RTT group, but it was found to be based on a paper technical variance (TV) form that spoke to outdated practices. Incidents from these TV forms would be periodically circulated to the RTTs for shared learning. At the same time, there also existed a duty to report into the broader hospital Patient Safety Reporting System (PSRS). This system consisted of generic fields that did not fit the needs of the radiotherapy language or incident type. This double reporting was found to lead to underreporting, as approximately 300 TV were filed in a given year, as compared to only 15 PSRS forms. In addition, there was no formalized quality review process, and no facilitation of learning from incidents for the larger multidisciplinary team. It was felt important to approach the implementation of a new model in a strategic and evidence-based manner, and this was done using the principles of the Deming Cycle (Figure 9.4).

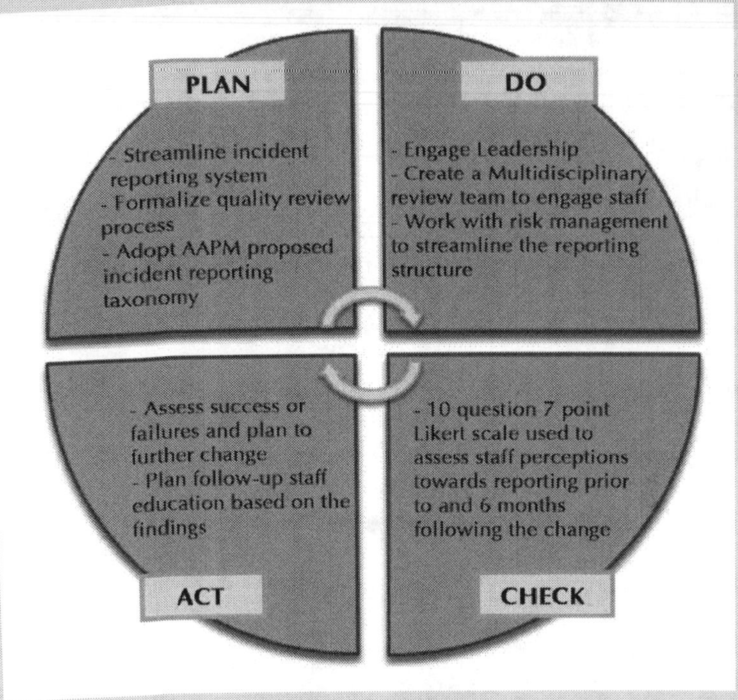

FIGURE 9.4 Deming Cycle as applied to implementation of novel incident reporting structure and program.

The process of implementation took place first with multiple presentations to leadership, and the recruitment of staff for the new multidisciplinary review team, where practices could be revised and approved. Once the new processes were ready, a questionnaire was administered to all staff to assess current reporting attitudes. A series of multidisciplinary education sessions on the formalized quality review process were held, with discussions on the future of national reporting and showcasing the redesigned hospital PSRS.

The key element to the success of our project was the engagement and buy-in of the multidisciplinary leadership and staff. The conceptual support of leadership came very early on as the planned changes were approved by the risk management and legal departments, as it was argued that implementation of a more robust system would bring the radiation therapy department more in line with the goals of the hospital with respect to incident management. True practical engagement did not take hold until the preliminary system was in place and incidents began to be reported by front-line staff. RTTs adopted the new structure quite readily, as they already had a long-standing history of reporting, and the new system proved to be more streamlined and standardized. Additionally, there was comfort in knowing that for the first time, contributing factors would be investigated. For the other members of the multidisciplinary team who had not been accustomed to reporting using the previous system, buy-in required some encouragement and assurance of the value of the process. This was accomplished with education and reinforcement of how collaborative and structured reporting was able to drive positive change within the department. In total, the planning, implementation, and evaluation of the project took 18 months to complete, using limited funding and resources, but with high departmental impact as staff are increasingly well-versed in the use and value of the system (Figure 9.5).

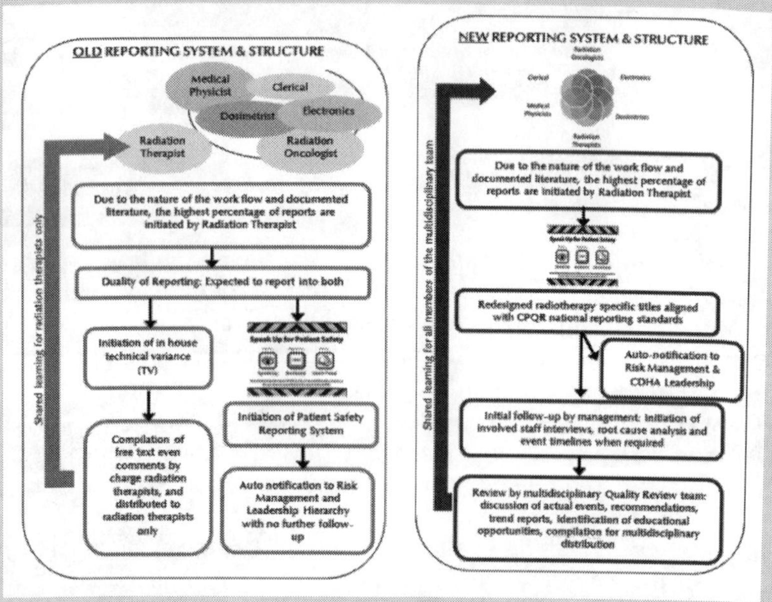

FIGURE 9.5 Old and New Incident Reporting System and Structure in the Radiation Therapy Department at the Nova Scotia Cancer Centre, Queen Elizabeth II Health Sciences Centre in Halifax.

Incentive strategies as a policy lever to implement something specific such as a program, policy, or clinical treatment protocol, are also a meaningful area of research. Specific data related to such incentives include public reporting of performance data and pay-for-performance, which seeks to promote accountability through financial incentives.[55,56]

This chapter has demonstrated that HSR is a field of research that allows for the examination of issues that impact the health system as a whole, or aspects of it. There are various methods that can be used to conduct this type of research, and the scope can range from micro level departmental programs or initiatives to macro level national or international policy or strategy. For the radiation therapy research, taking a formal and rigourous approach to evaluating a local program or generating efficiencies in clinical workflow can lead to reliable and informed outcomes.

KEYWORDS

- Delphi process
- Program implementation
- Program evaluation
- Total quality management
- Change process theory
- Cost effectiveness analysis

REFERENCES

1. Lohr, K. N.; Steinwachs, D. M. Health services research: an evolving definition of the field. Health Serv. Res. **2002,** *37(1)*, 7–9.
2. Oxman, A. D. L., John, N.; Lewin, S.; Fretheim, A. SUPPORT Tools for evidence-informed health Policymaking (STP) I: What is evidence-informed policymaking? Health Res. Policy Syst. **2009,** *7(S1)*, 1–7.
3. Howlett, M.; Ramesh, M.; Perl, A. Studying Public Policy: Policy Cycles and Policy Subsystems. Oxford University Press: Oxford, 2009.
4. Creswell, J. W. Research design: Qualitative, quantitative, and mixed methods approaches. Sage Publications: Thousand Oaks, CA, 2013.

5. Kim, C. S.; Hayman, J. A.; Billi, J. E.; Lash, K.; Lawrence, T. S. The application of lean thinking to the care of patients with bone and brain metastasis with radiation therapy. *J. Oncol. Pract.* **2007,** *3(4)*, 189–193.
6. Donabedian, A. The quality of care. *Arch. Pathol. Lab. Med.* **1997,** *121*, 11.
7. Joosten, T.; Bongers, I.; Janssen, R. Application of lean thinking to health care: issues and observations. *Int. J. Qual. Health Care.* **2009,** *21(5)*, 341–347.
8. Kollberg, B.; Dahlgaard, J. J.; Brehmer, P.-O., Measuring lean initiatives in health care services: issues and findings. *Int. J. Prod. Performance Manage.* **2006,** *56(1),* 7–24.
9. Chang, A. M.; Gardner, G. E.; Duffield, C.; Ramis, M. A. A Delphi study to validate an advanced practice nursing tool. *J. Adv. Nurs.* **2010,** *66(10),* 2320–2330.
10. Danielson, B.; Brundage, M.; Pearcey, R.; Bass, B.; Pickles, T.; Bahary, J.-P.; Foley, K.; Mackillop, W. Development of indicators of the quality of radiotherapy for localized prostate cancer. *Radiother. Oncol.* **2011,** *99(1),* 29–36.
11. Hudson, A. R. *Report of the Cancer Services Implementation Committee*. Ontario Ministry of Health and Long-Term Care, Toronto, 2001.
12. McGowan, T., Private management of a public service: what can be learned from the CROS experience? *Hosp. Q.* **2003,** *6(4),* 33–8.
13. Rogers, E. M. Diffusion of innovations 4th ed. Free Press: New York, 1995.
14. Greenhalgh, T.; Robert, G.; Macfarlane, F.; Bate, P.; Kyriakidou, O. Diffusion of innovations in service organizations: systematic review and recommendations. *Milbank Q.* **2004,** *82(4),* 581–629.
15. Dirksen, C. D.; Ament, A. H.; Go, P. Diffusion of six surgical endoscopic procedures in the Netherlands. Stimulating and restraining factors. *Health policy.* **1996,** *37(2)*, 91–104.
16. Van de Ven, A. H.; Polley, D. E.; Garud, R.; Venkataraman, S. The Innovation Journey. Oxford University Press: New York, 1999.
17. Maxwell, R. J. Quality assessment in health. *BMJ.* **1984,** *288(6428),* 1470.
18. Hopkins, A.; Costain, D. Measuring the Outcomes of Medical Care. Royal College of Physicians of London: London, 1990.
19. Cleary, P. D., The increasing importance of patient surveys: now that sound methods exist, patient surveys can facilitate improvement. *BMJ.* **1999,** *319(7212)*, 720.
20. Canadian Partnership for Quality Radiotherapy. Quality Assurance Guidance for Canadian Radiation Treatment Programs. Canadian Partnership for Quality Radiotherapy: Toronto, 2011.
21. French, J.; McGahan, C. Measuring patient satisfaction with radiation therapy service delivery, *Healthc. Manage. Forum*, **2010**, *22(4),* 40–50.
22. French, J. The use of patient satisfaction data to drive quality improvement. *Can. J. Med. Radiat. Technol.* **2004,** *35(2)*, 14–24.
23. Vuori, H. Patient satisfaction—does it matter? *Int. J. Qual. Health Care.* **1991,** *3(3)*, 183–189.
24. Bak, K.; Dobrow, M. J.; Hodgson, D.; Whitton, A. Factors affecting the implementation of complex and evolving technologies: multiple case study of intensity-modulated radiation therapy (IMRT) in Ontario, Canada. *BMC Health Serv. Res.* **2011,** *11*, 178.
25. Klefsjö, B.; Bergquist, B.; Garvare, R. Quality management and business excellence, customers and stakeholders: do we agree on what we are talking about, and does it matter? *TQM J.* **2008,** *20(2),* 120–129.

26. Svensson, G.; Wood, G. Corporate ethics in TQM: management versus employee expectations and perceptions. *TQM Magazine*. **2005,** *17(2),* 137–149.
27. Huq, Z. Managing change: a barrier to TQM implementation in service industries. *Managing Service Quality.* **2005,** *15(5),* 452 469.
28. Patel, P.; Mitera, G. A Systematic Scoping Literature Review of Incorporating a Total Quality Culture Within Radiotherapy Staffing Models: A Management Strategy to Improve Patient Safety and Quality of Care in Radiation Therapy Departments. *J. Med. Imag. Radiat. Sci.* **2011,** *42(2)*, 81–85.
29. Mitera, G.; Whitton, A.; Gutierrez, E.; Robson, S., Total quality culture in radiotherapy departments across Ontario. *Radiother. Oncol.* **2011,** *99(1)*, 90–93.
30. Langley, G. J.; Moen, R.; Nolan, K. M.; Nolan, T. W.; Norman, C. L.; Provost, L. P. The improvement guide: a practical approach to enhancing organizational performance. Jossey-Bass: San Francisco CA, 2009.
31. van Lent, W. A.; Goedbloed, N.; Van Harten, W. Improving the efficiency of a chemotherapy day unit: Applying a business approach to oncology. *Eur. J. Cancer.* **2009,** *45(5),* 800–806.
32. Kim, C. S.; Lukela, M. P.; Parekh, V. I.; Mangrulkar, R. S.; Del Valle, J.; Spahlinger, D. A.; Billi, J. E. Teaching internal medicine residents quality improvement and patient safety: a lean thinking approach. Am. J. Med. Qual. **2010,** *25(3),* 211–217.
33. Pencheon, D. The good indicators guide: understanding how to use and choose indicators. NHS Institute for Innovation and Improvement: 2008.
34. Al-Araidah, O.; Momani, A.; Khasawneh, M.; Momani, M., Lead-time reduction using lean tools applied to healthcare: the inpatient pharmacy at a local hospital. J. Healthc. Qual. **2010,** *32(1),* 59–66.
35. Potter, R.; Haie-Meder, C.; Van Limbergen, E.; Barillot, I.; De Brabandere, M.; Dimopoulos, J.; Dumas, I.; Erickson, B.; Lang, S.; Nulens, A.; Petrow, P.; Rownd, J.; Kirisits, C. Recommendations from gynecological (GYN) GEC ESTRO working group (II): concepts and terms in 3D image-based treatment planning in cervix cancer brachytherapy-3D dose volume parameters and aspects of 3D image-based anatomy, radiation physics, radiobiology. Radiother. Oncol. **2006,** *78(1),* 67–77.
36. Potter, R.; Kirisits, C.; Fidarova, E. F.; Dimopoulos, J. C.; Berger, D.; Tanderup, K.; Lindegaard, J. C. Present status and future of high-precision image guided adaptive brachytherapy for cervix carcinoma. Acta Oncol. **2008,** *47(7),* 1325–1336.
37. Chan, K.; Rosewall, T.; Kenefick, B.; Milosevic, M. MRI-guided brachytherapy process for cervical cancer: identify procedure time and opportunities for efficiencies. Radiother. Oncol. **2012,** *104(S2),* S50.
38. Bush, R. W. Reducing waste in US health care systems. *JAMA.* **2007,** *297(8),* 871–874.
39. Kotter, J.P. Leading Change. Harvard Business Review Press: Cambridge, 2012.
40. Neuten, J. J.; Rubinson, L. Research techniques for the health sciences 3rd ed.; Pearson Education Inc: San Francisco, 2002.
41. Berwick, D. M., A user's manual for the IOM's "Quality Chasm" report. Health aff. **2002,** *21(3),* 80–90.
42. Taylor-Powell, E.; Steele, S. Collecting evaluation data: An overview of sources and methods. University of Wisconsin Cooperative Extension Service. *Cir. G3658-4,* 1996.

43. Drummond, M. F.; O'Brien, B.; Stoddart, G. L.; Torrance, G. W. Methods for the economic evaluation of health care programs. Oxford: Oxford University Press: Oxford, UK, 2005.
44. Laupacis, A. Economic evaluations in the Canadian common drug review. *Pharmacoeconomics,* **2006,** *24(11),* 1157–1162.
45. Williams, I.; Mclver, S.; Moore, D.; Bryan, S. The use of economic evaluations in NHS decision making: a review and empirical investigation. *Health Technol. Assess.* **2008,** *12(7),* 1–175.
46. Yong, J. H.; Beca, J.; O'Sullivan, B.; Huang, S. H.; McGowan, T.; Warde, P.; Hoch, J. S. Cost-effectiveness of intensity-modulated radiotherapy in oropharyngeal cancer. *Clin. Oncol.* **2012,** *24(7),* 532–538.
47. Yong, J. H.; Beca, J.; McGowan, T.; Bremner, K. E.; Warde, P.; Hoch, J. S. Cost-effectiveness of intensity-modulated radiotherapy in prostate cancer. *Clin. Oncol.* **2012,** *24(7),* 521–531.
48. Mitera, G.; Swaminath, A.; Rudoler, D.; Seereeram, C.; Giuliani, M.; Leighl, N.; Gutierrez, E.; Dobrow, M.; Coyte, P.; Yung, T.; Bezjak, A.; Hope, A. Cost-effectiveness analysis comparing conventional versus stereotactic body radiotherapy for surgically ineligible stage I nonsmall cell lung cancer. (*Submitted for publication*).
49. Straus, S. E.; Tetroe, J. M.; Graham, I. D. Knowledge translation is the use of knowledge in health care decision making. *J. Clin. Epidemiol.* **2011,** *64(1),* 6–10.
50. Graham, I. D.; Logan, J.; Harrison, M. B.; Straus, S. E.; Tetroe, J.; Caswell, W.; Robinson, N., Lost in knowledge translation: time for a map? *J. Contin. Educ. Health Prof.* **2006,** *26(1),* 13–24.
51. West, E.; Barron, D. N.; Dowsett, J.; Newton, J. N. Hierarchies and cliques in the social networks of health care professionals: implications for the design of dissemination strategies. *Social Sci. Med.* **1999,** *48(5),* 633–646.
52. Curran, G. M.; Thrush, C. R.; Smith, J. L.; Owen, R. R.; Ritchie, M.; Chadwick, D. Implementing research findings into practice using clinical opinion leaders: barriers and lessons learned. *Jt. Comm. J. Qual. Patient Saf.* **2005,** *31(12),* 7.
53. Street, Jr. R. L.; Makoul, G.; Arora, N. K.; Epstein, R. M. How does communication heal? Pathways linking clinician–patient communication to health outcomes. *Patient Educ. Couns.* **2009,** *74(3),* 295–301.
54. Lemieux-Charles, L.; McGuire, W. L. What do we know about health care team effectiveness? A review of the literature. *Med. Care Res. Rev.* **2006,** *63(3),* 263–300.
55. Mehrotra, A.; Damberg, C. L.; Sorbero, M. E.; Teleki, S. S. Pay for performance in the hospital setting: what is the state of the evidence? *Am. J. Med. Qual.* **2009,** *24(1),* 19–28.
56. Jamtvedt, G.; Young, J. M.; Kristoffersen, D. T.; O'Brien, M. A.; Oxman, A. D. Does telling people what they have been doing change what they do? A systematic review of the effects of audit and feedback. *Qual. Saf. Health Care.* **2006,** *15*(6), 433–436.

CHAPTER 10

INNOVATION AND INVENTION

COLLEEN DICKIE MRT(T) MRT(MR) MSc

Radiation Therapist, Radiation Medicine Program, Princess Margaret Cancer Centre, Toronto Canada
Assistant Professor, Department of Radiation Oncology, University of Toronto, Toronto Canada

AMY PARENT MRT(T) BSc CMD

Radiation Therapist, Radiation Medicine Program, Princess Margaret Cancer Centre, Toronto Canada

CONTENTS

This chapter addresses key components to successful implementation of change in practice through innovation and invention, and provides clarity to the use of terms that are commonly at play in these conversations. It builds on concepts introduced in Chapter 9 (Health Services Research and Program Evaluation) that relate to the strategies for exploring and adopting change, such as the Deming Cycle.

Whether the goal is to effect change through innovation by optimizing an aspect of practice, or to be a lead investigator of a research study, radiation therapists (RTTs) can be critical to the eventual success of an innovation. RTTs have a unique perspective and opportunity to apply their front line experience in the identification of clinical problems, shortcomings in practice, and other areas of need. Change can involve a product, program, practice, or process.

10.1 PRINCIPLES OF INNOVATION

Several interrelated terms are relevant to the discussion of change as it concerns innovation. Innovation is the optimization of an existing entity, not to be confused with invention which is the creation of a product or process for the first time. Intellectual property is the assignment of ownership to the expertise that informed the innovation or invention. Patenting is the formal, legal means by which to protect intellectual property. A thorough understanding of each of these terms can set the stage for engaging in change.

10.1.1 INNOVATION

Innovation is "the intentional introduction and application within a role, group, or organization, of ideas, processes, products or procedures, new to the relevant unit of adoption, designed to significantly benefit the individual, the group, or wider society" and can encompasses any improvement or significant contribution to an existing product, process or service.[1] In healthcare, it can be seen as the effort to balance cost and quality of healthcare and can involve two broad categories:[2]

Product innovation: development or improvement of physical goods, devices, or services locally and occasionally for the wider market

Process innovation: enhancement of the steps or approach in delivery of goods, devices, or services, to improve access, quality, or efficiency

Innovation is often the product of a desire to address an identified need or deficiency, but it must extend beyond the idea itself and encompass the realization of that idea and the subsequent benefit to a recipient or stakeholder in the system. The impact of an innovation can be defined by how it is seen to change the existing environment, as either disruptive or sustaining in nature.

10.1.1.1 DISRUPTIVE INNOVATION

A disruptive innovation is one that is revolutionary or radical. It fundamentally changes a system through necessitating a change in roles or practices to accommodate the innovation, thus marginalizing the previous system. Computed tomography-based simulation, intensity-modulated radiation therapy (IMRT), and cone-beam computed tomography are all disruptive innovations, as they forced radiation medicine professionals to assume different roles, structures for communication, and effectively change practice.

10.1.1.2 SUSTAINING INNOVATION

Sustaining innovations or technologies are those that improve performance of existing products or processes, and tend to be incremental rather than radical.[3] The introduction of volumetric arc radiation therapy can be seen as a sustaining innovation. This delivery approach can generate efficiencies through decreasing treatment time, and offers additional tools to boost dose to deep-seated tumours, but essentially it capitalizes on existing practices and workflows.

According to Omachonu and Einspruch, healthcare innovation in any of the domains described can be focused within the realm of treatment and diagnosis, education, outreach, or prevention, and can serve to improve quality, safety, outcomes, efficiency, or costs.[2] Case example 10.1 explores the success of a process innovation in education – SPICE (Students Partnering in

Interprofessional Care and Education) – which was designed to enhance the value and nature of interprofessional practice in the inpatient oncology setting.

CASE EXAMPLE 10.1

SPICE (Students Partnering in Interprofessional Care and Education): Innovation in Education

Tracey Hill MRT(T) BSc MEd
Radiation Therapist, Regional Cancer Care and Interprofessional Educator, Thunder Bay Regional Health Sciences Centre, Thunder Bay, Canada

An exciting and innovative project evolved from the desire to advance interprofessional education and collaborative care in the inpatient setting of palliative care and oncology. With assistance from *Health Force Ontario*, a partnership developed between the Thunder Bay Regional Health Sciences Centre, the Northern Ontario School of Medicine and the St. Joseph's Care Group. The SPICE (Students Partnering in Interprofessional Care and Education) Project involved senior level healthcare students from numerous different disciplines including radiation therapy, diagnostic imaging, nursing, social work, dietetics, medical laboratory, cardio-respiratory, physiotherapy and occupational therapy.

Clinical bedside teaching is a conventional teaching method used by medical, nursing, and other health professions. The SPICE Project invited healthcare students, many who are traditionally educated in a highly technical setting with minimal interaction with other learners, to join their professional peers at the bedside. This collaborative model of learning was very different from the uniprofessional environment most of these students were coming from. The focus was on the patient with cancer and students gained insight into the realities and challenges of providing care for these patients in an oncology inpatient setting. Teams were provided with experiential and reflective learning opportunities both with patients at the bedside and in simulation settings, and guided by trained clinical facilitators. This learning included listening to patients, listening and questioning peers and improving understanding of oncology treatments and patient experiences. Students learned with, from, and about each other, while providing collaborative care for shared patients.

The impact of interprofessional teaching and learning through SPICE translated into new ways of caring for and educating patients across the continuum of their treatment and care. Preliminary evaluation data indicated that student-driven interprofessional learning objectives and innovative opportunities increased the satisfaction of the experiences, as well as the learning outcomes.

Acknowledgement to M. Addison, Lecturer, Division of Clinical Sciences, Northern Ontario School of Medicine; S. Berry, Assistant Professor, Division of Clinical Sciences, Northern Ontario School of Medicine; L. Sihvonen, Project Lead, Students Partnering in Interprofessional Care and Education.

10.1.2 INVENTION

Invention is a type of product innovation that can be defined as the creation of a product or introduction of a process for the first time.[3] In some cases, it can be a breakthrough invention that represents a significant advance in global healthcare, such as the discovery and implementation of the X-ray in 1895, while in other situations it can represent a refinement of an existing technology that serves or facilitates a novel use.[4] The stethoscope, band aid, artificial pacemaker, and in vitro fertilization are varied examples of what are often considered the most important medical advances through invention.[5]

Both invention and innovation are crucial to change.

Case example 10.2 introduces an invention that has provided a novel method of effective immobilization of extremities for the radiation therapy treatment of soft tissue sarcoma.

CASE EXAMPLE 10.2

A novel immobilization solution for extremity soft tissue sarcoma: the RT-6060 T-Form Extremity Immobilizer System (Part 1: Invention)

As the radiation therapy treatment paradigm changed for extremity soft tissue sarcoma patients from a conventional parallel-opposed beam arrangement to intensity-modulated radiation therapy (IMRT), the need for more accurate patient positioning was recognized. In the past, the soft tissue sarcoma program within the Princess Margaret Cancer Centre used a thermoplastic shell secured to a Perspex base for extremity immobilization (Figure 10.1). This was inexpensive and adaptable to many anatomic locations, but did not attach to the linear accelerator couch top, which allowed for unacceptable patient movement during radiation delivery and variable interfraction patient positioning.

An extensive product search concluded that currently available limb immobilization did not meet the needs of the sarcoma site group. Most accessible products on the market were expensive, only available for either upper or lower extremities (not both), provided immobilization within the radiotherapy volume (introducing concerns about increased skin dose), and only attached to one type of radiotherapy couch top, which was not suitable for large centres with many different brands of linear accelerator. An innovative prototype developed in-house overcame all of these challenges (Figure 10.2). It was inexpensive, adaptable to upper and lower extremities as well as right and left sided disease, effective, efficient, reproducible, adjustable to various linear accelerator couch tops, and most importantly, comfortable for the patient.

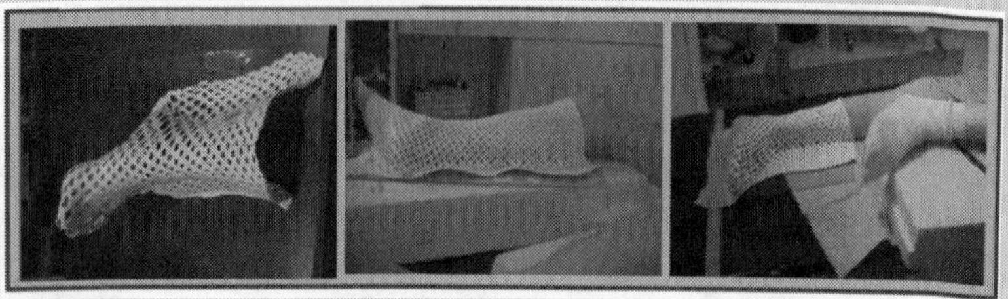

FIGURE 10.1 Example of previously used soft tissue sarcoma immobilization

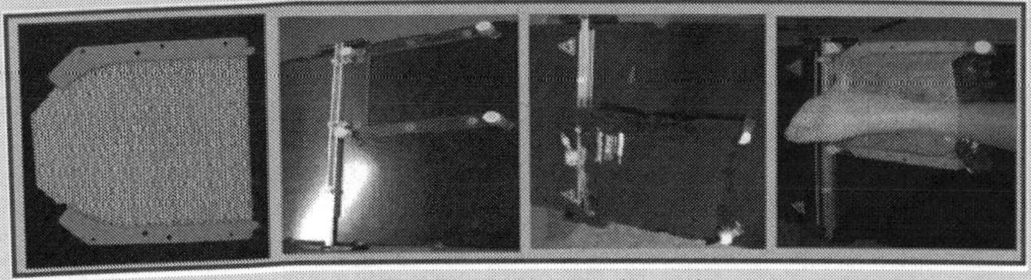

FIGURE 10.2 Example of reinvented in-house immobilization device.

Staff presentations and training took place prior to implementation in the clinical environment. Front line staff readily took on the challenge of identifying the benefits and downfalls of the invention, and also solicited and conveyed valuable patient input for design improvements. Frequent communication with the departmental machine shop staff and the various manufacturers occurred to ensure the necessary changes were implemented and to enhance the broader marketability of the device.

10.1.3 INTELLECTUAL PROPERTY

Innovation and invention are the realization of an idea, and that idea is considered to be the property of the inventor. Intellectual property (IP) is a legal concept which refers to the protection of creations of the mind, be they inventions, discoveries, expressive works of art, or any other nontangible entities created by a human being.[6] IP may result from activity in the industrial, scientific, literary and artistic fields, and its generation, protection, and implementation are of increasing value and interest in the area of medical innovation.

10.1.4 PATENT

Patents, copyrights, and trademarks form legal protection of IP and define the exclusive rights associated with the invention or innovation of IP. A patent is protection or a right granted by the government to exclude others from making, using, or selling the invention in the country where the patient is issued.[7] Any creation of IP within healthcare, whether it is innovative or inventive, may be protected by a patent if it meets certain criteria. As defined by the Canadian Patent Act, an invention can be considered for a patent if:[8]

- it is novel (never existed before)
- it demonstrates utility (functional, operative, and valuable to the market)
- it is ingenious (nonobvious to someone with expertise in the area)

The decision of whether or not to patent has no real influence on the clinical success of the end product within the researcher's own environment. Without a patent, however, it is unlikely that other hospitals will benefit from the same invention as a patent broadens exposure as well as protects the integrity of the original design. If a product patent application is to be considered, a more comprehensive analysis is required and all information can be gathered from the Canadian Government's Intellectual Property Office.[7]

A question that commonly arises relates to whether or not to patent a product or service, even if it is thought to meet the minimum criteria. Patenting of IP involves a significant amount of time, effort and money. An initial patent expense can cost approximately $15,000, and only increases from that point depending upon whether an international application is required. If patenting across borders, a rough investment of $50,000 to $100,000 may be necessary for translation and maintenance fees.[2] Therefore, it may not be worth the expense of protecting a creation with a patent. To stimulate change in one's immediate clinical setting, collaboration with a team of experts within the individual institution may provide more tangible results. Awareness of this potentially exorbitant patenting expense is not meant to discourage future entrepreneurs, but rather to contribute to an informed decision. The process can also take a prolonged period of time that can be prohibitive and impact on the decision to patent.

Some general questions must be considered before making the decision to file a patent application. These might include:

- does the product or process have commercial value?

- will it be obsolete before the patent application is issued in a rapidly evolving healthcare field such as radiation therapy?
- will it appeal to a large population with a potential for profit?

These are questions that may not seem significant to the researcher but weigh heavily on whether or not the commercial industry, clinical practice, or education environment will adopt the finished product, which of course is the overriding incentive to patent. These questions were explored by the inventors of the sarcoma extremity immobilization device in their decision to patent their invention (*see* Case example 10.3).

CASE EXAMPLE 10.3

Novel immobilization solution for soft tissue sarcoma of the extremities: the RT-6060 T-Form Extremity Immobilizer System (Part 2: Patenting and Evaluation)

Following in-house development of the novel immobilization device, it become apparent that there could be broader application based on the efficiency and effectiveness of the device, including use with lymphomas and various bone and soft-tissue metastases. The potential appeal to other clinical institutions was recognized due to its adaptability to larger patient populations and different anatomical areas, thus effectively replacing a multitude of immobilization devices with a single innovative solution.

For these reasons, it was thought that the increased applicability would be of interest to companies who might be in a position to invest in the product. A patent application was submitted for the in-house device by the Technology Development and Commercialization Department within the University Health Network. The device's clinical benefits were presented to various industrial partners over the course of one year by the RTTs who invented it and senior physicist who supported this invention. The institutional commercialization department negotiated the final contract on behalf of the inventors, and a codevelopment agreement was reached between the purchasing company and the original inventors (Figure 10.3). The RT-6060 T-Form extremity immobilizer was initially introduced following both phantom and volunteer testing.

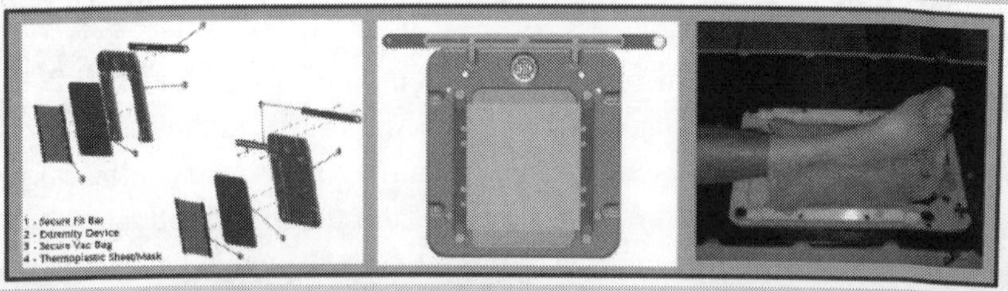

FIGURE 10.3 Example of the Commercial Product.

The device was hypothesized to improve departmental workflow measures and sarcoma patient stability for radiation therapy treatment, but it was important to test this formally and to disseminate results to strengthen the argument for the value of the device. The custom-made extremity immobilizer was thus compared to an established standard that was internationally used and accepted (the polystyrene filled vacuum cradle).[9] Ninety two patients were immobilized with the custom device and 98 with the vacuum cradle. Patient setup times, conformal RT versus IMRT, and 2D versus 3D image guidance were compared for these cohorts. It was found that use of the custom device improved patient throughput and reduced the average patient set up time by 2–6 min. The timesavings in setup were most prominent for patients treated with IMRT for soft tissue sarcoma of the thigh. Random and systematic patient setup errors were also significantly reduced using the custom device with 3D image guidance. This study demonstrated that the error margin surrounding the RT target volume could be safely reduced by 2–4 mm.[9]

This study then led to a second study analyzing the patient set up uncertainty during RT and between RT fractions (intra and interfractional set up error) using the custom device for 3D image guided IMRT.[10] A 775 cone beam computed tomography image datasets were analyzed for 31 lower extremity sarcoma patients and the translational and rotational setup errors were calculated. It was determined that a 5 mm planning target volume error margin could be safely implemented for sarcoma treatment which replaced the existing 1 cm error margin. This evidence-based error margin was implemented clinically in 2005, thus further attesting to the value of the patented device, as it supported toxicity-sparing measures in treatment planning.

10.2 IMPLEMENTING INNOVATION

The implementation of innovation requires advanced planning and consideration of how best to ensure the success of the change, as valuable innovations can fail if not integrated into practice in a strategic manner. Local barriers to implementation should be explored and preempted where possible. The interaction between the novel practice or product and the existing environment must be considered, as well as the need to generate buy-in from those expected to make use of the innovation. In implementing change, there is often an inherent tendency to revert to what is familiar and resist change. Unless stakeholders can be convinced of the value of an innovation, and have the necessary support and resource framework to implement it, it can fail.[11]

10.2.1 INNOVATION ADOPTION LIFECYCLE

The Innovation Adoption Lifecycle (Figure 10.4) suggests that people will come on board with the acceptance of an innovation at different times. Greater effort and time will be required to gain the support of the majority than is necessary for an initial small cohort of the population.[12] In implementing an innovation, it is important to recognize where efforts will need to be expended to ensure the success of the innovation. The first to engage in the adoption process are the innovators; those who are often part of the innovation process, generating novel ideas, and actively engaging in the implementation. Early adopters will readily support an innovation and often provide feedback on the initial experiences with it, encouraging the early majority to adopt and benefit as well. The late majority tends to require the evidence of success provided by the critical mass, and will adopt a new product or process only if it has already become fairly ensconced in practice. Finally, the laggards can be considered the resisters to change, or those who are critical of novelty, whether because of the effort required to become competent in using the innovation, or a firm belief in the "old way." These various roles can be assumed by individuals within a department, different professions within an institution, or different institutions within a healthcare system.

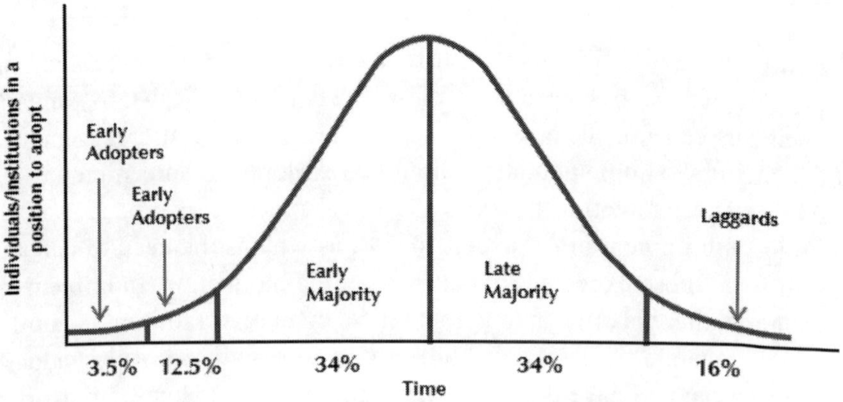

FIGURE 10.4 Innovation Adoption Lifecycle (adapted from Rogers[12]).

Several principles and frameworks discussed elsewhere in this book (*see* Chapter 9: Health Services Research and Program Evaluation, and Chapter 11: Knowledge Dissemination: Value and Approaches) provide further insight into approaching change. This includes consideration of the Deming Cycle, which can be readily applied to the generation and dissemination of innovation. Through the iterative process of planning, implementing, evaluating, and acting on feedback, innovation can be developed and refined to ensure that it meets the needs of the user and will gain the necessary support for a change in practice (*see* Figure 10.5).

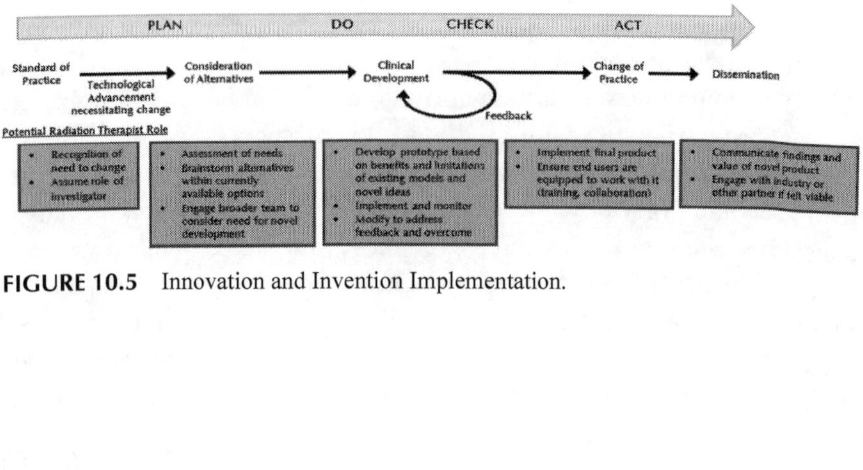

FIGURE 10.5 Innovation and Invention Implementation.

RTTs can be both the adopters of innovations developed by others, and also, as already discussed in this chapter, the instigators of novel innovations. Case example 10.4 highlights the process innovations that have revolutionized the role of RTTs in the implementation of cone-beam computed tomography (CBCT) technology at the Princess Margaret Cancer Centre.

CASE EXAMPLE 10.4

Leading Process Innovation in Volumetric Image-Guided Radiation Therapy

Winnie Li MRT(T) BSc MSc(c)
Radiation Therapist, Radiation Medicine Program, Princess Margaret Cancer Centre, Toronto, Canada
Lecturer, Department of Radiation Oncology, University of Toronto, Toronto, Canada

Advances in image-guided radiation therapy (IGRT) have been facilitated by the availability of 3-dimensional kilovoltage CBCT guidance systems.[13,14] As more information became immediately available to front line users of the technology, IGRT through CBCT disrupted the traditional radiation medicine practice model, significantly impacting the role of the RTT, necessitating role adaptation.[15] It was identified at the early stages of CBCT implementation that novel strategies were required to ensure seamless clinical integration of the technology. This required timely knowledge transfer and innovative training strategies. To ensure therapists were readily equipped to manage daily decision making regarding patient setups, various processes were implemented through RTTs at the Princess Margaret Cancer Centre to support the CBCT-IGRT platform.

Process Innovations:
Imaging Specialist – A research RTT was identified to assist in the multidisciplinary collaboration between RTTs, physicists, and oncologists. Enabling consistent communication, the RTT was involved in technology testing, development and implementation of procedures and protocols and staff education.

Protocol Design – To ensure clear information was exchanged between all disciplines, workflows and protocols were designed with a multidisciplinary approach. Dependent on the treatment sites of IGRT, protocols were devised using various surrogates for target registration, action levels, and when further investigation was required. Region of interest delineation guidelines for image registration were also developed to decrease interobserver variation among RTTs.

Initial Staff Education – Staff training, education, and support have been recognized as essential components to the development and growth of an IGRT program.[16–18] At the onset of clinical implementation of CBCT technology at our institution, to ensure RTTs were readily equipped to manage daily decision making regarding patient setups, a two-level training program was designed and executed.[16] The in-house training program was developed to ensure adequate preparation for CBCT clinical rotations, and to increase competency during 3D image matching.

Continuous Staff Education – To maintain critical thinking and decision-making skills by RTTs in the environment of volumetric IGRT, continuous training is essential. Based and structured upon evidence-based concepts, the electronic online module was developed to enable yearly refresher training to ensure IGRT concepts are understood and enforced.[19] The electronic module focused on the technical aspects and fundamental theory of CBCT acquisition, ensuring RTTs bridge concepts with clinical practice and refreshing their knowledge and confidence in image fusion and assessment.

Facilitated by CBCT, RTTs are readily making online decisions about patient setups through education, well-defined processes, and critical analysis skills. RTT-led process initiatives ensured safe implementation of this novel technology at a large radiation therapy centre. It should be recognized that mastery of skills and baseline knowledge contributes to increased comfort for image assessment, facilitating the forthcoming era of adaptive radiation therapy. At the Princess Margaret, the innovative leadership role of the RTT was central to the successful CBCT implementation.

10.3 PROJECT MANAGEMENT

The development of innovations and inventions should be approached from a broader context of project management. The innovator or inventor needs to take on a project manager or lead investigator role to achieve the end result – the safe and successful implementation of the novel product or process. The following steps provide a road map to researchers within radiation medicine who have recognized a need for innovation and are just embarking on the journey. These steps have been drawn from the authors' experiences of introducing novel products/ processes to the clinical setting. They parallel concepts introduced earlier in the implementation and briefly discuss staff reaction as outlined in the Innovation Adoption Lifecycle (Figures 10.4 and 10.5). Steps to increase the likelihood of successful implementation of innovation or invention are:

1. Performing due diligence
2. Recognizing the clinical advantage
3. Knowing the population that may benefit
4. Having an execution plan
5. Introduction to the clinical environment
6. Being adaptable
7. Critical analysis for evidence-based practice
8. Knowledge dissemination

Many models for project management exist. These are some of the common elements of a good project plan.

10.3.1 PERFORMING DUE DILIGENCE

Abiding by the "plan" part of the Deming Cycle, the researcher should identify whether or not a product or process exists that addresses the need for change by performing an extensive product or literature search (*see* Chapter 2: Literature Reviews). It should also be ascertained whether an existing product or process could be modified or implemented in a different context to suit a new purpose. For example, if a new staffing model for RTTs working in brachytherapy is required, it may be valuable to build upon an existing nursing model that has been extensively tested. If a solution is not readily available or an existing product or model is discovered that needs modification, the researcher has identified a clinical problem that can be addressed. Brainstorming alternatives that are innovative or inventive is a critical undertaking in the initial planning stage.

10.3.2 RECOGNIZING THE CLINICAL ADVANTAGE

Still a part of the planning process, if nothing is present in the marketplace in terms of products or models that can fulfill the clinical requisites of the researcher, there is an opportunity for invention or innovation of a product or process that will satisfy all desired criteria. The innovation should offer a unique competitive advantage in comparison to what is available for purchase. The competitive advantage could be clinical (e.g., to benefit a particular patient population or increase the effectiveness or efficiency of workflows) or could provide a monetary benefit (e.g., more affordable than what is currently available or provides a broader scope in terms of application). Assessing the advantages of the novel idea, as well as noting the limitations of existing products/processes can aid in the development of a robust prototype.

10.3.3 KNOWING THE POPULATION TO BENEFIT

Becoming familiar with the stakeholders who will benefit from the innovation is paramount. Customers for a clinical innovation may include patients, staff, other hospitals, or other cancer programs. Researchers or product developers would be well served by aligning their vision to what is valued by the "recipient of change" to ensure the eventual success of the product. Value can increase if worth is determined and ingrained in the design at the onset of innovation.

10.3.4 HAVING AN EXECUTION PLAN

Respecting the "do" part of the implementation cycle, development of an execution plan can involve many aspects of project management. Identifying resources, processes, risks, key team players, suppliers, partners, clinical expertise, and mechanical expertise upfront is essential. Convincing pivotal team members of the value of the innovation and aligning colleagues with the aims and goals of clinical implementation is imperative for success and will ensure that the early adopters and early majority encourage efficient implementation. Organizing meetings and involving key team players in the workflow discussion before process or product use is critical to achieving successful implementation into the clinical setting.

Once the advantages of a new product or process have been clearly identified and communicated, the project team will need to develop a business case that will help "sell" the target audience on the value of adopting the innovation in favor of existing processes or devices. Transparency of the project's vision and aims may increase acceptance and engage relevant staff or team members.

10.3.5 INTRODUCTION OF THE PRODUCT TO THE CLINICAL ENVIRONMENT

Following implementation of the execution plan, careful monitoring of the process is crucial. Before adoption, comprehensive education and training must be provided to each of the clinical areas that are potentially impacted by the change. For example, when introducing the novel sarcoma immobilization device to the radiation medicine setting, key team members needed to endorse the products use, and disseminate its potential clinical advantages. Radiation oncology team leaders were involved with advocating product use, CT simulation staff embraced product use, and treatment unit staff needed to develop confidence in the product's ability to realize the anticipated benefits. This progression may require multiple training presentations on multiple occasions, and refresher training designed at set periods of time. A mock procedure may help to determine any roadblocks in a developed workflow, and may also provide valuable feedback for improvements in the efficiency of processes and procedures relating to the novel innovation or invention.

10.3.6 BEING ADAPTABLE

Inventors and innovators need to be adaptable to change and remain open to constructive criticism of their IP. Any feedback is useful and devices and processes should incorporate user input where appropriate. "Checking" or "studying" the clinical development of the product or process strengthens general acceptance and use in the clinical setting. This type of collaboration can build and maintain "buy-in" to ensure a continually viable product. The researcher should be open to modifications of their product or process, and be prepared to learn from the experience. Success on the first attempt is rare. If a product or process does not work the first time, valuable lessons may be learned and the invention or innovation can be modified to result in eventual success.

10.3.7 CRITICAL ANALYSIS FOR EVIDENCE BASED PRACTICE

In accordance with the "check" step of the Deming Cycle, if the product or process impacts or influences the clinical environment, the effect should be measured. Ideally, it should be published. Critically analyzing the invention or innovation contributes to evidence- based change in clinical practice, and can further support buy-in from those who might not readily acknowledge the anticipated benefits of the change. This "act" step may provide the significant incentive for change from the late majority and even laggards. Example 10.3 demonstrates two research projects that resulted from one invention implementation.

This is why it is imperative that one should analyze their invention or innovation critically in a scientific manner. Measure the effect of the invention or innovation with an unbiased approach and publish if possible to disseminate the information to other centres that may benefit. It is difficult to criticize a study and refuse adoption of a product or model that demonstrates sound scientific rigor.

10.3.8 KNOWLEDGE DISSEMINATION

Publication and presentation of the innovation are fundamental forms of knowledge dissemination. If the radiation medicine community does not know that a product exists, no one will use it. The results of the research should be presented at national and international forums to expand potential consumer base (*see* Chapter 11: Knowledge Dissemination: Value and Approaches). It is valuable to attend national and international conferences. Talking to vendors and attending pertinent lectures will educate the researcher on what others feel is most important to realize in their clinical setting, which can reinforce the aforementioned steps of recognizing the clinical advantage and knowing the population to benefit.

Revisiting steps in the project management process and gathering information is fundamental if the research intent is to include national and international exposure. Small changes in the radiation medicine environment may have a large clinical impact so do not disregard any modification or idea of invention or innovation.

Throughout the research process, project management will never follow the outlined steps in a sequential manner. It will most likely be an iterative process of modifying and implementing, and as technology changes so rapidly in radiation medicine, further product modifications will likely ensue.

The strength behind some of the most successful invention or innovation implementation is in the support network provided by fellow colleagues, and in the relentless pursuit of perfection by the researcher. In every step of the process, many obstacles will impede progress. These obstacles may be directly related to the performance of the innovation or invention, or may be user-based. Negative perceptions can be overcome by incorporating user input and training relevant staff. Knowledge is the key to acceptance.

Innovation and invention are key ingredients in the evolution of radiation therapy, and the drive to provide the highest quality care. While it may not always involve a formal research project or approach, innovation is nonetheless founded on the scientific principles of identifying and addressing a gap or need in one's environment. To be successful, innovation must afford an improvement, which can be represented by greater effectiveness, efficiency, satisfaction, or cost reduction. The nature of this improvement must also be articulated to stakeholders, especially those expected to make use of the novel process, product, or practice. Whether change involves innovation such as the invention, implementation, and patenting of a clinical device, or the modification of a departmental process, it will be most successful if approached in a systematic and strategic manner, beginning with the end in mind.

KEYWORDS

- Disruptive innovation
- Sustaining innovation
- Patenting
- Intellectual property
- Innovation adoption lifecycle
- Project management

REFERENCES

1. West, M. A. The Social Psychology of Innovation in Groups. In: Innovation and Creativity at Work: Psychological and Organizational Strategies Chichester, West, M. A.; Farr, J. L. (Eds.), UK: Wiley, 1990, pp. 309–334.
2. Omachonu, V. K.; Einspruch, N. G. Innovation in healthcare delivery systems: a conceptual framework. *Innov. J.*, **2010,** *15(1).*
3. Christensen, C. M. The innovator's dilemma: when new technologies cause great firms to fail. Harvard Business Press: Cambridge MA, 1997.
4. Raab, G. G.; Parr, D. H. From medical invention to clinical practice: the reimbursement challenge facing new device procedures and technology – Part 1: issues in medical device assessment. *J. Am. Coll. Radiol.* **2006,** *3,* 694–702.
5. Healthcare Global. Top ten: medical inventions and discoveries. http://www.healthcareglobal.com/top_ten/top-10-business/top-10-medical-inventions-and-discoveries. (accessed October 19, 2013).
6. Landes, W. M.; Posner, R. A. The economic structure of intellectual property law. Harvard University Press: Cambridge MA, 2003.
7. The Canadian Intellectual Property Office. What is Intellectual Property? http://www.cipo.ic.gc.ca/eic/site/cipointernet-internetopic.nsf/eng/Home (accessed July 25, 2013).

8. The Canadian Intellectual Property Office. A Guide to Patents. http://www.cipo.ic.gc.ca/eic/site/cipointernet-internetopic.nsf/eng/h_wr03652.html. (accessed July 25, 2013).
9. Dickie, C. I.; Parent, A.; Griffin, A.; Craig, T.; Catton, C.; Chung, P.; Panzarella, T.; O'Sullivan, B.; Sharpe, M. A device and procedure for immobilization of patients receiving limb-preserving radiotherapy for soft tissue sarcoma. *Med. Dosim.* **2009,** *34(3),* 243–249.
10. Dickie, C. I.; Parent, A. L.; Chung, P. W.; Catton, C. N.; Craig, T.; Griffin, A. M.; Panzarella, T.; Ferguson, P. C.; Wunder, J. S.; Bell, R. S.; Sharpe, M. B.; O'Sullivan, B. Measuring interfractional and intrafractional motion with cone beam computed tomography and an optical localization system for lower extremity soft tissue sarcoma patients treated with preoperative intensity-modulated radiation therapy. *In. J. Radiat. Oncol. Biol. Phys.* **2010,** *78(5),* 1437–1444.
11. Kotter, J. P. Leading Change. Harvard Business Review Press: Cambridge, 2012.
12. Rogers, E. M. *Diffusion of Innovations*, Glencoe: Free Press. 1962.
13. Jaffray, D. A.; Siewerdsen, J. H.; Wong, J. W., et al. Flat-panel cone-beam computed tomography for image-guided radiation therapy. *Int. J. Radiat. Oncol. Biol. Phys.* **2002**, *53*, 1337–1349.
14. Jaffray, D. A. Emergent technologies for 3-dimensional image-guided radiation delivery. *Semin. Radiat. Oncol.* **2005,** *15*, 208–216.
15. White, E.; Kane, G. Radiation medicine practice in the image-guided radiation therapy era: new roles and new opportunities. *Semin. Radiat. Oncol.* **2007**, *17*, 298–305.
16. Li, W.; Harnett, N.; Moseley, D. J.; Higgins, J.; Chan, K.; Jaffray, D. A. Investigating user perspective on training and clinical implementation of volumetric imaging. *J. Med. Imag. Radiat. Sci.* **2010**, *41*, 57–65.
17. Foroudi, F.; Wong, J.; Kron, T.; Roxby, P.; Haworth, A.; Bailey, A.; Duchesne, G. Development and evaluation of a training program for therapeutic radiographers as a basis for online adaptive radiation therapy for bladder carcinoma. *Radiography* **2010,** *16*, 14–20.
18. Liszewski, B.; DiProspero, L.; Bagley, R.; Osmar, K.; D'Alimonte, L. A preliminary evaluation of a clinical training program for volumetric imaging. *J. Med. Imag. Radiat. Sci.* **2012,** *43(Suppl),* p. S31.
19. Li, W.; Moseley, D.; Cashell, A.; Foxcroft, S.; Wenz, J. Development and Implementation of an Electronic Education Tool for Volumetric Image Guided Radiation Therapy. *J. Med. Imag. Radiat. Sci.* **2013,** *44(1)*, p. 45.

PART 4

REPORTING RESEARCH

CHAPTER 11

KNOWLEDGE DISSEMINATION: VALUE AND APPROACHES

KATHERINE JENSEN MRT(T) ACT BA

Clinical Instructor Alberta School of Radiation Therapy, Tom Baker Cancer Centre, Calgary Canada

BRIAN LISZEWSKI MRT(T) BSc

Quality Assurance Coordinator, Odette Cancer Centre, Sunnybrook Health Sciences Centre, Toronto Canada

Research Affiliate, Canadian Partnership for Quality Radiotherapy

CAITLIN GILLAN MRT(T) BSc MEd FCAMRT

Radiation Therapist, Radiation Medicine Program, Princess Margaret Cancer Centre, Toronto Canada

Assistant Professor, Department of Radiation Oncology, University of Toronto, Toronto Canada

CONTENTS

Radiation therapists' (RTTs') involvement in research or leading research initiatives is crucial to the production of new knowledge in the medically and technically advancing field of radiation medicine, but their involvement in research is not enough. To contribute to the collective knowledge, results of radiation therapy research must be communicated to those who might benefit from it, and then implemented in practice as necessary. Knowledge dissemination can take many forms, and the selection of a forum to present research results can be as crucial to successful dissemination as the content itself. Armed with an understanding of the basic principles and considerations in knowledge translation, the researcher can navigate the world of departmental lunch-and-learns, professional conferences, policy, and peer-reviewed journals, to ensure the efforts dedicated to conducting the research are not wasted by not being disseminated to an appropriate audience and translated into practice where indicated as dictated by evidence-based practice.

11.1 PRINCIPLES OF KNOWLEDGE TRANSLATION

The Canadian Institutes for Health Research define knowledge translation (KT) as "a dynamic and iterative process that includes the synthesis, dissemination, exchange, and ethically sound application of knowledge to improve the health of Canadians, provide more effective health services and products, and strengthen the healthcare system.[1]" It can thus be seen to extend beyond the unidirectional transfer of information from the researcher to another, but also the implementation of the new understandings and insights gleaned from that research to effect an improvement in the system.

KT can thus be considered to encompass two primary realms – communication of information, and implementation of change. In fact, many terms are used interchangeably to convey the same "knowledge to practice" concept, including knowledge transfer or exchange, dissemination, diffusion, change management, implementation, or integration.[1]

Without effective KT, potentially valuable discoveries and insights to improving standards of care cannot be translated into practice. Even currently accepted standards of care are not always being provided in all contexts and jurisdictions, due in part to a lack of awareness.[2] Implementation of research findings has been known to be slow and inconsistent.[1] The Institute of Medicine's 2001 report entitled "Crossing the Quality Chasm: A Health System for the 21st Century" suggests that the chasm identified in the title is the gap between what is known and what is practiced, commonly referred to as the "knowledge gap.[1,3]" While the broader healthcare system can have inherent challenges to implementation (*see* Chapter 9: Health Services Research / Program Evaluation), there are also more microlevel barriers of which researchers and clinical professionals should be aware.

11.1.1 BARRIERS TO RESEARCH UTILIZATION4

- Lack of organizational commitment (health human resource and financial support)
- Concerns about quality/validity of research, and consequences of premature implementation of unwarranted change
- Beliefs about role limitations and lack of research skills of professionals believing the change to be necessary
- Poor communication (limited access to or understanding of novel research findings)

Regardless of barriers, a cost-benefit analysis of the value of a change should always be performed, as not all research findings should be implemented. Graham argues the importance of avoiding the "KT imperative," or the tendency to change practice despite lack of proof of relevance or appropriateness for a given desired effect, population, setting, or set of resources.[1]

Strategies for overcoming barriers to knowledge utilization or assessing the potential benefit of change are beyond the scope of this book, but can be sought in the change management and KT literature.[5,6] The remainder of this chapter will be dedicated to the primary task of the researcher in KT – communication and dissemination of results.

HOT TIP

While it is always more "exciting" to highlight work that demonstrates the relative value or effectiveness of an intervention (the acceptance of the alternate or research hypothesis), it is often equally as important to disseminate negative findings. Letting others know that you found no effect or relationship in a given investigation can save them from needlessly undertaking the same investigation.

11.2 CONSIDERATIONS IN DISSEMINATION

There are many ways in which research findings can be disseminated, and it is important to consider the objectives of dissemination, the audience that might benefit from the knowledge, the resources available to support dissemination, and the timelines within which the researcher is operating. These factors may depend on the content, scope, and methodology of the research itself or on the circumstances under which it was conducted (e.g., if the research was funded through grant capture). The basic considerations are presented in Table 11.1 and will be discussed in contextual detail in the following sections.

TABLE 11.1 Considerations in Selecting a Forum for Dissemination.

Considerations	Information to consider about the research	Information to seek about the forum	Examples
Content (What?)	magnitude and rigour of work and results status of results (preliminary data vs. full analysis) potential impact of the new knowledge	competitiveness of call for abstracts submission categories (e.g., works-in-progress oral presentations, options for opinion or review pieces in journals etc.) journal impact factor or rejection rate	*Opinion/Review* – letter to editor, white paper *Preliminary/Small-Scale* – lunch-and-learn, poster *Full Analysis/Rigourous/Novel* – journal publication

TABLE 11.1 *(Continued)*

Consider-ations	Information to consider about the research	Information to seek about the forum	Examples
Objectives (Why?)	What is attempting to be accomplished (change front-line practice, affect policy, highlight new resource/program)	aims of a conference/journal committee terms of reference committee/organization /agency mission and values	*Change Practice* – journal publication, presentation, poster *Policy* – policy brief, business case, management presentation *Highlight Novel Resource* – presentation (lunch-and-learn or conference), newsletter
Cost and Resources (How?)	available funds to support registrations, flights, publication fees, poster printing restrictions/limitations on funding provided by department or granting agency (e.g., registrations only, time limit, reimbursement vs. covering in advance)	poster printing costs conference registrations and associated fees open-access publication fees (*see* Chapter 12: Preparing and Submitting a Manuscript for Publication)	*Minimal Costs* – lunch-and-learn, publication (not open access) *Moderate Costs* – local conference, poster printing *High Costs* – international and large-scale conferences, open access publication
Audience (To Whom?)	target group – RTT only, broader radiation oncology, cancer professionals, educators breadth/jurisdiction – beneficial only to local department, senior management, generalizable nationally or internationally responsibilities to stakeholders or funding agencies	membership of conference hosting association /organization regular attendee list of rounds or lunch-and-learns scope of conference (local versus national or international) reported target audience of publication or commonly published designation of authors	*RTTs*- CAMRT Annual General Conference, RTi3 Conference, *Journal of Medical Imaging and Radiation Sciences* *Radiation Oncology* – Canadian Association of Radiation Oncology (CARO) Annual Scientific Meeting, *International Journal of Radiation Oncology*Biology*Physics* *Local* – lunch-and-learn, staff meeting, department newsletter *International* – International Society of Radiographers and Radiological Technologists (ISRRT) World Congress, American Society for Radiation Oncology (ASTRO) conference

TABLE 11.1 *(Continued)*

Considerations	Information to consider about the research	Information to seek about the forum	Examples
Timelines (When?)	benefit of rapid dissemination requirements to be within funding period of a granting agency length of time between submission and presentation	reference to abstract submission deadline reported time to publication (or communication with editor) investigation of grant funding expiry for use of funds	*Shortest Period of Time* – lunch-and-learn, newsletter *Moderate Period of Time* – conference oral or poster presentation *Longest Period of Time* – journal publication

Once the considerations are addressed relating to why, when, and to whom research results will be disseminated, the researcher can then use this information to select the appropriate format(s). A singular mode or often a combination of methods can effectively communicate a researcher's findings to the radiation therapy community. Case examples 11.1 and 11.2 highlight the importance of knowledge dissemination in making information accessible to relevant populations, encouraging further sharing, and ultimately impacting practice.

CASE EXAMPLE 11.1

Implementation of the Canadian Association of Medical Radiation Technologists' Best Practice Guidelines

Chelsea Soga RTT BSc MA(c)
Radiation Therapist, Prince Edward Island Cancer Treatment Centre, Queen Elizabeth Hospital, Charlottetown, Canada

The Best Practice Guidelines (BPG) project developed out of the Canadian Association of Radiation Technologists (CAMRT)'s strategic plan as a means to update outdated standards. Best practice clinical guidelines are "systematically developed statements to assist practitioner and patient decisions about appropriate healthcare for specific clinical circumstances.[7]"

The three-year BPG Development project concentrated on creating rigourously developed evidence-based recommendations to serve as an accessible resource for all members of the professional association. Development of BPGs relied on a committee that represented the diversity and unique areas of expertise of the membership. Guidelines were based on the best possible evidence using the most current scientific literature and opinions from content experts. The resulting set of guidelines will encourage all medical radiation technologists (MRTs) to continue to evaluate and increase knowledge to better serve their patients.

MRTs work in very busy environments and for a tool such at the BPGs to be a useful resource it must be readily accessible. The committee decided the best way to share the guidelines with the membership was not through a static publication or white paper, but through the CAMRT website. A webpage specific to the BPGs was thus created, featuring five main headings that expand with one click to show the main topics and guidelines within. Guidelines are easily located either using the topics and headings or the search feature, to allow efficient access to required information.

Plans for knowledge dissemination, to ensure guidelines were accessible and known to the membership were an important consideration from the beginning of the project. The CAMRT newsletter, provincial association meetings, and informational sessions were initial forums for dissemination, coordinated by committee members and CAMRT. These created awareness and interest among the membership. The project was then launched at the CAMRT Annual General Conference through an oral presentation. The website was also set up on multiple computers in the exhibit area, and members were encouraged to test the functionality and explore the content. This provided hands-on experience and an opportunity for members to provide feedback which further increased interest in the project, and increased the likelihood that members would further disseminate the new knowledge of the BPGs at their home institutions. The project is dynamic, and as content will continue to evolve with changing practice and the needs of the professions, it was felt important to approach the provision of knowledge in this way.

The CAMRT's BPG are available at: https://ww2.camrt.ca/bpg/

CASE EXAMPLE 11.2

Comparison of Spine, Carina and Tumour as Registration Landmarks for Volumetric Image-Guided Lung Radiotherapy[8]

Jane Higgins MRT(T) BSc CIA
Radiation Therapist, Radiation Medicine Program, Princess Margaret Cancer Centre, Toronto, Canada
Instructor, Department of Radiation Oncology, University of Toronto, Toronto, Canada

Gaps between current practice and best practice are the foundation to a research question, but this is only one part of the research puzzle. Dissemination of research is just as crucial to ensure the findings reach a maximum number of professionals within the healthcare community thus allowing best practice to be considered, discussed and possibly implemented.

In 2007, daily volumetric image-guidance was deployed across a large radiation therapy institution. As a rapid change in practice, it quickly became evident that many options were available for image-guidance (IG) methods in patients receiving thoracic radiotherapy. Moving from a 2-dimensional to 3-dimensional imaging era required reexploration of imaging techniques that had not previously been available.

The timeline for this study was of high priority with respect to finding the most efficient and most accurate volumetric IG method. In 2008, after adequate data had been acquired, the retrospective study commenced. Thirty consecutive lung cancer patients were selected and volumetric imaging data examined. The study goals were to investigate the feasibility, reproducibility and geometric accuracy of three different landmarks for image registration (spine, carina and target) using two IG methods (automatic and manual registration) to establish and implement best practice and inform the modification of local policies and procedure for this site group.

In late 2008, this study was presented at in-house lung site group rounds and hospital grand rounds – where local practice decisions were to be made. This marked the first stages of knowledge dissemination. Following this, the study was then presented at multiple national and international conferences. The study findings were disseminated using multiple formats; poster presentation, oral presentation and workshops which all took place prior to publication. One positive aspect to presenting the study findings multiple times en-route to publication was that it created the platform for broader discussion, which strengthened the overall outcome and impact of the manuscript.

In 2009, all data had been analyzed and the manuscript was complete. The paper was sent to an international journal for review and consideration for publication. It took approximately 4 months for the manuscript to be accepted and published. Post-publication, the findings were presented again at several national conferences and thus knowledge dissemination continued. Most importantly though, best practice was established and implemented locally – automatic bone registration followed by visual inspection of carina and visible target. Volumetric IG methods for thoracic radiotherapy were selected and formally written into departmental imaging workflows, policies and procedures.

11.2.1 ABSTRACT

While not a method of dissemination in itself, the abstract is a necessary precursor or element of conference presentations and publications, the primary formal methods available to a researcher to disseminate knowledge.[9] A requirement prior to acceptance to one of these venues is the submission of an abstract or short summary of the researcher's work for review by the conference or journal's selection committee. The abstract is an essential component of research writing and because it follows a specific format. The abstract serves to pull together the most important elements of the research. It also helps to clarify the substantive components of the researcher's work and provides a concise summary of the research findings, written to persuade the audience to read the research paper or attend the presentation for which the abstract was written.

The specific requirements of a given abstract will vary, and it is important that the researcher identify these requirements before writing. Conferences and journals will have guidelines that should be accessible to potential authors. Most abstracts will follow a similar format, including a title, and background, methods, and results sections.

HOT TIP

An abstract is not meant to convey all the information related to a given body of work. It is intended as a summary of the highlights of the work, encouraging those who might be interested in the topic to seek out the presentation or publication for complete background, methodology, results, and critical analysis.

Abstract writing is a skill that must be developed and honed over time. Don't expect to be able to draft an acceptable version in your first try. When embarking on peer-reviewed submissions, engage a mentor with experience in abstract writing to assist you with the process. Also, expect many comments and revisions – even the most expert abstract writers will not get it right the first time.

When titling the body of work, the researcher should focus on being clear and concise. The title should reflect both the voice of the work, the intended audience, and the conference or publication to which it is being submitted. The focus of an abstract should be the methods and results, as the latter are the reason the abstract is being submitted, and the former suggest how the results were achieved. Not all results will be reported here, but key statistics or points should be stated. Graphs or tables are not appropriate, and it is often a challenge to reflect the key contents in words. This is especially so when one acknowledges the limitations on the length of most abstracts. Depending on the conference or publication, a word limit (or even a character limit) will be defined, and this tends to hover around 300 words, though some forums are more generous. These restrictions reinforce the importance of using persuasive language that avoids any extraneous thoughts or words. An example of a clear and concise scientific abstract is included as case example 11.3.

CASE EXAMPLE 11.3

Evaluation of variability in seroma delineation between clinical specialist radiation therapist and radiation oncologist for adjuvant breast irradiation[10]

Grace Lee MRT(T) BSc MHSc
Clinical Specialist Radiation Therapist, Radiation Medicine Program, Princess Margaret Cancer Centre, Toronto, Canada

Purpose

Breast cancer is managed by a multidisciplinary team with a goal for the timely provision of high quality care. Given radiation oncologist (RO) time constraints, an opportunity arises for task delegation of breast seroma target delineation to an advanced practice clinical specialist radiation therapist (CSRT) with clinical and technical expertise to facilitate treatment planning. To explore this further, we quantitatively evaluated the variability in postsurgical seroma delineation between the CSRT and ROs.

Methods

Specialized site specific training was provided to the CSRT, who, with 7 ROs, independently contoured the seroma and graded its clarity, using the cavity visualization score (CVS), for 20 patients with clinical stage Tis-2N0 breast tumours. The conformity indices were analyzed for all possible pairs of delineations. The estimated "true" seroma contour was derived from the RO contours using the simultaneous truth and performance level estimation algorithm. Generalized kappa coefficient and centre of mass metrics were used to examine the performance level of the CSRT in seroma delineations.

Results

The CVS of the CSRT correlated well with the mean RO-group CVS, (Spearman $\rho = 0.87$, $P < .05$). The mean seroma conformity index for the RO group was 0.61 and 0.65 for the CSRT; a strong correlation was observed between the RO and CSRT conformity indices (Spearman $\rho = 0.95$, $P < .05$). Almost perfect agreement levels were observed between the CSRT contours and the STAPLE RO consensus contours, with an overall kappa statistic of 0.81 ($P < .0001$). The average centre of mass shift between the CSRT and RO consensus contour was 1.69 ± 1.13 mm.

Conclusions

Following specialized education and training, the CSRT delineated seroma targets clinically comparable with those of the radiation oncologists in women with early breast tumours suitable for accelerated partial breast or whole breast radiotherapy following lumpectomy. This study provides support for potential task delegation of breast seroma delineation to the CSRT in our current multidisciplinary environment. Further study is needed to assess the impact of this role expansion on radiotherapy system efficiency.

Reference

Lee, G.; Fyles, A.; Cho, B.; Easson, A. M.; Fenkell, L. L.; Harnett, N.; Manchul, L.; Tran, P. K.; Wang, W.; Craig, T., Evaluation of variability in seroma delineation between clinical specialist radiation therapist and radiation oncologist for adjuvant breast irradiation. *Practical Radiation Oncology* **2012,** *2(2),* 114–121.

HOT TIP

Word counts are strict, and care should be taken to follow them. In many cases, online submission portals will cut off any text that exceeds the stated limit. Sentence structure should be simple, and extraneous words, such as "the" can often be eliminated. Abbreviations can be used after being spelled out the first time.

Also, try to avoid the tendency to use unnecessarily big words that can be replaced easily with simple words (e.g., "employ" versus "use"). These tactics can save you many critical words and characters.

Given the strict requirements and limited word count, abstracts will generally require several drafts, and the process of preparing an abstract should thus be started well in advance of any deadlines. All authors included on the work should be given a chance to review and edit the abstract prior to submission. In the case of an abstract for a journal publication, the abstract is often the last element to be drafted, as wording can be borrowed from the broader text, and shortened and modified as necessary.

11.3 METHODS AND FORUMS FOR DISSEMINATION

11.3.1 CONFERENCES

Conferences offer a variety of benefits with respect to knowledge translation. The interaction with colleagues creates a dynamic environment within which information synthesis, dissemination, exchange can occur. Therefore it is important to consider many factors when deciding upon the appropriate venue in which to present. Consideration of the audience is the key component when deciding where to present one's findings. A predominantly radiation therapy-related subject might be presented at a venue such as the RTi3 Radiation Therapy Conference, CAMRT Annual General Conference or ASRT Conference, whereas findings relevant to a broader radiation medicine audience may be more appropriately presented at conferences hosted by CARO or ASTRO. Topics that relate to education, technology, or the broader healthcare system might also find an audience outside of radiation medicine altogether. Travel and registration costs, time away from work, available bursaries and per diems must be taken into account when selecting the appropriate conference.

Once the appropriate conference has been identified, the researcher should consider the ideal method of presentation. Most conferences give presenters an option of the mode of presentation, often either poster presentation or oral presentation. In general, the more mature, rigourous and relevant research is selected to be presented through oral presentations with more emerging work being chosen for poster presentations. Oral presentations provide the researcher the opportunity to showcase material in a more focused manner, yet requires stronger public speaking skills. Conversely, posters allow the researcher to present information in greater detail, in a more one-on-one fashion to attendees with specific interest in the topic, but posters add cost to conference attendance and are often not given an opportunity to be highlighted to the wider conference audience.

11.3.2 ORAL PRESENTATION

RTTs have many opportunities to disseminate their research, quality assurance findings and unique quality control initiatives, results of team projects or pilot studies and individual innovative practice ideas and results through an oral presentation venue. Oral presentations afford the researcher the opportunity to interact with the audience, infuse their work with their own personality, and generate discussion, but require a level of confidence and skill in oral delivery.[7] Preparing for a good oral presentation is an iterative process that requires time, patience and experience. When done properly, presentations can meet both the goals of the researcher (and team) for accurate communication of the work and findings, and of the audience in terms of learning needs.

When considering an oral presentation one must take into account two equally important aspects of the presentation itself: the first being the technical considerations relating to the PowerPoint™ preparation, venue room constraints and logistics of presenting; the second, the expertise and preparation of the speaker to deliver and effectively disseminate the intended knowledge.

In general, there are three main categories of presentations, each with its specific opportunities and challenges.

11.3.2.1 SCIENTIFIC PRESENTATION

Scientific presentations are scheduled in a topic-related grouping of rigourous research presentations that run 10–155 min in length followed by two to three minutes for questions and comments. The format is usually adheres to strict timing and provides a mechanism for attendees to be exposed to a large cross-section of relevant research activities in a specific area of interest.

11.3.2.2 EDUCATIONAL PRESENTATION

Educational sessions are generally longer in length (30–500 min) and focus more on teaching or educating attendees about a new and proven idea, concept or approach. These presentations are generally built around a set of clear learning objectives and can be more interactive then the scientific presentation.

11.3.2.3 WORKSHOP

The workshop format is a much more interactive format that actually affords the attendees an opportunity to try their hand as one or more elements of an emerging concept, approach or process. Presenters will develop activities – individual or group – that get attendees engaged in the content to help them more easily adopt or adapt a new technique, process or other concept. Workshops can range from an hour to more than 2 hours depending on the focus, content and intention.

There are several more novel options for presentations. These include round table discussions, panel discussions, fireside chats, practice-sharing sessions and poster highlight presentations. While these formats are not covered here in detail, researchers may encounter these options when considering dissemination methods at conferences and scientific meetings.

11.3.2.4 KEYS TO AN EFFECTIVE ORAL PRESENTATION

1. CONTENT

STRUCTURE

Ensure the presentation has a logical progression. Similar to a narrative, it should have a beginning, middle, and end, and a structure that would include: introduction and background, methods, results, discussion and conclusions. In addition, it benefits the audience for the researcher to provide objectives and an outline at the outset, for example, to explain at the start of the presentation that the objective of the session is "to understand the application of fewer tattoos in the tangential breast setup." This helps to guide the audience along the path of the presentation, and to appreciate what knowledge will be gained through attending the session.

VISUAL AIDS

Charts, graphs and other visual aids can be useful cues to guide the presenter through the talk, and to summarize findings in a logical manner. It is important, however, to be cognizant of allotted time and to focus on the most important elements. Bourne suggests that "if you have more than one visual for each minute you are talking, you have too many and you will run over time.[11]" Visual aids can provide the presenter an opportunity to present a large volume of data on one slide, drawing the audience's attention to key aspects. It is also critical that graph axes and table columns be clearly labeled to allow for the audience to interpret them.

ACKNOWLEDGEMENTS

It is academically responsible to acknowledge those who contribute to the research being presented. This might include colleagues, research assistants, or students who may have assisted in recruitment or data collection and analysis, but who did not meet the criteria for coauthorship. Funding agencies and supporting departments should also be credited for their roles. However, unnecessary or excessive acknowledgements should be avoided. A slide can be prepared with relevant names, but does not need to be read out to the audience. Instead, if necessary, contributors can be acknowledged orally at the point in the presentation where their contribution is being discussed, thus providing a more meaningful acknowledgement and not detracting from the flow of the presentation.[12]

HOT TIP

Avoid gimmicks! Excessive PowerPoint™ animations, sound-effects, and complicated colour schemes are not necessary. Instead, they can detract from quality research. Instead, focus on the content and delivery – the true star of the presentation! Similarly, attempts at being exceedingly humorous cloud the underlying message. A singular anecdote can break the ice, but delivery should be clear and professional.

2 PREPARATION AND DELIVERY

AUDIENCE

When delivering an oral presentation, the speaker drives the presentation and sets the tone for the interaction. However, consideration must be made for audience. It is therefore important to tailor the content of the talk to the expertise, experience, and interests of the individuals to which it is presented. If the conference is a predominantly radiation therapy-related audience, the researcher can speak directly to the implications to radiation therapy practice. If the audience is more varied, the researcher should suggest the commonalities beyond the scope of the radiation therapy context in which the research was conducted. For example, at a patient safety-related conference, highlight the implications to patient safety, to facilitate the audience's translation of findings to their own contexts.

DELIVERY

The average adult has an attention span of approximately 18–20 min. Reciting a paper or Powerpoint™ presentation verbatim will quickly lose the audience's attention to the topic. An oral presentation should speak to the audience, discussing the project with the "take home message" of the research or educational content being woven throughout and reiterated at the end. While the act of presenting can be daunting, the speaker should be an expert on the topic and has likely been immersed in the details for a significant period of time. Focus on the content and the intent of the presentation should help the presenter to stay on track and to convey the necessary information.

PRACTICE

Presenters should appear prepared for a talk, but excessive preparation or memorization can make a presentation appear lifeless and will cause the audience to disengage. Practicing in front of a less daunting audience, such as the broader research group or other trusted colleagues, in advance of the formal presentation, may be valuable. Feedback and suggestions

HOT TIP

Rehearsing the talk privately is instrumental in getting the presenter used to the flow of the slides and creating the transition language to be used from one slide to the next. While practicing, presenters will notice changes to be made and stop rehearsal to make the change then start at the beginning again. This usually results in the early part of the presentation being very well prepared and the end of the presentation being less well rehearsed. Be sure the later part of the presentation is given as much attention as the early part when practicing.

about content and presentation style can be solicited, and potential audience questions can be identified and prepared for.

QUESTIONS

Audience questions and comments after the presentation offer both the chance for interaction with the audience and the chance for some anxiety for the presenter! If faced with a question to which the presenter does not have a ready answer or a comment that identifies a limitation of the work, it is better to opt for honesty. Suggesting that something had not been considered, that further investigation might be required, and that the insight is appreciated is preferred to avoiding the question or glossing over a

HOT TIP

Always assume that you are speaking to the world expert on the subject. Speaking down to the audience can appear disrespectful. Similarly, overcompensating by using technical terms and "showboating" can have the same effect. Balance the talk with an intelligent, but non-expert view.

HOT TIP

Computers can fail, PowerPoint™ presentations can corrupt, the USB might not have the right presentation on it, but the show must go on. If this happens, do not dwell on the glitch and stall the presentation – all is not lost! If you have rehearsed your presentation well enough, you should know your subject and presentation, allowing you to speak intelligibly about it. The audience is there to hear what you have to say and will be quite understanding. It is possible to "wing" a presentation without technology, and overcoming any hiccups can actually endear an audience and create a uniquely memorable presentation.

methodological oversight. Questions offer the chance to gauge the level of acceptance and/or interest in the work and to inform modifications to the work, thus benefitting both the audience and the researcher.

11.3.3 POSTER PRESENTATION

As compared to an oral presentation, which might only reach the individuals able to attend the single session at which it is presented, posters allow the researcher to reach a wider audience. This forum also allows the researcher to present specifically targeted information in greater detail. "Posters are a hybrid form—more detailed than a speech but less than a paper, more interactive than either.[11]" The major advantage of selecting a poster to disseminate the research findings lies in its strength of visual appeal. Researchers can capitalize on the visual appeal and the poster as a medium to draw the attention of conference attendees. Posters are designed to be hung in a common area at a conference, often grouped by topic. Some conferences will organize dedicated time for poster viewing, when researchers are encouraged to stand by their work and engage with other attendees. More creative means of highlighting posters are also emerging, including hosting of sessions that include one-minute oral presentations to generate interest in poster content, guided poster tours and poster discussions facilitated by an expert in a given field.

Preparing and presenting a poster has many advantages for the researcher. This forum can offer an interactive opportunity for the researcher and participants to share ideas, often generating a valuable exchange of information. Given the format, a poster is also an exercise in brevity, forcing the researcher to identify the key points of the work, and to lay them out in a logical manner.

Poster preparation is an art, but there are a few guidelines that should be followed (*see* Figure 11.1 for an example):

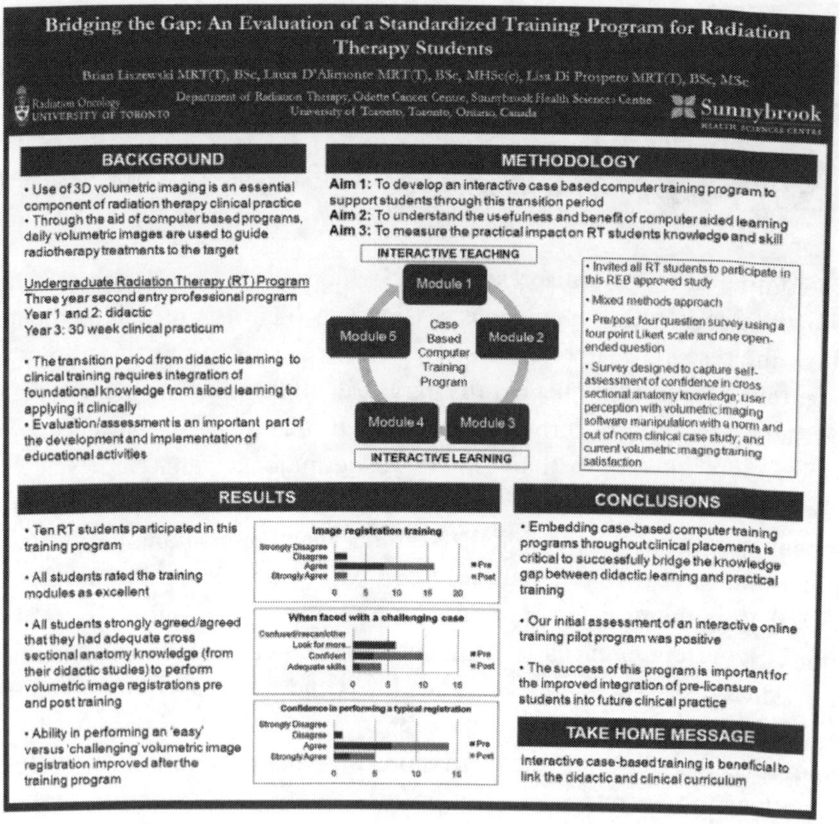

FIGURE 11.1 Scientific Poster.

11.3.3.1 CONTENT

Each poster should have at the top the title of the paper, the name(s) of the author(s) and their affiliation(s). Relevant institutional logos are also recommended. The suggested headings to be used within the poster will depend on the content of the presentation, but may include: Background/ Introduction, Methods, Results, Conclusions. Full sentences or point form can be used, or a combination of the two, depending on the layout and the amount of content to be included. Figures and tables are recommended where feasible, and should be clear and simple, laid out in an aesthetically pleasing manner within the poster, labeled appropriately. References do not normally need to bc included on the poster, but should be available upon request Acknowledgements and contact information should be included, as appropriate, often at the bottom of the poster in a coloured text box to keep them separate from the research content.

11.3.3.2 DESIGN

Posters can be designed in programs such as Powerpoint™, using a single slide. The page setup can be modified to the poster size required by the conference (for example, height = 36″, width = 42″). Poster backgrounds should be simple, using solid and nondistracting colours. Healthcare institutions and academic programs will often have poster templates that they encourage researchers to use. The size of the characters for the title should be at least 2.56 cm (approx. 1 inch high) to ensure readability from a distance of three to four feet. Care should be taken to make sure all content text, including that employed in figures and tables, is clear. Between three and four columns are normally used to lay out the content, with the size of the characters in the text being about half that of the title characters.

Figures and tables can be interspersed throughout, and attention should be given to balancing text and graphics. Images or text copied and pasted from another program may appear crisp when seen on the computer screen, but when blown up to the size of a poster may be blurry. It is sometimes necessary to print a draft of a poster to ensure any figures are clear.

Posters can be printed on single sheets of heavy cardstock, and laminated if desired. This can be done at most print shops, and some clinical and academic institutions will have in-house services that specialize in poster printing.

HOT TIP

It is important to know how long the printer requires to prepare the poster, especially if a high volume is expected in advance of a popular conference. The researcher should also request to see a proof of the poster in advance of printing, often in a smaller form, to ensure that fonts, colours, and figures will print appropriately.

HOT TIP

If you cannot find funding for professionally printed poster, you can create a poster-like presentation using standard letter sized paper. The guidelines remain the same as for a professionally printed poster but you can break the content up per page and arrange them in a logical and interesting manner on the poster board. You can add visual interest by backing the printed pages with coloured paper.

11.3.4 JOURNAL PUBLICATION

Publication in a peer-reviewed journal is one of the most effective ways to:

- communicate new knowledge to the profession
- inform evidence-based practice that ultimately improves the care of patients
- obtain important writing experience that will be critically reviewed and appraised by experts

While the details of navigating the publication process will be addressed in the following chapter (Chapter 12: Preparing and Submitting a Manuscript for Publication) some key points can be considered here in juxtaposition with the other means of dissemination. Publication is often considered the pinnacle of research, however the writing and publication process are time and resource intensive, and not all research warrants publication. If it is deemed important to disseminate work in this way, based on the rigour of the work, the perceived value to the target community, and the availability of necessary time, expertise, and funding, publication can be a rewarding experience for the researcher.

A publication is the most detailed means of disseminating knowledge, and requires the most comprehensive reporting of the methods undertaken, and the most thorough reporting and critical analysis of the results, limitations, and implications. While a poster or oral presentation can focus only on the highlights or summative elements of the work, a manuscript is not forgiving of gaps in analysis, and will likely lead to rejection by journal reviewers or editors. For the same reasons, however, a manuscript provides the opportunity for the researcher to articulate the full scope of the work, and to engage in an evidence-based and supported discussion of the findings. It is common for a researcher to first present work as a poster or oral presentation in the interim prior to completing the necessary analysis and manuscript for publication.

Just as the consideration of a conference audience is important in determining where to submit a poster or oral presentation proposal, the vast array of peer-reviewed journals each serve a distinct audience and purpose. Objectives, impact factors, publication formats, and publication time are all important factors to consider in selecting a journal, and these are discussed in Chapter 12 (Preparing and Submitting a Manuscript for Publication), along with a detailed explanation of the process of preparing a manuscript for a selected journal. Case example 11.4 provides insight to the considerations made when preparing a manuscript about the use of filmcards by RTTs.

CASE EXAMPLE 11.4

The anatomy of an abstract: "Filmcards Used in Radiation Therapy? Are They a Potential Source of Cross Infection?"

Katherine Jensen MRT(T) ACT BA
Clinical Instructor Alberta School of Radiation Therapy, Tom Baker Cancer Centre, Calgary, Canada

Publishing research findings in a journal meets the goals of addressing the questions of the "who" and "why" of dissemination. By carefully selecting a journal that is well matched to the research subject and content allows the authors to target and select the audience (who), while simultaneously meeting the goal of improving patient care (why). Lawlor et al. selected the Journal of Medical Imaging and Radiation Sciences (JMIRS) because they were interested in targeting radiation therapists in Canada.[12] JMIRS is a well-respected and peer-reviewed journal subscribed to by a large number of RTTs in Canada and internationally. The goal of the authors' research was to determine whether filmcards can harbour bacteria and given this information would then allow RTTs to make decisions as to how and when to use the filmcards in their day-to-day practice. The article provides a good example of how a final manuscript would appear in a journal.

The title accurately describes the topic of research, and is followed by the names, credentials, and affiliations of the authors. The credentials of each author allow the reader to understand that this was a multidisciplinary team of researchers with specific expertise and their expertise reinforces the weight of the research findings. The abstract adheres to the journal's guidelines and includes four headings, less than 500 words, no references, graphs, figures or tables. It highlights the critical findings of the filmcard experiment, providing not only a provincial recommendation, but also a national call for all radiation therapy centres to set infection control policies that endorse a one-time per patient filmcard use. Any RTT reading this article would understand immediately the implications of this recommendation and would be able to assess the impact of the recommended change to practice.

The introduction provides a concise explanation of the composition of filmcards and a description of how they are used in radiation therapy. Because very little previous research had been done on filmcards the authors then draw a parallel between the use of filmcards and stethoscopes. When disseminating research findings it is important for authors to relate their work and connect their work to other researchers who have performed similar work.

When reporting a scientific investigation, the materials and methods section must be comprehensive, and authors here used a figure to outline the study design, ensuring that anyone who wanted to repeat the experiments would have sufficient details to do so. This act positively enforces the weight and transparency of the research process that was undertaken.

The results section presented the findings and organized and supported them using tables and photographs. The discussion section then summarizes the implications of the findings and includes a paragraph on the limitations of the study with an explanation of how the authors' managed those limitations. The conclusion is very short and restates the main research findings.

It is recommended that new authors take time to carefully select the venue to be used to disseminate their research findings. Disseminating research findings in a journal has the advantage of reaching a large specific readership while reassuring the reader through peer review that there is sufficient merit in the process and findings.

There are several other methods for disseminating information depending on the intention of the message. Information derived from research can be used to develop white papers, guidelines and recommendations, policy development and task group deliberations. These will not be covered in this chapter, but are avenues that researchers can consider to aid in the translation of knowledge to practice.

11.4 HARNESSING TECHNOLOGY IN DISSEMINATION

While not necessarily a means of dissemination in and of itself, in the age of advancing technology RTTs must consider the value of disseminating the knowledge they are producing electronically. Many journals are moving towards e-access as the sole format of publication, and conferences are finding electronic poster-boards to be a cost-efficient and impactful alternative to paper on poster display boards.

Webinars are also creating a new niche in KT, with the advantage of reaching many people with timely information, with all the benefits of oral presentation. Online software such as GoToWebinar can provide a forum to host an online presentation that can be accessed by anyone with a link, with options for free access or a requirement for preregistration. Functionalities of the software can allow webinar attendees to see the speaker and the presentation content, and also to interact through raising their hands, asking questions, and responding to evaluation surveys, all through the single platform. While there is an initial learning curve to both setting up and presenting a webinar, it is an effective and increasingly efficient means of dissemination. Many conferences and organizations are finding it a valuable tool to keep a target audience engaged in the time between face-to-face meetings, and to ensure timely dissemination of pertinent research findings.

The constellation of online technologies and platforms commonly known as "Web 2.0" also warrants consideration here. Web 2.0 technologies further change the focus of dissemination to revolve around users' information needs. Audio podcast and video presentations can be quickly and widely disseminated through online platforms such as YouTube, Slideshare and blogs. Examples of this type of dissemination can be found in the National Cancer Institute Cancer Control Plan, Link, Act, Network with Evidence Based Tools (P.L.A.N.E.T.) "Research to Reality" cyber seminar series. Many peer-reviewed journals have also embraced the concept of 360° marketing where domains such as Twitter and Facebook are being used to disseminate information and formulate interactive discussions on research findings that have been distributed online. Web 2.0 applications such as this have the potential to develop networks of multiple organizations that can communicate more easily and can share information rapidly and more cost-effectively.

The potential opportunities for dissemination of RTTs' research and other work through technology-driven forums is staggering and will continue to advance, both as individual approaches and as a means of augmenting traditional formats.

Upon completion of research, it is vital that the RTT communicate findings to the relevant community. KT involves not only the communication of information, but also the implementation of change. This chapter illustrated the many ways in which research knowledge can be disseminated, and the important considerations required when selecting the mode with which to circulate one's findings, including the target audience, available resources, and information to be presented. Often a combination of methods is used, as capturing and sharing RTT research findings through multiple venues can increase dissemination to the appropriate audience.

KEYWORDS

- Knowledge translation
- Research utilization
- Dissemination
- Abstract
- Oral presentation
- Poster
- Publication

REFERENCES

1. Graham, I. D.; Tetroe, J. Some theoretical underpinnings of knowledge translation. Acad. Emerg. Med. **2007,** *14(11)*, 936–41.
2. Lang, E. S.; Wyer, P. C.; Haynes, R. B. Knowledge translation: closing the evidence-to-practice gap. *Ann. Emerg. Med.* **2007,** *49(3),* 355–63.
3. Institute of Medicine. Crossing the Quality Chasm: a new health system for the 21st century. The National Academies Press: Washington D.C., 2001.
4. Hutchinson, A. M.; Johnston, L. Bridging the divide: a survey of nurses' opinions regarding barriers to, and facilitators of, research utilization in the practice setting. *J. Clin. Nurs.* **2004,** *13(3),* 304–15.
5. Miles, G.; Miles, R. E.; Perrone, V.; Edvinsson, L. Some conceptual and research barriers to the utilization of knowledge. *Calif. Manage. Rev.* **1998,** *40(3)*, 281.
6. Kotter, J. P., Leading change: Why transformation efforts fail. *Harv. Bus. Rev*. **1995,** *73(2)*, 59–67.
7. Field, M.; Lohr, K. Institute of Medicine Committee to Advise the Public Health Service on Clinical Practice Guidelines. Clinical practice guidelines: directions for a new program. National Academy Press: Washington, D.C., 1990.
8. Higgins, J.; Bezjak, A.; Franks, K.; Le, L. W.; Cho, B.; Payne, D.; Bissonnette, J.P. Comparison of spine, carina, and tumour as registration landmarks for volumetric image-guided lung radiotherapy. *Int. J. Radiat. Oncol. Biol. Phys.* **2009,** *73(5),* 1404–1413.
9. Coad, J.; Devitt, P. Research dissemination: The art of writing an abstract for conferences. *Nurse Educ. Pract.* **2006,** *6(2),* 112–116.
10. Lee, G.; Fyles, A.; Cho, B.; Easson, A. M.; Fenkell, L. L.; Harnett, N.; Manchul, L.; Tran, P. K.; Wang, W.; Craig, T. Evaluation of variability in seroma delineation between clinical specialist radiation therapist and radiation oncologist for adjuvant breast irradiation. *Pract. Radiat. Oncol*. **2012,** *2(2),* 114–121.
11. Miller, J. E. Preparing and presenting effective research posters. *Health Serv. Res.* **2007,** *42* (1 Pt 1), 311–328.
12. Bourne, P. E., Ten simple rules for making good oral presentations. *PLoS Comput. Biol.* **2007,** *3(4),* e77.
13. Lawlor, D.; Cannon, K.; Duan, Q.; Jensen, K., Filmcards Used in Radiation Therapy: Are They a Potential Source of Cross-infection? *J. Med. Imag. Radiat. Sci.* **2012,** *43(1),* 52–59.

CHAPTER 12

PREPARING AND SUBMITTING A MANUSCRIPT FOR PUBLICATION

JOHN FRENCH RTT MSc FCAMRT CHE

Senior Director, Operations, Business and Strategic Planning, Radiation Therapy, Vancouver Centre, British Columbia Cancer Agency, Vancouver Canada

CONTENTS

This chapter will discuss the process of preparing and submitting a manuscript for publication. It will be written from the perspective of a journal editor and a published author, and will attempt to describe what an editor and editorial board look for when receiving a manuscript for consideration; how authors can increase acceptance rates by appropriate journal selection; the process of preparing a manuscript for publication; and what happens once a manuscript is submitted and how to work successfully and collaboratively with manuscript reviewers.

12.1 THE EDITOR'S PERSPECTIVE

Understanding how to successfully take a manuscript to publication requires an understanding of the perspective of the journal editor. The Journal Editor has many responsibilities. These may vary by journal but the key responsibilities include the initial review of submitted manuscripts for publication and the management of the peer review process. The latter includes the selection of reviewers and often the adjudication of conflicting reviews. An important point to note is that the editorial role is normally a volunteer role – this means that editors are taking on additional work on top of their existing positions. Editors are generally busy people who are taking on more work for intrinsic rather than extrinsic rewards, so it follows that prospective authors should try and make the job of the editor easier rather than harder. This is not difficult to do. It also follows that by making the work of the editor easier an author is more likely to be successful in getting work published.

It follows that understanding what an editor looks for when a new manuscript turns up on his or her desk is an important part of a strategy for getting published, in the same way that understanding what a recruiter is looking for is an important determinant of a successful job hunt. By assuming the perspective of an editor, a budding author can make the life of an editor easier, and increase the likelihood of getting published.

12.1.1 WHAT THE EDITOR LOOKS FOR IN A MANUSCRIPT

The editor is most likely the person that will make the initial decision as to whether the paper will be suitable for publication in a given journal. In general, a publisher will most likely be looking at the following qualities of the paper:

- research quality
- relevance
- originality
- readability
- structure

Although it cannot be gauged from the original submission, editors are also hoping for one other quality – an author who is receptive to feedback and willing to work with them to get the paper published. This characteristic increases the likelihood that a paper will move smoothly through the review and publication process.

12.1.2 RESEARCH QUALITY

The overall quality of the research described in the paper impacts its value to an editor. Simply put, poorly conducted research is less likely to get published than well done research. Thus, a research paper that uses survey results from ten subjects may be of lower quality than one which reports on results from 1000 respondents. Research that has been previously conducted and reported may also be seen to be of less value than novel research. A literature search that misses some of the key papers on the subject may be of less value than one that is comprehensive. Poor statistical analysis makes a paper less publishable than a robust analysis.

The lesson here is simple. Potential authors should ensure from the start that the research they are doing has a robust methodology, that they are familiar with the existing work on the subject, that they are adding to knowledge in the field, that they are not repeating what others have done, and that they have a means to analyse data properly.

12.1.3 RELEVANCE

An editor will then grade the relevance of the paper to the aims and objectives of the journal. The aims and objectives generally describe the audience the journal wants to reach, so it is important to research this aspect of journals before submitting. As one can imagine, a journal with an audience that consists primarily of veterinarians in the United States is unlikely to publish a paper on the job satisfaction of nurses in China. Yet, many authors seem to fail to consider how relevant their work is to the journal in which they are hoping to publish. Even if a paper is relevant to the journals aims and objective, it still needs to be relevant with respect to the current state-of-the-art or science in the field in which it is published. For example, a paper aimed at a radiation therapy journal and describing a treatment modality using wedges and compensators is unlikely to get published in a Canadian radiation therapy journal if this technique is no longer used anywhere in Canada. However, it may be publishable in another country's journal, where infrastructure, equipment, and techniques may not be as advanced.

12.1.4 ORIGINALITY

Editors want to publish original work. This of course means that work should not be plagiarized, but more importantly it means that the work should present new research or findings on a subject. Originality does not mean that the work has to be entirely new, but it should add something to the existing body of knowledge on the subject. As an example, if the journal in which the researcher hopes to publish has recently published a literature review on radiation reactions to the large bowel it is unlikely that this journal will want to publish a similar review on the subject shortly thereafter. Similarly, trying to publish a paper on the use of cone beam CT for prostate radiation therapy, a topic that has been well-documented, will require ensuring that the work adds new knowledge to the area, rather than repeating previously published work with similar findings that have been well-reported elsewhere.

12.1.5 READABILITY

A writer has just one single, albeit difficult, job, and that is to make it easy for the reader to make use of the research. The more readable a paper is, the more likely it is to be published. Readability is the extent to which the paper tells the story to the reader. It is a function of how the paper is structured, how it is written, and how data and information is presented. In the scientific literature it is includes both the writing and the use of images, illustrations and graphs. In general authors should ensure that anything they submit has been read and critiqued by others, and attention paid to how easily the work can be understood by the reader.

12.1.6 STRUCTURE

The structure of a paper should always meet the guidelines of the journal. If there is a 3000 word limit in the journal there is little point in submitting a 40,000 word thesis, even if it is the result of three years of dedicated and hard work. If the journal wants APA style for referencing, then use APA style. In general scientific publications follow more or less the same format, namely: Abstract, Introduction, Methodology, Results, Discussion, Conclusion, and References. Some journals will have slight variations on this theme, and it is important to make the work fit the required structure of the journal. So if a journal has Discussion and Conclusion as one section then it is wise to adapt the work to fit the structure, rather than making the editor have the work of requesting it.

12.1.7 ENGAGED AUTHORS

What editors really look for is a proactive and receptive author. This is someone who will take the time to research the journal before submitting and ensure that the work meets the aims, objectives and guidelines of the journal. It is also the responsibility of the author to submit the work in the correct format and following the guidelines laid out by the journal. The submitting or corresponding author is also expected to respond to the feedback received from the editor or reviewers, to be prepared to make the suggested changes. The feedback process should be seen as a collaborative effort that improves the work, not as a criticism of the work.

12.2 SELECTING A JOURNAL

One of the most important considerations in getting published is the selection of a journal. Publication is an investment of time and energy in a researcher's work. A published paper is an achievement – a project finished, a line on a resume, an increased chance for promotion, an academic necessity, an enhancement to the body of knowledge in the field. Yet getting published is hard work. It does take time and effort, and few authors get published without having to do a lot of work preparing, editing, submitting, then revising and resubmitting papers. Manuscript production and acceptance is an iterative process and the author must be prepared to engage openly in this process. The following are some tips for selecting a journal in which to publish.

12.2.1 RESEARCH THE JOURNAL

Studying journals in terms of the type of papers they publish, reputation, impact factor, key audience, publisher, and composition of editorial board will provide a good understanding of whether the work will fit a particular journal, and also a good understanding of the market for both current and future work. See Appendix for a list of journals relevant to common topic areas in radiation therapy.

12.2.1.1 PUBLISHER

A journal that is published by a professional publisher may be preferential to one that is self-published by a professional society.

12.2.1.2 IMPACT FACTOR

The impact factor measures the degree to which work in the journal is recognized by others. A higher impact factor means that a paper in the journal is more likely to be noticed than in a journal with a lower impact factor.

The impact factor is a function of the number of times an article in that journal was cited in another article as compared to the number of articles published by that journal in the two preceding years. For example, the impact factor for the *International Journal of Radiation Oncology, Biology, Physics* was 4.524 for 2012. This suggests that for every article published by the journal in 2012, there were almost five articles from this journal in 2010 or 2011 that were cited elsewhere since. This number would have been made available in 2013.

12.2.1.3 DATABASE INDEXES

The number and reach of the databases in which the journal is indexed is another measure of the visibility of any work published in the journal. A journal that is indexed in PubMed has the highest visibility. To be selected for indexing, a journal must be reviewed and rated against such criteria as the scope and quality of the content published, the geographical representation of the work, and the editorial and production quality of the journal.

12.2.1.4 REPUTATION

Reputation is not easily measured objectively, but it is known that some journals have a better reputation in a given field than others. The impact factor will provide a preliminary assessment of reputation, but discussion with colleagues can often add valuable insight as to the appropriateness of a given journal.

12.2.1.5 EDITORIAL BOARD

The composition of the editorial board is a good measure of the credibility of a journal, and should be considered when determining to which journal an article should be submitted.

12.2.1.6 PUBLICATION FREQUENCY AND TURNAROUND TIMES

Be it based on volume of content or other production factors, the publication frequency is the number of times a journal is published per year. Journal turnaround times, such as the time from initial submission to notification of acceptance are important. These two elements can provide an indication of how quickly papers are published online and are important factors when determining where to submit.

12.2.1.7 READERSHIP

As discussed previously, it is important to consider the audience most likely to access work published in a given journal. This can be informed by subscribership, which could be aligned with membership in a professional association that is affiliated with a journal.

12.2.2 BE REALISTIC

Possibly, the work of a novice researcher will be so important and well-written that it will be publishable in the New England Journal of Medicine at the first attempt – possible but unlikely. Aiming for this journal may be an unrealistic goal. Similarly, the department newsletter may be unattractive as it does not reach beyond the level of a local institution and is not indexed in searchable databases. It is thus important to be realistic and cognizant of the strengths of the work and the most desirable audience, to pitch it with the greatest likelihood of success.

12.2.3 HAVE A STRATEGY

Finding the right balance between getting published in the most prestigious journal possible and not continually rewriting and submitting work is hard. Many authors have a strategy of selecting several journals before submitting, and are prepared to resubmit to the second journal if the work is rejected from the first choice journal. *See* case example 12.1 for an experience of the author's in finding success in a second submission.

CASE EXAMPLE 12.1

A paper was initially submitted to a high profile European Radiotherapy journal. After a few weeks the following notice was received:

"Thank you for submitting your paper "XXXXX" to the journal. It has been evaluated by the editors and I regret having to inform you that we have found that it may be rather descriptive of a local regional practice, but may have limited scientific information for our readers as such.
Although it has certain global important information about the indications and use of radiotherapy for a specific disease, we do not find that it fulfills the requirements for publication relative to other papers submitted to the journal. Thank you for giving us the opportunity to evaluate this material."

This was clearly a rejection letter. The authors reviewed and discussed and elected to submit to an equally high profile North American Radiotherapy journal, rather that aiming for a less prestigious journal The paper was sent for peer review and several comments received, which were subsequently addressed, and finally the following notice received:

"Your manuscript has been reviewed by experts in the field, and I am pleased to inform you that it has been accepted for publication in the Journal of ...."

The lesson here is clear. Firstly, do not give up on a paper – rejection is common and any work that is initially submitted and rejected can and should be submitted elsewhere.

12.3 PREPARING A MANUSCRIPT FOR PUBLICATION

Preparing a manuscript for publication requires a skill set in communication, diligence, and attention to detail. As mentioned earlier, the job of a writer is to make it easy for the reader to understand the work that was done, why it was done, and what was learned as a result. Scientific writing is relatively straightforward as it is based around a common structure and format. As mentioned above, individual journals will have guidelines for authors that will specify the required length of the submission, the formatting in a standard word processor, the headings required, and the convention to be followed for referencing. It is important to follow these guidelines, as a submission may be rejected outright if it does not appear to be formatted appropriately. In general, each element of a scientific paper can be addressed as follows:

12.3.1 ABSTRACT

The abstract is a short summary of the contents of the paper. An abstract is often only between 50–200 words long. Its importance is that it attracts readers to the paper. It is the first thing that people will read, and will either encourage or discourage them from accessing and reading the full paper. In essence it is an advertisement for the overall work. For this reason, an abstract is often the last part of a paper that is written, and it needs to contain the main details of methods, results, and conclusions of the work. Collapsing a full research study into 200 words is no small feat!

12.3.2 INTRODUCTION

The introduction should contain an overview of the related work in the field, which is derived from a summary of the existing literature on the subject (*see* Chapter 2: Literature Reviews) and what new questions the paper seeks to answer, and why these are important.

12.3.3 METHODOLOGY

The methodology, sometimes known as “materials and methods” simply describes what was done. This is a factual description of how the experiment, literature search, or analysis was conducted and how results were analysed (including which statistical tests were performed). The main purpose of the methodology section is to illustrate what was done, to the extent that the readers could replicate the study in their own environment if they chose to do so.

12.3.4 RESULTS

The results section describes, often with the use of graphs and tables, what results were obtained. It does not attempt to explain the results, or interpret them, and should be free from bias in reporting both positive and negative findings. Most data can be more easily understood by the reader by being presented in graphical or tabular format, so these are often used in the results section to make it easier for the reader to understand the data obtained from the work. Many journals have a limit on the number of graphs or tables that can be included in a submission, so it is important to adhere to these limits. However, a figure can convey information in a much more succinct and understandable manner than can text, so the use of figures is encouraged. As the intent of a figure is to make it easier for the reader to understand the results, the author should ensure that an appropriate type of graph or table is used, with clear labelling of titles and axes where necessary.

12.3.5 DISCUSSION

The discussion is the author's interpretation of the results, contextualised within the broader scope of existing knowledge on the subject and comparable work and findings. This is the section the authors use to describe to the reader why they think they got the results that they did, and what the results might mean. Areas where the results are consistent with the findings from other studies can also be highlighted, as well as where they might be in disagreement with previous work. As research design is rarely perfect the author will generally include a description of the limitations and shortcomings of the work, and how these might have impacted the results obtained.

Finally, it is important to highlight directions where further research may be useful.

12.3.6 CONCLUSION

The conclusion section, which is often included as the final paragraph of the Discussion, is basically a reiteration of the main points of the work; what was done and what was found as a result. It is often an abbreviated version of the abstract, and therefore is often one of the final pieces written.

12.3.7 REFERENCES

The references are simply a list of others' work that was referred to throughout the research project, linked in a formal and standardized way to the body of the paper. Each journal will have a preferred convention for referencing and will usually provide resources that will guide the author in the appropriate style, ordering, and formatting of references. This should be followed strictly. Any unreferenced mention of findings, ideas, or other work published elsewhere is considered plagiarism if not directly referenced. Chapter 2 (Literature Reviews) provides further insight on approaches to referencing that can facilitate the process.

By breaking down the format into the key blocks it is possible to make the writing process easier and more manageable. A typical manuscript is between 3,000 and 5,000 words long, with between three and five figures, which can be tables, diagrams or charts. Writing 5,000 words may be a daunting task, but writing 300–500 words often seems to be less so. Therefore many authors focus on writing each section as an independent piece of small writing, rather than trying to work on the comprehensive final product. In fact, it is often easiest to tackle the sections in a different order. The methods are often the most straightforward to write, followed by the results and then the introduction and discussion. It can be seen that by breaking down each section of a paper into a manageable section, the task of preparing a paper becomes easier.

Before submitting it is highly advisable to have others review the manuscript carefully and provide editing assistance.

12.4 AUTHORSHIP

Assigning authorship to a manuscript can be a complex and difficult process. As authors generally work in the same institution or field there is a risk of causing offense and damaging working relationships if someone feels they have been denied an authorship, been placed incorrectly in the list of authors, or someone has been included as an author who should not have been. Good advice is to assign authorship at the beginning of the research study, and then to review it at the point of submission. In addition, it is important to ensure that those who helped with the work, but do not merit an authorship, should be suitably acknowledged. Many journals publish guidelines that describe authorship and require all authors to attest that they have fulfilled authorship requirements as a part of the submission process. Authoring protocol can vary between professional fields, but in general the following rules and guidelines apply to determining who is considered to be an author and the sequence of authorship.

12.4.1 *CRITERIA FOR AUTHORSHIP*

Most journals follow the Vancouver Guidelines for authorship, as noted by the International Committee of Medical Journal Editors.[1] These guidelines were established by an informal meeting of journal editors in Vancouver, Canada in 1978. In general, the following three conditions must all be met for an individual to be considered for authorship:

1. An author must have made "substantial contributions" to the design of the study or the acquisition or analysis of data collected through this design. This would include framing the study objectives and hypothesis, defining and executing the experimental design and

selection of appropriate methodologies and statistical tests, and interpretation and presentation of results.

2. An author must also have contributed intellectually to the drafting or revision of the article. This would include contribution to the preparation of at least one section of the manuscript, and contextualization of the paper within the broader scope of published literature.
3. An author must have had access to and approved the final, submitted version of the manuscript. In this capacity, authors are all responsible for the integrity of the work, both in its initial submitted version and after any revisions required prior to acceptance for publication.

In many cases, there will be people who contributed significantly to the research but who do not meet the criteria for authorship. This might include those who provide technical help (such as data extraction or manipulation), data collection support (such as interviewers or those collecting surveys from patients), or supervisory or organizational support. These individuals should be credited in an Acknowledgements section that articulates the individual contributions made.

12.4.2 SEQUENCING OF AUTHORS

The convention for the sequence in which authors are listed can vary. Some professional domains list authors in alphabetic order. In some cases the final listed author is deemed to have had a supervisory role, while in others this is not the case. It is important that the authorship is listed in a manner that follows the tradition in the academic area in which the work is to be published. More importantly, it is advisable to agree on the sequencing of authorship before work is commenced. In general, the following guidelines may apply to the sequencing of authorship for work published in the health sciences domain:

First author – the author who did the bulk of the work related to the publication, and who contributed at all stages of the design, execution, interpretation, and writing of the research.

Corresponding author – the author who corresponds with the journal regarding the review process and who will be contacted by those who read the final work for any further information. This is traditionally a responsibility assumed by the first author, but may not be appropriate in instances where the first author will not have as ready access to the rest of the team (for example, a radiation oncology fellow who is first author may no longer be affiliated with the institution where the research was conducted at the time of submission or publication).

Last author: the author who had the supervisory role in the work, and who provided guidance throughout the process. This individual is often referred to as the "senior author."

Other authors: any other author who met the authorship criteria. These authors are generally listed in the order of the magnitude of their contribution, or in alphabetical order if their is contribution is not easily determined or differentiated.

12.5 WHAT HAPPENS WHEN A PAPER IS SUBMITTED

The exact steps a paper will undergo when submitted will vary from journal to journal, but the same general process can be expected to occur. Firstly, the paper will be reviewed for any evidence of plagiarism or having been published elsewhere. If there is a possibility of this, and most journal editors or managers have software tools that can help detect issues, the paper will likely be rejected. Secondly, the paper will be reviewed for suitability by an editor. This involves a preliminary review to determine if the paper is potentially suitable for the journal, and worthy of a more detailed peer review, as outlined above.

12.5.1 PEER REVIEW

If a paper passes the first two review processes it will be sent out for peer review. The editor will select many professionals with expertise on the subject to review the paper and provide detailed feedback on its suitability for publication and any suggestions for strengthening the paper in preparation for publication. Once the reviewers have done this, generally a process that requires several weeks, the editor will compile the feedback and send it to the author with a decision about its suitability for publication. The peer review process is normally blinded, where the reviewers are not provided the identities of the authors or the specific site where the study was conducted, and authors are not informed as to who reviewed their work. Alternatively, the review process can be open, where the identities are known. Some online journals publish the original submission, the reviewers' comments, and the final version of the paper.

The peer review process is a critical part of the scientific process. Peer reviewers offer their time and expertise, for little reward, to help strengthen a paper and ensure the sustained reputation of the journal. Successful authors realise this fact and take the time to incorporate reviewers' suggestions into their work. This process invariably makes the revised version of the paper much stronger than the originally submission. Acting as a peer reviewer is itself a valuable experience, and one that many researchers take on at some point in their careers.

It is important for an author to know how to respond when notice is received about a submitted paper. Case example 12.2 provides a modified version of a notice received by the author, suggesting the type of response that might be received for a submission, and how best to respond.

CASE EXAMPLE 12.2

The following was received from the editor of the author's first choice journal for publication. Note that while an initial read suggests the paper has been rejected it is in fact an offer of publication subject to addressing the concerns of the reviewers.

"The reviewers have commented on your above section. They indicated that it is not acceptable for publication in its present form. However, if you feel that you can suitably address the reviewers' comments, I invite you to revise and resubmit your manuscript. Please carefully address the issues raised in the comments. If you are submitting a revised manuscript, please also:

(a) outline each change made (point by point) as raised in the reviewer comments AND/OR
(b) provide a suitable rebuttal to each reviewer comment not addressed"

The authors subsequently provided a structured response in a timely fashion. Most comments were addressed directly, reflected as tracked changes in the original manuscript, and accompanied by a "Response to Reviewers" letter itemizing the changes. For any feedback not addressed, a respectful comment was provided to justify the lack of response. Within a few weeks of the submission of revisions to the editor, the work published in the first choice journal.

12.6 PUBLICATION

Once accepted for publication, authors can breathe a sigh of relief, but the process is not quite complete. At this point, the article is considered to be "in-press" and can be referenced as such in a citation in a curriculum vitae or in a subsequent paper. As a draft of the manuscript is formatted and typeset for publication, authors will be afforded an opportunity to review what is known as the "proof." This is not the time to make edits to the content of the manuscript, but rather to address any concerns with typographical errors, formatting of tables or figures, or other issues with the conversion from a word-processed document to the final format for publication.

The manuscript will then be slated for publication in an upcoming issue of the journal. In advance of this, articles are often made available online, often referenced as being "e-published ahead of print." Increasingly, as publishers move away from printed hardcopy journals, e-publication is the sole means of publication. If this is the case, a volume and issue number will nonetheless be assigned to provide a full citation to facilitate access.

This chapter has described some of the considerations to be made when trying to get a paper published. It is hoped that it will be helpful in this regard. Ultimately, successful authors are those who choose journals wisely, follow journal guidelines, respond to the suggestions of reviewers and put in the required effort to make their work readable by their audience.

KEYWORDS

- Authorship
- Originality
- Relevance
- Impact factor
- Peer review process

REFERENCES

1. International Committee of Medical Journal Editors. Uniform requirements for manuscripts submitted to biomedical journals: ethical considerations in the conduct and reporting of research: authorship and contributorship. http://www.icmje.org/ethical_1author.html (Accessed September 15, 2013).

PART 5

RESEARCH CULTURE

CHAPTER 13

ACADEMIA AND SCHOLARSHIP

NICOLE HARNETT MRT(T) ACT BSc MEd

Director, Graduate Programs, Medical Radiation Sciences Program & Assistant Professor, Department of Radiation Oncology, University of Toronto, Toronto Canada

CONTENTS

This chapter builds on a peer-reviewed article by Harnett et al. entitled "The scholarly radiation therapist. Part one: charting the territory" published in the Journal of Radiotherapy in Practice.[1] *Excerpts are incorporated with permission.*

"Originality is the essence of true scholarship. Creativity is the soul of the true scholar."

— Nnamdi Azikiwe

It should be clear to the reader by now that there is a strong movement across Canada to foster the research agenda in the radiation therapy profession. Each of the case studies found in these chapters tells an individual story of the "what" and "how" of conducting research in hopes that it might resonate with individual practitioners and ignite a desire to be part of the movement. But perhaps it is time to address the one remaining unanswered question – "why research?"

The rationale for ensuring that research is a fundamental aspect of radiation therapy practice is multifaceted. Healthcare takes place at the intersection of numerous jurisdictions – academic, political, financial – all of which impact on the practice of the professions involved in the provision of care to patients. In this chapter, the concepts and terminology related to research, scholarship and professionalization will be reviewed to inform the reader of the theoretical, historical and practice trends that have brought radiation therapy practice to its current state.

13.1 BACKGROUND

In radiation medicine, as in many medical specialties, interprofessional collaborative practice has emerged in the last decade as the best model for contemporary patient care where individual practitioners work in a cooperative, team-based and less hierarchical structure.[2] Professional boundaries overlap and synergize to ensure a harmonized, more seamless team approach. This model of collaborative practice is more patient-focused as all members of the team contribute their professional competence (knowledge, skills and judgment) to the continuum of care and scopes-of-practice begin to blur. In radiation medicine, radiation therapy treatment is prescribed, planned and delivered by three very distinct yet interdependent professional disciplines; radiation oncology, medical physics, and radiation therapy. The direct care of patients who are receiving, or have received, radiation therapy also includes a fourth, and important, profession – nursing. As the disciplines integrate to provide a more fluid model of care, the commonalities amongst and the differences between the respective professions begin to surface. One of the key aspects of practice where radiation therapists (RTTs) differ from their radiation medicine counterparts is in the area of research, scholarship and academic activity. RTTs are relative newcomers to this arena and may not be familiar with the scholarship that is intrinsic to the mores of the other professions.[1]

13.2 PROFESSION AND PROFESSIONALIZATION

In fact, the term "profession" is difficult to pin down. It has been defined many ways, but as it relates to radiation therapy, the term can best be defined as a calling requiring specialized knowledge and often long and intensive academic preparation.[3] More focused review of the literature on the concept clearly articulates that research is a fundamental activity within a given profession. While RTTs have likely always engaged in some kind of informal practice enquiry, it has been primarily in the past two decades where RTTs have begun entering the world of formal research – from conducting chart audits to participation in multicentre clinical trials. Historically, the nature of RTTs' experience in research activities was working for or collaboratively with medical physicists or radiation oncologists rather than conducting their own practice-based research.[4] In addition, while the experiences were likely rewarding and educational (and helped to propel the research agenda forward), they rarely fully harnessed the unique expertise of the RTTs as members of a legitimate professional group. The definition of a profession relies, to a large degree, on ownership and development of the specific professional knowledge base through applied research.[5,6] It has been argued that the knowledge base for radiation therapy has been developed primarily through the research activities of other disciplines and, as such, RTTs have had a limited contribution to their own practice development and may not, therefore, have been fully regarded as a profession.[7]

The origin of radiation therapy as a profession is quite similar to other allied health professions where the need for a new professional group arises out of a significant evolution in the practice of medicine or through the discovery of a new way of treating or curing diseases. In general, these novel healthcare professional roles did not surface instantly as complete, well defined professional scopes, but rather grew organically and evolved over time to a point where it was recognized that a distinct and definable practice domain was identifiable – such is the case for radiation therapy. As with many other professional groups before, the process of "professionalization," which includes the establishment of standards of practice, creation of common educational expectations and self-regulation, continues today.[1] One of the most important recent developments in this ongoing process is the adoption of evidence-based practice as the gold standard across the healthcare sector (*see* Chapter 1: Evidence-Based Medicine and the Scientific Method). With this paradigm shift, many more RTTs are integrating research more fully into their daily practice as "an integral part of routine work.[8]"

13.3 EDUCATIONAL EVOLUTION

As the demands of the radiation therapy professional continue to evolve and escalate, so must the educational preparation evolve to equip practitioners with the necessary competence and judgment to function as expected in the academic, interprofessional environment. Since the identification of radiation therapy as a distinct practice discipline almost 100 years ago, the educational preparation has evolved from an "apprenticeship" or "on the job training" model where the focus was on "what to do" to a structured, in-depth curriculum that focuses more on the "why it needs to be done.[1]" Emphasis has evolved to higher order outcomes built upon a broader curriculum that provides "…comparable training in the relevant social sciences – the type of education that will inform graduates about the social, economic and political forces that continually impact on the health-care environment.[4]" For the first time, in some jurisdictions, radiation therapy education falls within the academically focused university culture (*see* Figure 13.1). Literature reviews have demonstrated a positive correlation between upgrading entry-level requirements and subsequent participation in research activities.[9] Thus, this educational shift represents an important step in the professionalization of radiation therapy as the concepts of original enquiry and scholarship become embedded in the educational process. This phenomenon provides important insight that further allows the RTT to contribute as an equal partner in research within the radiation medicine domain. And in fact, in the last decade, in line with the many advancements in clinical practice as well as increasing educational preparation, research involvement has increased dramatically as more RTTs become involved in basic and translational research.[10] Many RTTs are now gaining employment as researchers in radiation treatment programs that are evolving to capitalize on the intellectual capital that exists in the radiation therapy department. More so than ever before, RTTs are innovating, enquiring and contributing fully to the advancement of the science of radiation therapy and the practice of radiation medicine overall.

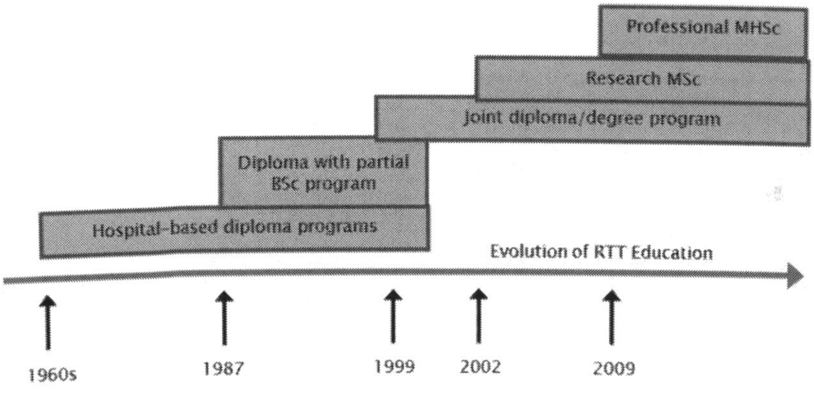

FIGURE 13.1 Evolution of education in Radiation Therapy in Ontario.[1]

13.4 SCHOLARSHIP

As mentioned above, the concept of "scholarship" is relatively new to radiation therapy as a profession, but is a concept that must be understood and embraced if the profession is to continue its growth and recognition as a legitimate professional group. Traditionally, in academic circles, the term "scholar" was reserved for those individuals who were strongly or solely focused on research and publication.[11] In the field of radiation medicine, physicians (as well as physicists and nurses) have conventionally been the members of the team that are engaged in scholarly work. This involvement in research is a fundamental and natural outcome of the academic environment where university-based preparatory education is provided for these groups and is also usually accompanied by a university appointment, with its overtly stated expectations for research, grant capture and publication.[1]

13.4.1 BOYER'S MODEL

While scholarship has been traditionally associated with basic research and publication (and, more marginally, teaching), Ernest Boyer has framed the elements of modern day scholarly activity more broadly according to the following:[12]

- the scholarship of discovery
- the scholarship of integration
- the scholarship of application
- the scholarship of teaching

In general, Boyer felt that there are many valuable activities taking place outside the pure academic arena that warranted note and recognition for their contribution to the advancement of existing bodies of knowledge (*See* Table 13.1). This broader definition has changed the way healthcare professions think about scholarly contribution and may also be a valuable way of looking at scholarship in radiation therapy, especially for a profession that was originally envisioned as "service-driven" and primarily vocational in nature.

TABLE 13.1 An overview of Boyer's scholarship framework.[13]

Category	Description	Sample Activities
Discovery	Original enquiry and building new knowledge	Performing the activities that result in creating new knowledge Peer-reviewed presentations, publications
Integration	Taking existing knowledge and interpreting it outside the original domain	Adapting information for broader contexts Working with an interprofessional team to devise guidelines for department-wide practice change
Application	Service-based activities that serve the public, patients and/or professions	Volunteering as part of the leadership of a professional organization Serving on governmental working groups to address current issues
Teaching	Developing novel methods of teaching to enhance learning and comprehension	Developing and evaluating new curricular materials and/or methods Research supervision Conducting educational research

The historical view of scholarship generally conjures up visions of researchers researching simply for the sake of new knowledge – independent of context and free of intention. Knowledge was sought as its own reward. With this newer interpretation of what scholarship looks like, it becomes easier for healthcare professionals to envision themselves as active participants in the translation of new knowledge (disseminated through scientific means): into local practice, the adoption of a new approach or technique, or in the education of students or professionals about new ways of working and thinking. This new way of looking at scholarship allows clinicians to have a goal of their scholarly activities – primarily that of improving the quality of care that is provided to their patients. As RTTs claim higher professional standing, they will undoubtedly become increasingly responsible for contributing to the radiation therapy knowledge base through the standard scholarly activities of research and publication.[7] Yet, the profession also needs to look beyond the traditional (and often quite rigid) "publish or perish" mentality of scholarship and adopt a more flexible definition that works.

13.5 NEW WAYS OF WORKING

In order to fully incorporate scholarly practice into the professional consciousness, strategies for remodeling daily practice and departmental structure need to be developed. If we look to other more established professions and how they structure the incorporation of scholarship into their practice model, we find a variety of approaches that capture the various elements put forth by Boyer. For example, the use of terms like "clinician-educator" or "clinician-scientist" to categorize team members and allot the time (also known as protected time) required for them to dedicate to activities and expectations appropriately, would help to organize department workloads (*See* Table 13.2). The development of such a model in radiation therapy practice will take creativity and commitment, as the usual approach of machine-based scheduling is difficult to modify in this way. The inclusion of scholarship-related activities within an accepted staffing standard would represent the first step in the journey to a model that would accommodate increased academic production from the radiation therapy profession.

TABLE 13.2 Sample model of career paths that incorporate varying academic activities.[14]

	Primary commitment	Clinical	Education	Research	Other
Clinician-Teacher	Clinical service. There is significant contribution to the delivery of service teaching and promoting and advancing excellence in clinical care.	70–90%	10–30%		10–30%
Clinician-Educator	Clinical service and education, educational administration and activities related to education, including educational research. They may take on roles such as preceptor, lecturer, or mentor.	25–75%	15–50%	10–30%	10–30%

TABLE 13.2 *(Continued)*

	Primary commitment	Clinical	Education	Research	Other
Clinician-Investigator	Clinical service and research. Research may include basic, clinical, or translational and they may be cross-appointed to a Research Institute or basic science department.	15–50%	10–20%	30–70%	10–20%
Clinician-Scientist	Research and clinical service. Research may include basic, clinical, and translational and they are primarily or cross-appointed to a Research Institute or basic science department.	10–15%	10–15%	70–80%	10–15%
Scientist	Research, which may be basic science, translational or educational, with no clinical responsibilities. Educational and/or administrative involvement only as it relates to educational research or scholarly activity.	–	10–25%	75–80%	10–25%

There are examples of departments that have created a vision that incorporates the further "professionalization" of the radiation therapy profession and the resulting practice models have demonstrated the ability to elevate RTTs' scholarly contribution and production.[15] Many other examples can be drawn from the allied health professional literature.

In the profession of radiation therapy, there has been movement into novel areas of clinical work as new technology forcing new ways of working in an interprofessional team, often resulting in overlap and sharing of activities that were traditionally the sole domain of medical or physics colleagues. This observed advancing practice is often associated with the expectation of increased educational preparation and comes with an increase in professional autonomy and responsibility. While this does not always include a formal division of clinical and academic responsibilities, as outlined in the models above, it has become apparent that with a more autonomous practice and development of new knowledge comes the potential for scholarly work in the form of research and its dissemination in a similar manner to the other members of the treatment team.[15] In these instances, departments have begun to formally recognize the contribution of the respective RTTs by creating job descriptions that include protected time for such activities. This may represent one of first forays into a new model of practice within the radiation therapy profession and, if successful, could provide the springboard for its adoption or adaption in other jurisdictions.

13.6 VISION FOR CONTINUED ADVANCEMENT THROUGH RESEARCH

Many tips and tools for nurturing an academic, scholarly research culture are discussed in detail in Chapter 14 (Getting Started: Building a Research and Evidence-Based Culture). However, there are some broad points that cannot be overlooked in a conceptual discussion about the rationale for RTT research. The value of research and academic contribution by RTTs needs to be continually articulated and fostered by employers and by the professional bodies that represent the profession and further emulated and embraced by RTTs in daily practice. It is critical that these values remain hinged to excellence in patient care and align with the strategic directions of practice environments.

The onus is on the radiation therapy community to understand how the profession can contribute to the advancement of these organizational and jurisdictional goals. It is also important to ensure that prelicensure training, continuing education and professional development opportunities include exposure to and opportunities to develop skills in the world of scholarship and research practice such that a profession-wide standard of research competence can be realized.

As well as providing practical resources for scholarship, professional development should incorporate the cultivation of "cognitive growth and perceived self-competency" with respect to the research agenda.[16] Opportunities for the analysis of and reflection on daily practice – such as collegial discussions, mentoring and teaching – are crucial to the advancement of RTTs' contribution to the knowledge base for radiation therapy.[17] These kinds of activities should be built into a new practice model as has been the case in other healthcare professions. Essentially, the purpose of all these activities is to create more empowered practitioners that may "question the status quo, share thoughts and engage in scholarly discourse.[18]" Only through an ongoing initiative to raise our collective research and academic competence can we continue to be invited to the tables of knowledge creation and translation, and be seen as equal partners in the radiation medicine domain and members of a bonafide and vital profession.

KEYWORDS

- Professionalization
- Educational preparation
- Academia
- Boyer's Model

REFERENCES

1. Harnett, N.; Palmer, C.; Bolderston, A.; Wenz, J.; Catton, P. The scholarly radiation therapist. Part one: charting the territory. *J. Radiother. Prac.* **2008,** *7(2)*, 99–104.
2. Pearson, P.; Jones, K. The primary health care nonteam? *BMJ*, **1994**, *309,* 1387–1388.
3. Merriam Webster. Profession. http://www.merriam-webster.com/dictionary/profession. (Accessed October 15, 2013).
4. Baird, M. Evolution of a degree program: the Australian example. *Radiol. Technol.* **1992,** *63,* 404–409.
5. Schon, D. Educating the reflective practitioner. Jossey-Bass: San Francisco, 1987.
6. Manning, D.; Bentley, H. B. The consultant radiographer and a doctorate degree. *Radiography*, **2003,** *9,* 3–5.
7. Nixon, S. Professionalism in radiography. *Radiography*, **2001,** *7,* 31–35.
8. Harris, R. Find and deliver: research and practice in therapeutic radiography. *Radiography*, **2000,** *6,* 225–226.
9. Canadian Association of Medical Radiation Technologists. Degree education for medical radiation technologists: the facts and the fiction behind CAMRT's education plans. CAMRT: Ottawa, 1998.
10. Snaith, B. A. Peer-review publication patterns: a comparison of international radiography journals. *J. Med. Imag. Radiat. Sci.* **2013**, *44,* 37–43.
11. Smith, M. J.; Liehr, P. Story theory: advancing nursing practice scholarship. *Holist. Nurse Pract.* **2005**, *19(6),* 272–276.

12. Boyer, E. L. Scholarship reconsidered: priorities of the professoriate. Carnegie Foundation for the Advancement of Teaching: Princeton NH, 1990.
13. Neumann University. Convivium. http://www.neumann.edu/academics/Convivium.asp (Accessed: October 15, 2013).
14. University of Ottawa Faculty of Medicine, Office of Professional Affairs. Faculty career paths. http://www.med.uottawa.ca/ProfessionalAffairs/eng/faculty_career_paths.html (Accessed: October 15, 2013).
15. Bolderston, A.; Harnett, N.; Palmer, C.; Wenz, J.; Catton, P. The scholarly radiation therapist. Part two: developing an academic practice—the Princess Margaret Hospital experience. *J. Radiother. Pract.* **2008,** *7(2)*, 105–111.
16. Diers, D. Clinical scholarship. *J. Prof. Nurs.* **1995**, *11,* 24–30.
17. Elberson, K. L.; Williams, S. A. Innovative strategies for promoting clinical scholarship: a holistic approach. *Holist. Nurs. Pract.* **1996**, *10(3),* 33–40.
18. Meisenhelder, J. B. Cultivating scholarship in the clinical setting. *J. Nurs. Staff Dev.* **1994,** *10(2),* 87–90.

CHAPTER 14

GETTING STARTED: BUILDING A RESEARCH AND EVIDENCE-BASED CULTURE

LISA DI PROSPERO MRT(T) MSc

Manager, Education and Research, Radiation Therapy, Odette Cancer Centre, Sunnybrook Health Sciences Centre, Toronto Canada Lecturer, Department of Radiation Oncology, University of Toronto, Toronto Canada

CAROL-ANNE DAVIS RTT ACT MSc

Clinical Educator, Radiation Therapy Services, Nova Scotia Cancer Centre, Queen Elizabeth II Health Sciences Centre, Halifax Canada

CONTENTS

OPENING REMARKS

Rachel Harris MSc PgD PgCCE DCR(T) DClinRes

Professional Officer for Research, Society and College of Radiographers, London, United Kingdom

I am delighted that this book has been devoted to the need for research for the profession.

Research is integral to everyday radiation therapy as it aids in both building an evidence base for practice and helps ensure continuous service improvement. It is no longer acceptable to continue with practice based largely on tradition. Patients expect and should receive the best evidenced-based care available.

To sustain best practice, radiation therapists must accept that research is an essential part of their role and not simply an optional extra activity. We need to promote a culture where all of us are both research users and research-aware. We should reevaluate regularly and strive to improve our practice using the latest research findings. Some of us will need to be research doers and some research leaders, ensuring we are building on the current evidence base.

With such a pivotal role in the care of patients undergoing cancer treatments, radiation therapists should ensure they work and research collaboratively with each other, both across centres and with other health professional colleagues. Everyone needs to be part of the research effort.

Sharing of findings through publications and presentations is another key part of research. Advances in best practice need to be communicated to the rest of the profession, so we should all be proactive in building on our unique body of knowledge in this field.

In this chapter Lisa and Carol-Anne give a flavour of how to get started in research. They provide some really useful tips and pointers. Research can seem daunting at first, but we can do it, and we must do it if we are to advance as a profession. Start small and build on your confidence and skills. You can do this. Together we must embrace research and support others in its implementation.

Integrating research into clinical practice provides the conduit for seeing research as not an "add on" but an expectation of professional practice.[1–3] The barriers, organizational and individual, to conducting research are not unique to radiation therapy.[4–6] Practitioners must be "motivated to learn the new skills and organizations will need to facilitate required knowledge and skills.[7]" As such, establishing support through collaborations and possessing self-awareness of one's own strengths is essential to a sustained and impactful research portfolio.

Being successful in research can be supported by both intrinsic (individual) and extrinsic (departmental) factors. Intrinsic factors involve elements the individual researcher can focus on to ensure success: motivation, mentorship, building of a strong team, and the foundational skill base. Empowered with these tools the radiation therapist (RTT) is well placed to begin defining his or her own research portfolio. In terms of extrinsic factors, success in research relies heavily on the environment in which RTTs practice and interact. RTTs practice in a range of settings from large, academic institutions with a strong research culture and mandate to smaller institutions lacking many of the resources and supports required to facilitate engagement. The departmental culture is critical to the success of a capacity-building and sustainable research program.

This chapter is designed to provide some insight to the individual researcher and the broader radiation therapy department (big or small) regarding the ingredients necessary to support research, and the means by which these ingredients can be brought together.

14.1 INTRINSIC FACTORS IN RESEARCH SUCCESS

14.1.1 BE MOTIVATED: WHAT ARE YOU CURIOUS ABOUT?

Embarking on research has many rewards and challenges and is often motivated by both a thought-provoking problem and the curiosity to investigate it. Alternatively, and frequently in parallel, the undertaking of research can be triggered by personal motivations such as professional contribution and personal satisfaction. Regardless of the source, motivation is the catalyst for taking a simple question to formal inquiry. There are many unanswered questions in healthcare, especially in a technologically charged field like radiation therapy; technology is increasing exponentially and roles are rapidly changing and evolving. As such, and as any field, radiation therapy knowledge has gaps and potential for improvement, providing opportunities to inform best practice. From entry level to experienced RTTs, problems are identified on a daily basis with the potential to be feasible research studies. Despite the plethora of questions to be answered, many agree that getting started is the hardest part.

HOT TIP

Everything and anything is questionable, and these questions make way for research.[8]

From inception to completion, research can be a complicated, time-consuming and an inherently challenging undertaking. Motivation and self-satisfaction will support and sustain the novice researcher especially if the area being researched is of interest and significance to the researcher. Choosing a research topic from a personal perspective is therefore important to the novice RTT researcher. A passion for the research topic may be the motivating factor and a determinant as to whether the researcher is willing to devote the necessary time and effort to the project. When time-frames are tight and data accrual and analysis are difficult, the enthusiasm for the research topic is critical.

As important as choosing a topic of interest to an individual is the issue of relevance in general. In undertaking research, one must establish if the study being contemplated has relevance: what is the significance of the study? To be worthwhile, there must be potential for the results to provide new knowledge and be meaningful.[9]

To assist RTTs in getting started with research, five key questions may be of assistance:[10]

1. How motivated are you to undertake this research?
2. Does the research topic pique your interest...are you curious about it?
3. How relevant is the research to your practice; to the broader practice of radiation oncology?
4. Is the research project feasible?
5. What does the literature say about the topic?

A research career can begin by simply finding a topic that is of interest. The completion of one project of interest lends itself to future work, which then naturally builds a research portfolio that is unique to the individual RTT. Generating that initial question can start with reflecting on daily practice – "why do we do what we do?." Chapter 1 (Evidence-Based Medicine and the Scientific Method) discusses the formal development of a research question in greater detail.

HOT TIP

Remember, if research were easy, everyone would do it! It may not be easy, but many RTTs do it!

14.1.2 FINDING A MENTOR

Prelicensure education provides the knowledge and skills for successful clinical practice. However, the current academic framework in radiation therapy in Canada is such that the knowledge, skills, and confidence to carry out research activities must be acquired experientially or through further formal education postlicensure. The majority of training programs lack the necessary curricular elements to provide the basis of sound research skills, as the focus is on fundamental entry-to-practice competencies that have not traditionally included research. Building of research skills is thus most readily accomplished through the partnership and guidance of a mentor, who can provide insight regarding research methods and direction, and a sounding board in navigating the intricacies of a research team.[10]

Choosing a mentor, in itself, requires a form of research process.[11] A research mentorship can either evolve naturally or require the focused effort of the novice researcher. If seeking a formal mentorship relationship, the researcher should meet with potential candidates, identified through recommendation or by common research interest, to ensure an appropriate fit. This initial meeting can serve to determine if a connection exists between mentee and mentor. A mentor will not only provide expertise but can act as a confidante for discussion, and provide strategic guidance, ongoing encouragement, and often valuable networking opportunities.[12] A successful partnership can be of benefit to both mentee and mentor as it allows the mentee to learn from the expertise borne of experience and to be initiated into an established research community. For the mentor, the relationship can encourage a reexamination of one's own knowledge and skill, and to deconstruct the research process to its basic framework. It may also provide a necessary teaching interaction to meet requirements of academic appointment or another professional engagement and even lay the groundwork for future projects together.

HOT TIP

Do not be hesitant to ask, even the most seasoned researcher, to be your mentor. In my own experience, the majority of researchers love collaborations, at all levels. Mentorship and collaborative relationships is of great benefit to them – increasing their own research productivity and fulfilling a requirement of their own teaching dossier. They will welcome the invitation or connect you to one of their colleagues.

14.1.3 BUILDING A TEAM

Forming and managing a research team, as with any successful groups, relies in capitalizing on individual strengths, contributions and commitment of members to reach a common goal.[13,14] Appropriate thought should be given to the development of a research team, including consideration of areas of expertise necessary for various elements of the project. This might include insight to a review of the literature or the proposed methodological approach, familiarity with the target population or study environment, varying professional backgrounds, and ability to navigate research ethics and the broader research process. Librarians and statisticians are two sets of professionals who can be of incredible value as members of the research team, either as formal collaborators or as experts consulted at relevant points in the research process (*see* Chapters 2: Literature Reviews and 5: Quantitative Methodologies and Analysis for more information about consulting these professionals). Case example 14.1 provides a novice researcher's account of the challenges in engaging a statistician.

Once the team is identified and invitations accepted for participation, roles must be defined as well as expectations of each team member. The primary investigator should be clear with expectations, timelines and goals of the work. This is also a great discussion point for establishment of authorship order and what constitutes authorship.[15,16] Team rules or a charter can be used or simply a documentation of discussion through the use of minutes and actions – this provides transparency and accountability to all team members.

CASE EXAMPLE 14.1

Statistical Support: A Novice Researcher's Experience

Carol-Anne Davis RTT ACT MSc
Clinical Educator, Radiation Therapy Services, Nova Scotia Cancer Centre, Queen Elizabeth II Health Sciences Centre, Halifax, Canada

The last phase of my master's degree involved the undertaking of a research project to meet the dissertation portion of the program. With a keen interest in PET-CT (and knowing that a topic of personal interest and curiosity would be a strong motivator during my research!), I sought a supervisor and mentor locally with radiation oncology, research and publication experience.

With intent to investigate how PET-CT impacts high-risk target volumes, my supervisor and I met frequently to hone my research question and methodology. Navigating this new research world and coordinating meetings with my supervisors locally and at the university was certainly a challenge. Despite a lot of hard work, persistence and dedication from the team of local experts that I had assembled, almost nine months passed until I had a solid proposal for my project and was ready to head to the local ethics board for approval. Everything was in place: my research question, the study population, the methodology and even an initial description of the statistics to be used as part of the data analysis. To complete my research proposal, I needed my sample size...something that no member of my team was able to help me with.

Without the support of a strong research culture for RTTs locally, finding statistical support was difficult. On the advice of my local supervisor I contacted a statistician who had collaborated previously on a study in our diagnostic imaging department. At our first meeting I handed him my research proposal and asked if he could generate my sample size, something he was able to quickly do after I gave him a synopsis of my research question and methodology. To my surprise, I was informed that I required a sample size of 380 patients. When I questioned why such a large sample size was required, the statistician replied that my research question (a derivate of a "yes" "no" form of question) dictated the sample size. If my research question asked if PET-CT had an impact, and the answer could be yes or no, then the odds of the research findings would be similar to flipping a coin. Thus, I required a massive sample size.

Dismayed, I felt I had to abandon my research project (11 months of work) and take on a smaller, more manageable project. Time was passing and I already had one extension granted from the university. I contacted the statistician again, this time for advice and guidance. My original proposal was set aside and he asked me a simple question. He asked, "what is the story you'd like your research to tell"? In layman's terms I described what I wanted to find out about PET-CT. We dusted off my original proposal and from the original question to the hypothesis, methodology and analysis he and I, as a team, rebuilt my project. He taught me that in research, often the methodology builds on? the question. As well, I learned that the inclusion of a statistician early in the research process is crucial. Instead of using statistical support as the last step in my research study development, I developed a relationship with my statistician where he became a true collaborator on my team.

> My research eventually began, the results significant. In the end, my sample size ended up being 186 patients and ....my statistician was second author on my publication submission!

14.1.4 BUILDING A SUPPORTIVE NETWORK OF PEERS

Any researcher benefits from discussion with peers about potential research opportunities. While it will help inform and shape a research direction it may also generate interest from others to participate. It has been shown that healthcare professionals feel more confident approaching a research project with a group of peers.[17] Undertaking a research study as a group may alleviate many fears and challenges often encountered by single novice researchers and may contribute to the project's success.[18]

In addition to seeking support of others in the workplace, novice researchers should investigate the possibility of support from peer professionals nationally and internationally. Networking with peers through internet searches and key contacts in other similar hospital and clinic departments may yield a vast and rich list of resources that the novice researcher can tap into.

HOT TIP

Use electronic media to your advantage! Early in your research process, contact key professional associations. Many professional organizations have lists of resources and content experts for member support. Utilize the organization's listerv options so that your inquiry can be sent nationally for support, feedback and collaboration. As well, linked to many professional associations' websites are powerful social media tools: use them to get your need for support and resources out there! Chapter 11 (Knowledge Dissemination: Value and Approaches) also provides insight regarding harnessing technology for the purposes for research dissemination.

14.1.5 LEARNING AND REFINING KEY SKILLS

Successful research is simply a product of a set of developed skills. While many of these relate directly to the ability to implement the scientific method, there are important softer skills that are valuable assets in conducting research. Skills for success are:[19]

- Networking
- Communication
- Leadership
- Resilience

The ability to network provides the opportunity for brainstorming, discussion and moreover, and gathering of expertise. These connections that are built can then be harnessed for further collaborations and/or consultations.

Communication is key to successful research. It must be mastered in both the written and oral format.[16] Elegant, focused and clear writing is required not only for the final publication but early on in the execution of the proposal, preparing an ethics submission, the preparation of abstracts, and more importantly, in the competitive realm of funding calls. In writing, the context of the funding agency, the conference and the journal should direct reframing of the work so that the research is aligned with its target.

Effective presentation skills are also mandatory to any successful research as the impact of work is determined by the success of dissemination not only locally but on a wider stage. Communication although a quality in most, can be learned, as it is also a skill that can be mastered with intentional practice. Chapter 11 (Knowledge Dissemination: Value and Approaches) discusses oral presentation skills and considerations in greater detail.

HOT TIP

Practice, practice, and practice – most people are uncomfortable while presenting to their colleagues and peers. Be confident, no one knows your research better than you do. It's your job to sell it. Do not be afraid to acknowledge a great question and say "great question, we have not considered that but I will bring it back to the team and would love to connect with you after the conference." You cannot think of everything.

The ability to navigate a team requires leadership – a toolbox that includes management skill that is delicately balanced with the skills to encourage, coach, problem solve and redirect. This goes hand in hand with being resilient throughout the research process; research is not easy and straightforward but can be a rewarding and educational experience. Many unexpected events and outcomes occur along the entire process from idea through to publication – all of which can be used as a learning experience.

14.1.6 FINDING A NICHE

Transitioning from point of interest to creation of a research portfolio requires a concerted effort to disseminate findings – to evidence the work that was conducted. Through dissemination, a natural linkage occurs between the topic and the researcher itself, whereby each is synonymous with the other. Findings which are not published are lost to a sea of data files, and in time the work is forgotten. Essential to building a research portfolio is evidence of the body of work that can be accessed and provide influence beyond an individual organization and moreover, one's immediate practice.

Although focusing a research portfolio does build expertise, it is worthwhile to expand partnerships to include other areas of interest. The exploration of "other" research can lead to insight, either intentional or not, that can impact future projects. This widened insight can provide an opportunity to think beyond the immediate lens of what is concretely seen and be influential to analysis, explanation and future work. Analogous to life experience, the move through professional practice comes with it a change in direction – a research portfolio will steer in other directions but at its core, early work will feed later work.

HOT TIP

Doing research in one's own department or institutions brings about some unique challenges which may be worthwhile investigating. If you are doing research within your own organization – a great resource is Doing Action Research In Your Own Organization (2009).[20] This text provides very helpful advice and strategies to move forward especially when research conclusions or recommendations may cause tension within the department.

14.2 EXTRINSIC FACTORS IN RESEARCH SUCCESS

14.2.1 BALANCING WORKPLACE AND RESEARCH DEMANDS

Healthcare professionals have identified numerous barriers to undertaking research, several which have a direct link to the workplace and work environment: workplace research culture, time, and support.[4] Whereas factors that encourage and support research include positive research attitude in the organization, and education and dedicated time for undertaking research.[17] Often, these factors are difficult to control and cause difficulty for even the most motivated RTT.

Increasingly, the healthcare workplace is becoming a more and more demanding setting where workload and complexity are increasing while resources and staffing are reducing.[21] For many, the ability to manage a heavy clinical workload and a research role requires careful attention to ensure that clinical responsibilities are maintained and research is not eroded. The importance of establishing dedicated research time, away from the front line and clinical duties is key. Even small amounts of protected time per week or negotiating more flexible work start and end hours may allow the researcher to stay on track and balance both their clinical and research responsibilities. There are many personal attributes of successful researchers and the ability to get along well in a team and manage time_effectively arc critical in balancing clinical and research realities, in essence time and team management.[22]

Integral to staying on target with deadlines and specific points in the research study is the RTT's ability to manage time effectively and be cognizant when and why deadlines are not met. Stress may be significantly reduced when deadlines are realistically and well laid out in advance, providing both guidance and reassurance that the project is progressing as planned. Additionally, the ability of a RTT to surround themselves with strong networks and solid mentors helps guide and support the researcher through the trials of the busy work place and the demands of the research.

Research is unique that when conducted as an add-on can easily be stretched and delayed – the downside is that a critical time-limited opportunity may be lost to competing researchers, or activities downstream of a missed deadline will be adversely affected.

14.2.2 SOLIDIFYING FUNDING

The demands of balancing both clinical and research demands can often be alleviated by the use of research assistants and associates. In reality, the cost associated with such a resource is prohibitive, especially when working in nonacademic centres or those with a nonresearch focus. Novice researchers should not shy away from seeking this type of assistance and should investigate venues for funding. Many professional associations, nonprofit organizations and hospital or health districts have research awards and funds available for exactly this type of assistance moreover, there are many partnerships with universities that provide enthusiastic students the opportunity for an experiential learning opportunity for little to no cost to the researcher.

HOT TIP

Do your homework…money is out there, get creative at finding it.

14.2.3 TRANSITIONING TO A RESEARCH CULTURE

Changing the workplace culture begins with changing the way individuals and peers think: many associate research with more traditional bench work and as such, these researchers are not involved with patient contact and clinical responsibilities.[22] Healthcare professionals must begin to think in terms of the inherent link between front line activities and basic research and the powerful combination of the two. The good news is that the combination of clinical experience and a sense of inquiry are ideally suited.

Successful research environments must be supportive, cooperative and visible and, as such, foster teamwork. Engaged individuals can come together to investigate a topic or area as a start for a research project.[17] Workplaces with a strong research culture will showcase research produced within their departments, and will consciously strive to generate excitement around radiation therapy research. Case example 14.2 highlights the value placed on professional recognition of research contributions by the Radiation Medicine Program at the Princess Margaret Cancer Centre.

CASE EXAMPLE 14.2

Professional Recognition for Research at the Princess Margaret Cancer Centre

Angela Cashell MRT(T) MSc
Clinical Educator, Radiation Medicine Program, Princess Margaret Cancer Centre, Toronto Canada
Lecturer, Department of Radiation Oncology, University of Toronto, Toronto Canada

The recognition of the research contributions and successes of RTTs at the Princess Margaret is seen as an important means of demonstrating support for research and fostering a culture of inquiry. Small gestures requiring little expense can go a long way to generate interest in research and encourage those engaged in it to continue.

At the Princess Margaret we organize a wine and cheese poster event during Medical Radiation Technologists' Week in November each year. We ask all staff who had been to a conference and presented their research within the last year, to bring their posters and to be available to chat with their colleagues. We also develop an abstract booklet that is posted on our intranet and available at the event, so that the information could be read and reviewed as needed. This provides an opportunity for oncologists, physicists and other allied health staff to appreciate the research that is on-going, and to discuss opportunities for future study. We are also exploring the possibility of setting up a permanent poster board within the department to provide a viewing venue for staff on a continuing basis.

We have a monthly email blast that goes out from our leadership group to recognize awards, publications or any other academic achievements. Our monthly Radiation Therapy Education and Research newsletter also highlights key publications and presentations, as the broader department is not always aware of the work being done by their colleagues, and the potential value it could have in the clinical setting.

The Radiation Medicine Program has also set up an annual research awards ceremony. This includes categories such as most influential publication, research productivity, research support etc., and staff receives a certificate of recognition and also a token gift or gift certificate. The awards recognize staff in all disciplines who have contributed to the research program, and separate categories have been developed for physics, oncology, and therapy, to ensure that members of each discipline are afforded an equal opportunity to be recognized.

Often, even in the absence of a strong research culture, all it takes is one person to get things started. A single individual can change the workplace culture. For example, a lunch-and-learn session where novice researchers can present their progress to date can serve to motivate both the researchers and the audience, thus generating enthusiasm amongst peers.[17] The successful accomplishments of one researcher may invigorate others to embark on their own research. There is a reciprocal benefit where the successful researcher experiences the power of knowledge transfer to novice researchers and in turn, the lessons learned have the power to motivate peers and colleagues.[17]

Creating enthusiasm and creating excitement related to research is fundamental to sustaining and maintaining a positive workplace research culture. Clinical research for each individual healthcare profession is needed to improve the quality of the specific profession's care and skill. Here, the concept of contributing to a body of knowledge is synonymous with owning the profession (*see* Chapter 13: Academia and Scholarship). The way a profession achieves best clinical practice is by acquiring new knowledge, and who better to acquire the knowledge than the profession who consumes it?

14.2.4 COLLABORATING INTERPROFESSIONALLY

Intra- and interprofessional partnerships between front-line clinicians and academic clinicians (faculty) are of benefit to support a research culture. These partnerships will innately provide the mentorship, learning and support required to further sustain a research culture.[23] Research is rarely a solo venture. It is also not often best undertaken uniprofessionally. Clinical practice in radiation medicine is dependent on the contributions of multiple professions, and research will often also benefit from interprofessional insight. The engagement of other professions can bring unique expertise and perspective to the development of a research question and study design, navigation of data collection in a clinical environment, and interpretation of results ensuring maximum relevance. It is essential in conducting research to have the buy-in of those whose support is necessary for the success of the project. For example, if recruiting patients at the time of initial radiation consult, it may be necessary for the radiation oncologist to flag an appropriate patient to be approached. Having an oncologist formally involved in the project can facilitate this, especially if this further generates support amongst his or her peers to cast a broader net for recruitment.

From the perspective of research culture, it is also important to acknowledge that some other professions in radiation medicine, especially radiation oncology and medical physics, have a long standing history of research engagement, as well as a stronger foundation in support, resources, and expertise relating to the conduct of research as it is often inherent to their clinical portfolio. RTTs can often benefit from capitalizing on these assets.

For a radiation therapy department first venturing into research, this may involve arguing for a model where oncologist or physicist principal investigators are encouraged to consider RTTs as research assistants or other junior participants in relevant clinical investigations. Not only does this build a cohort of RTTs with strong foundational research skills, it may also generate a buzz to other physicians and physicists that can be harnessed in the future to engage other RTTs in research activities.

Radiation medicine is inherently interprofessional, and this should apply equally to research as it does to clinical practice. That said, RTTs often feel the need to solve what is perceived to be their own questions and clinical issues within their own group. A strong departmental research culture relies on collaboration and mutual support between groups, and a case should be made for the involvement or consultation of all relevant professions in any given research study. While this is not a case that can be built overnight for a profession in its research infancy, demonstration of an interest, respect, and aptitude for research will begin to foster the necessary support from interprofessional colleagues.

14.2.5 BUILDING RESEARCH CAPACITY WITHIN A SUSTAINABLE MODEL

Building research capacity within professional practice requires raising an awareness among peers and colleagues that entices thinking and questioning. This intentional thinking will stimulate and challenge. In partnership with capacity is sustainability; one cannot be considered without the other. Of importance is to expand the "one" researcher to a small group of researchers who inspire and engage each other in discourse as they practice, teach and learn. The ability to build effective and positive relationships is a vital skill as well, especially for researchers who are performing research in an organization or department where the culture is not receptive. It is all about being able to influence others to see things from a research perspective.

Regardless of the passion of the RTT, the senior leadership must support a research culture within their organization that is modeled by their own philosophy and practice.[6] Minimal investment will result in great downstream return. Effective minimal investment can be realized as committed in-kind contributions to the research platform such as protected time for front-line clinicians.

Even more effective, is the creation of research clinician positions within an organization. Research clinician positions, similar to the physician model, will allow for the focused development of in-house expertise, mentorship and partnership to build research capacity. Physician models typically include dedicated time allocation (in relation to a full time equivalent position) to research and clinical activities that is stipulated in role profiles (*see* Chapter 13: Academia and Scholarship).

HOT TIP

Begin small, ask your administrator to commit to two hours per week so that you can work on your research. Show your results and celebrate your success with your administrator. This will set the stage for asking for more time and possibly could lead to a pilot research position which could then lead to permanent integration within the staff complement. Small gains are key to the buy-in process – be strategic in setting the stage.

The integration of advanced practice RTTs within organizations provides an ideal framework for capacity-building. As respected clinical leaders recognized for their research platform, their knowledge and skills can be harnessed in both capacity building as well as sustainability.[24]

In essence, building and sustaining research requires a culture shift of what research is and why it is needed; how it is embedded into practice; the foundational skills of inquiry as well as the support and expectation to carry it out to a recognized deliverable.[4–6,17] Some standard venues that facilitate inquiry include seminars, journal clubs, research committees, formalized research partnerships and mentorships to supporting the learning of the research process.

14.2.6 JOURNAL CLUBS: GENERATING AN INTEREST

To practice radiation therapy with an evidence-based focus, RTTs must be consumers of rigourous and clinically relevant research. Even within specialty areas, the number of journals and papers available has exploded exponentially making it difficult for healthcare professionals to keep up with the literature.[25] Journal clubs can be seen as a quick and efficient means of both reviewing the literature and learning in a group setting. Journal clubs have been used for many years by many types of health professionals as an education tool, a means to stay updated and as a component of the research utilization process.[26]

As defined by Kirchoff and Beck, research utilization is a process that begins when research findings are reviewed, critiqued and compared to current practice.[26] They further describe their own department's experience with journal clubs when research findings that are reviewed and found to be strong and represent a potential practice change, necessary steps are taken to change their practice.

When using journal clubs to take the step from research on paper to research in action (change in practice), caution should be employed in several key areas:[26,27]

- Structure the format of the journal club to focus on a single topic (as opposed to a single article or single journal)
- Employ strong critical appraisal skills (critique study design, bias, sample and conclusions)
- Assess trustworthiness and scientific merit of the data (how substantial is the evidence?)

- Examine the relevance to your practice or department (does the practice fit your environment?)
- Examine the feasibility of implementing the change (risk, readiness and resources)

For many, especially work places that lack any form of journal club, beginning small may be the best first step. By starting a journal club where the focus is an educational outcome allows the members to practice, learn and finesse their critical analysis skills and engage in entry to high-level discussions amongst peers. Evaluating research for integration into practice involves more than simply reading research. It entails critical appraisal.[27] Extend the invitation to all interested professional colleagues (especially those with experience in journal clubs). Both inter and intra-professional participation will further support the success of the journal club and foster richer and more comprehensive discussions from a range of lenses.

Despite the potential positive benefits that journal clubs offer as a means to practice evidence based radiation therapy, barriers to their implementation and success do exist. As with many research-based endeavors, support from administration and management is preferred to begin and sustain a journal club. Time will be required to properly prepare for each journal club and resources should be provided to allow RTTs to attend the journal club. For many departments, it may only be feasible to hold journal clubs under less resource-intense scenarios, such as holding journal clubs after hours. Think creatively in the age of digital connectivity – virtual journal clubs either synchronous or asynchronous can be as effective as the more traditional approach.

HOT TIP

A journal club is a great way to get started in research. All it needs is two interested RTTs, an article and a place to meet. The journal club, with a little care and nurturing, will evolve on its own.[4]

14.2.7 CRITICAL APPRAISAL

Building a solid knowledge base on how to critically assess research within the radiation therapy department may be a significant barrier for some departments. Not all RTTs have formal education in research or possess the required skills to judge the merit of a given paper. Consequently, many RTTs may be intimidated to join a journal club. Early stages of a journal club may entail an introduction to the fundamentals of research. In larger institutions, the researcher may find that a journal club already exists in the institution (physician, nurse, or allied health professional focus). This could provide a model for an RTT journal club, or even an opportunity to collaborate to highlight RTT research in an interprofessional environment. Novice research RTTs should not be daunted by the potential barriers for creating a journal club but instead be cognizant of them and use them to strengthen their process. There is no right or wrong format. Case example 14.3 reflects on the journal club model employed at the Odette Cancer Centre at Sunnybrook Health Sciences Centre in Toronto.

CASE EXAMPLE 14.3

Journal Clubs: The Odette Cancer Centre Experience

Angela Turner MRT(T) BA MHSc
Radiation Therapist, Odette Cancer Centre, Sunnybrook Health Sciences Centre, Toronto, Canada

The main objective of our journal club at the Odette Cancer Centre is to expose RTTs to recent published literature relevant to their practice. As well, through a facilitated group meeting, which is held once a month they learn about the various aspects involved in critiquing published literature, from examining methodology to the discussion of sample biases. This also serves as information, which will help them to navigate their own research projects in the future.

Each month a volunteer facilitator will choose a relevant, recent published article. The article is sent out via institutional e-mail with an invitation to attend the next scheduled journal club. Sessions are scheduled at the same time each month (e.g., first Tuesday at 1pm) so that staff can arrange their schedules if they want to attend. We also send out a critique template as the staff found this useful as a guideline when reading the article. Some hard copies of the articles are also posted on the "Journal Club" section of the notice board in the staff room.

Each session consists of a facilitated guide through the article using a standard PowerPoint™ template, which contains key aspects of published literature critique. Many of these types of templates can be accessed online and adapted to each journal club's format. Our sessions are kept informal and often discussions develop between staff who are not likely to have the opportunity to interact in any other setting. This knowledge exchange is another advantage of the journal club sessions, which we had not anticipated. It has also given novice presenters the opportunity to facilitate a peer group session in an informal setting as well as gain experience in conducting focused literature searches etc.

We ask participants to complete an evaluation after each session, which gives us feedback on aspects of the journal club such as content and scheduling that may be improved. A departmental survey is distributed annually to elicit feedback from other staff who do not regularly attend the sessions. From this survey we have found that many staff read and value the identified articles even without attending the sessions.

Our journal club has therefore provided an opportunity to develop skills and knowledge in research as well as encourage a culture of research awareness throughout the department.

14.2.8 BECOMING PART OF THE STRATEGIC DIRECTION

Ongoing support is realized not only as protected time and funding for research but by the adoption of this goal by leadership as part of the strategic "big picture" goals of the department. Expectations from both the leadership and the researcher include the endpoint deliverable of each project. This must include peer-reviewed publication to maximize impact of the research and as a measure of research productivity. But, it must also align with the greater goals of the organization – higher quality and more cost-effective care for patients. The perspective of a Radiation Therapy department manager on the development of a strong research culture is reported in case example 14.4.

Organizations that have built a successful research program have built processes to engage clinicians in an inquiry-based culture. What distinguishes effective from ineffective hospital research is the presence of departmental processes that unleash creativity of staff and involve them early on in the project, educate all staff by involving them at all levels of the research in all capacities, create internal expertise for research that can be harnessed to create, engage, excite and ignite a passion about inquiry, and finally celebrate successes that will be infectious to others encouraging them to participate and be part of change.[28]

HOT TIP

Integral to the establishment of the culture is the initial support of administrator colleagues. Given the economic constraints within the healthcare setting, researchers need to be able to articulate the value that radiation therapy research brings to the larger practice of radiation oncology and patient outcomes. Often researchers are faced with the task of efforts to convince administrators why research outside the physician researcher is of benefit.

CASE EXAMPLE 14.4

Developing a Research Program: Where to Start? A Manager's Perspective

Sheila M. Robson MRT(T) ACT BSc
Manager and Head, Radiation Therapy Department, Odette Cancer Centre Sunnybrook Health Sciences Centre, Toronto, Canada

Where did we start when RTTs were not traditionally seen as researchers? How did we convince people that RTTs are not only highly capable but have a valuable and unique contribution to make to research?

We leveraged every opportunity no matter how small or insignificant it seemed. The first opportunity came when the clinical trials department turned down an Oncologist's request for a nurse to assist with a trial of a medication designed to reduce skin reactions. We were approached (grudgingly!) to see if we could spare an RTT. We agreed and very carefully selected a therapist who we knew would excel. That Oncologist spoke to another and another and soon Radiation Therapists were in high demand to be part of projects. At this point we did two things. The first was to insist that radiation therapists be given full credit as coauthors on any papers; they were not just to be data collectors. The second was to hold a staff meeting where we sought buy-in from the therapists. If we were to have research program it had to be with full support from everyone, we could not pull therapists away from their research every time we were short staffed or we would lose all credibility as serious researchers. We got (and still have) their full support. We established a research and education fund to allow RTTs to attend professional development activities and the entire department fundraised enthusiastically to put this fund on a firm financial footing.

Once we had a cohort of staff with some research experience as collaborators we encouraged these people to mentor their colleagues and to start doing independent research, speaking at conferences, presenting posters and submitting papers. We then developed a departmental strategic plan that incorporated research, and a staffing plan that allowed for dedicated research time and operationalised the research program. We presented this to senior management and having a body of work made it much easier to promote our case. We were fortunate to have a very supportive senior leadership team and a core of equally supportive oncologists who actively encouraged and mentored RTTs.

From there we began to grow the program, dramatically increasing our research output, slowly adding extra research positions, hiring a Research and Education Manager, having RTTs appointed to the University of Toronto's Department of Radiation Oncology and having RTTs successfully apply for grants to support their work. We now have a very robust and well-recognized research program with broad involvement across the department. We started in a very small way but "from tiny acorns grow might oaks."

14.3 BEING THE CHANGE AGENT

14.3.1 FOSTER AN INQUIRY-BASED CULTURE – BECOME THE RESEARCH CHAMPION

Establishing a culture of research among a traditional practice that excludes research is simple – it requires one pioneer who generates excitement among colleagues to make research infectious. Historically, this pioneer is called a champion – a champion requires the foundational knowledge to support a given platform but more importantly, the skills to garner the support and engagement of colleagues to "want" to be involved in research activities. Becoming a champion is about being passionate about research and moreover, developing an ambassadorship for a department. This can infectiously build capacity. This is likened to the innovation adoption lifecycle (*see* Chapter 10: Innovation and Invention). In building a research program, it is critical to target the early adopters to recruit the early majority – who are open to new ideas but require some intentional prodding. The early majority are the influential pack that once onboard will add great support to the initiative. The goal is to have research integrated within the operations of daily clinical practice and to have both inter- and intra-professional colleagues want to research.

14.3.2 COMMUNITIES OF PRACTICE

Champions can be harnessed both internal and external to an organization, and RTTs can benefit from engaging with other professionals who are working with similar questions, populations, technologies and system constraints. In recent years, the role of the community of practice (CoP) has been explored on many levels, from institutional to provincial and even national and international. A community of practice is "a group of people who share a concern, problem or a passion about a topic, and who deepen their knowledge and expertise in this area by interacting on an ongoing basis.[29]" A CoP provides an ideal forum to create, discuss and share knowledge and moreover, foster the support, enthusiasm and engagement of like-minded individuals. Through group discussion of common issues, members of a CoP can build on both intellectual and social capital that crosses organizational, professional and geographical barriers. Simply, it is the benefit derived from the knowledge from both giver and seeker in addition to the benefit derived from the relationship of participants. Traditionally, a CoP meets face to face but technology has become the enabler of the virtual realm – CoPs are an old concept that has become resurrected in popularity.[30–32] Setting and working towards common aims can help with pooling of knowledge and experience to ensure the highest quality of care, and ultimately to standardization of practice.

A culture of continued inquiry is what sets the foundation for integrating research as part of practice. Integrating research into clinical practice provides the conduit for seeing research not as a hobby or "extra" commitment, but as an expectation of professional practice.[1,2] The barriers – organizational and individual – to conducting research are not unique to radiation therapy.[4–6] RTTs must be "motivated to learn the new skills and organizations will need to facilitate and encourage research.[7]" As such, having a self-awareness of one's own strengths and needs for additional learning, as well as establishing support through collaborations, is essential to a sustained and impactful research portfolio.

RTTs are slowly assuming responsibility for their own body of knowledge, and this is not the role of the few, sitting apart from the clinical environment, changing practice for their colleagues in the trenches. This is the undertaking of a profession, and it benefits all RTTs to be engaged in a culture of inquiry. For some, this will involve simply asking a question about whether something could be done in a more efficient or patient-centred manner, and browsing the published literature to determine if there is a more evidence-based approach to that particular technique or practice. For others, it will involve formal engagement in the world of research, contributing new knowledge to the field. Regardless of the level at which an RTT chooses to assume the role of researcher, it is important that peers, colleagues, leadership, and even patients and the public, be vested in the support of a research culture for RTTs.

HOT TIP

TOP 7 PEARLS FOR GETTING STARTED

1. Always ask yourself "why or why not?"
2. Gather greatness in forming your team
3. Course correct, nothing is perfect along any process
4. Be committed from start to finish, reenergize and reinvigorate
5. Don't overthink it – just get started, changes are always possible
6. Contribute to and build your body of knowledge – own your profession
7. Achieve best clinical practice by acquiring new knowledge

"Research is not just about an exciting discovery and the number of articles published, it's a rich and privileged journey into the lives of those with whom you work and the challenge of personal growth in the process.[33]*"*

KEYWORDS

- Motivation
- Research mentorship
- Inquiry-based research culture
- Interprofessional collaboration
- Journal clubs
- Communities of practice

REFERENCES

1. Gambling, T.; Brown, P.; Hogg, P. Research in our practice—a requirement not an option: discussion paper. *Radiography* **2003,** *9(1),* 71–76.
2. Reeves, P.; Wright, C.; Shelley, S.; Williams, P. The Society of Radiographers' research strategy. *Radiography* **2004,** *10(3)*, 229–233.
3. Harris, R. Research and the Radiography profession: A strategy for research 2010–2015. http://www.sor.org/learning/document-library/research-and-radiography-profession-strategy-research-2010–2015 (Accessed August 23, 2013).
4. Turner, A.; D'Alimonte, L.; Fitch, M. Promoting radiation therapy research: understanding perspectives, transforming culture. *J. Radiother. Pract.* **2013,** *12(2)*, 92–99.
5. Jolley, S. Raizing research awareness: a strategy for nurses. *Nurs. Stand.* **2002,** *16(33)*, 33–39.
6. Timmins, F.; McCabe, C.; McSherry, R. Research awareness: managerial challenges for nurses in the Republic of Ireland. J. Nurs. Manage. **2012,** *20* (2), 224–235.
7. Lapierre, E.; Ritchey, K.; Newhouse, R., Barriers to research use in the PACU. J. Perianesth. Nurs. **2004,** *19* (2), 78–83.
8. Sridharam, S. Research methodology: Motivation for research. http://research.vtu.ac.in/Downloads/materials/Research%20Methodology%20SNS%20(1).pdf (accessed June 3).
9. Balakumar, P.; Inamdar, M. N.; Jagadeesh, G. The critical steps for successful research: The research proposal and scientific writing: (A report on the preconference workshop held in conjunction with the 64th Annual Conference of the Indian Pharmaceutical Congress, 2012). *J. Pharmacol. Pharmacother* **2013.** *4(2),* 130–138.
10. Bauer-Wu, S.; Epshtein, A.; Reid Ponte, P. Promoting excellence in nursing research and scholarship in the clinical setting. *J. Nurs. Admin.* **2006,** *36(5)*, 224–227.
11. Steiner, J. F.; Curtis, P.; Lanphear, B. P.; Vu, K. O.; Main, D. S. Assessing the role of influential mentors in the research development of primary care fellows. *Acad. Med.* **2004,** *79(9)*, 865–872.
12. Keyzer, D. J.; Lakoski, J. M.; Lara-Cinisomo, S.; Schultz, D. J.; Williams, V. L.; Zellers, D. F.; Pincus, H. A. Advancing institutional efforts to support research mentorship: a conceptual framework and self-assessment tool. *Acad. Med.* **2008,** *83(3)*, 217–225.
13. Building and managing your own research team. http://newpi10.mcgill-cihr-ig.ca/guidebook/5 (accessed May 12).
14. Salas, E.; Wilson, K. A.; Murphy, C. E.; King, H.; Salisbury, M. Communicating, coordinating, and cooperating when lives depend on it: tips for teamwork. *Jt. Comm. J. Qual. Patient Saf.* **2008,** *34(6),* 333–341.
15. International Committee of Medical Journal Editors. Uniform requirements for manuscripts submitted to biomedical journals: ethical considerations in the conduct and reporting of research: authorship and contributorship. http://www.icmje.org/ethical_1author.html (Accessed September 15, 2013).
16. Coverdale, J. H.; Roberts, L. W.; Balon, R.; Beresin, E. V. Writing for academia: getting your research into print: *AMEE Guide No. 74. Med. Teach.* **2013,** *35(2),* e926–34.

17. Syme, R.; Stiles, C. Promoting nursing research and innovation by staff nurses. Appl. Nurs. Res. **2012,** *25* (1), 17–24.
18. Fitzgerald, M.; Milberger, P.; Tomlinson, P. S.; Peden-Mcalpine, C.; Meiers, S. J.; Sherman, S. Clinical nurse specialist participation on a collaborative research project. Barriers and benefits. *Clin. Nurse Spec.* **2003,** *17(1),* 44–49.
19. University of Manchester. Essential skills and qualities of a successful academic: networking, time management, resilience, presentation skills, writing skills, leadership and management. http://www.academiccareer.manchester.ac.uk/about/do/skills/ (Accessed May 12, 2013).
20. Coghlan, D.; Brannick, T. Doing Action Research in Your Own Organization. Sage Publications: Thousand Oaks, CA, 2009.
21. Grunfeld, E.; Zitzelsberger, L.; Coristine, M.; Whelan, T. J.; Aspelund, F.; Evans, W. K. Job stress and job satisfaction of cancer care workers. *Psychooncology.* **2005,** *14(1),* 61–69.
22. Cugini, M.; Charles, C.; Kinney, J. Getting started in clinical research. *J. Dent. Hyg.* **2012,** *86(1),* 26–27.
23. Balakas, K.; Bryant, T.; Jamerson, P. Collaborative research partnerships in support of nursing excellence. *Nurs. Clin. North Am.* **2011,** *46(1),* 123–128.
24. Gerrish, K.; Guillaume, L.; Kirshbaum, M.; McDonnell, A.; Tod, A.; Nolan, M. Factors influencing the contribution of advanced practice nurses to promoting evidence-based practice among front-line nurses: findings from a cross-sectional survey. *J. Adv. Nurs.* **2011,** *67(5),* 1079–1090.
25. Lee, A. G.; Boldt, H. C.; Golnik, K. C.; Arnold, A. C.; Oetting, T. A.; Beaver, H. A.; Olson, R. J.; Carter, K. Using the Journal Club to teach and assess competence in practice-based learning and improvement: a literature review and recommendation for implementation. *Surv. Ophthalmol.* **2005,** *50(6),* 542–548.
26. Kirchhoff, K. T.; Beck, S. L. Using the journal club as a component of the research utilization process. *Heart Lung.* **1995,** *24(3),* 246–250.
27. Tibbles, L.; Sanford, R. The research journal club: a mechanism for research utilization. *Clin. Nurs. Spec.* **1994,** *8(1),* 23–26.
28. Gawlinski, A. The power of clinical nursing research: engage clinicians, improve patients' lives, and forge a professional legacy. *Am. J. Crit. Care.* **2008,** *17(4),* 315–326; quiz 327.
29. Wenger, E.; McDermott, R.; Snyder, W. M. Cultivating Communities of Practice. Harvard Business School Publishing; Boston, MA, 2002.
30. Sharratt, M.; Usoro, A. Understanding knowledge-sharing in online communities of practice. *Elect. J. Knowledge Manage.* **2003,** *1(2),* 187–196.
31. Lesser, E. L.; Storck, J. Communities of practice and organizational performance. *IBM Sys. J.* **2001,** *40(4),* 831–841.
32. Majewski, G.; Usoro, A. Barriers of and incentives to knowledge sharing in (virtual) Communities of Practice: A critical literature review. *BU Acad. Rev.* **2011,** *10(1).*
33. Selby, S. Getting started: confessions of a novice researcher. *Aust. Fam. Physician.* **2005,** *34(12),* 1056.

GLOSSARY

Abstract: concise summary of the proposed or completed research, often between 200 and 300 words in length, often divided into background or introduction, methodology, results, discussion or conclusions

Accrual: the process of recruiting participants into an investigation; or the number of participants recruited

Accuracy: the degree of correctness of the measurement of a variable, and can reflect both the internal and external validity of a measure; increases as systematic error decreases

Alternative hypothesis (H_A): the hypothesis stated by the researcher, which proposes the likelihood of a relationship or effect between the study variables

Anchors: response options or points identified in scale-based surveys, often referring to belief or perception (i.e., "5 = Strongly agree")

Autonomy: fundamental ethical principle concerning a person's ability to make his or her own decisions; relates to the capacity to provide informed consent to treatment and/or to participate in research

Bias: is any force that could cause overall deviations from the truth, especially as it concerns an inclination to maintain a certain partial perspective, without considerations of other points of view or possibilities; can relate to behaviour or to statistical data-related bias

Binding: process of defining valuable elements for consideration in a qualitative case study, to focus on time, context, and place relevant to the phenomenon of interest

Blind (trial): study in which bias is minimized by not revealing to either the subject (single-blind) or both the subject and the researcher (double-blind) whether the subject is receiving the intervention (likely opposed to a placebo) in a randomized trial

Bonferroni correction: statistical method used to avoid type I error in situations of multiple comparisons, where it is increasingly likely to observe a rare event that might otherwise suggest the acceptance of the alternative hypotehsis

Boolean logic: set of rules (or operators) used by databases to allow combinations of terms and phrases that can facilitate interpretation by a database search engine; includes AND, OR, NOT, *, ?

Boyer's model: framework for professional scholarship that recognizes the contribution of discovery, integration, application, and teaching to the advancement of professional bodies of knowledge, moving beyond the idea of scholarship as research for the sake of research

Canada's Tri-Council Policy Statement (TCPS/TCPS-2): a joint policy of three federal research agencies which promotes the ethical conduct of research involving humans, and is considered the national standard

Canadian Institutes of Health Research (CIHR): Canada's federal funding agency for research; one of three federal agencies represented by Canada's Tri-Council Policy Statement

Capacity: the ability to understand the elements of information relating to a decision regarding consent to treatment or to participation in research, including appreciation of reasonably foreseeable consequences of consent or refusal; one of three components to consent

Case study: a report of a real-life scenario involving a single person, population or event used to draw evidence that can be applied to decision-making; can be used as an applied teaching or research methodology

Chi square test: a non-parametric statistical test for independence used to compare whether the frequencies of two outcomes, or differences in proportions, for two defined groups are statistically significant

Citation tracking: process of seeking instances of further reference of a given article, or of determining the number of times that article was cited in other articles; requires the use of online tools or functionalities which are often available through searchable databases

Clinical significance: the extent to which a therapy or intervention is of benefit to a target population in improving the state of health; often considered the practical counterpart to statistical significance, taking into consideration the effectiveness of an observed difference and feasibility of achieving this

Clinical trial: series of phases of study involving human participants, aimed to compare the effects of a health-related intenvention on a predetermined outcome or endpoint and held accountable through strict ethical guidelines; serve to generate safety and efficacy data to establish new treatment modalities and improve upon current standards of practice in the healthcare environment

Closed-ended question: quantitative type of survey item that provides a fixed list of response options for the respondent to choose from (e.g., mutliple choice questions)

Cluster random sampling: approach to sampling used when a simple random sample is not possible or feasible; involves breaking the total sample into smaller groups, called clusters, and sampling all member of the randomly selected cluster populations only

Cochrane collaboration: an international network of researchers that collaborates to produce systematic reviews of primary research in human health care and health policy, known as Cochrane Reviews; contributions, compiled in the Cochrane Library, inform clinical decision-making and evidence-based practice

Cochrane Library: *see* Cochrane Collaboration

Cochrane Review: *see* Cochrane Collaboration

Coding: process of organizing, categorizing, and analysing qualitative data to discover and highlight emergent themes

Cohen's Kappa: *see* reliability

Co-Investigator: formal collaborators on a research grant or investigation, working along with the principal investigator to conduct the research and take responsibility for the ethical, methodological, analytical, and financial aspects of the investigation

Community of practice: a group of professionals with a shared interest in a topic who interact regularly to broaden their knowledge and expertise relating to that topic

Compassionate use trials: a type of observational clinical trial whereby patients may be offered an intervention (drug, treatment, etc.) regardless of their eligibility for the full clinical trial

Confidentiality: is the protection of an individual's privacy, through a set of rules, laws or ethical guidelines protecting access to and safeguarding a research participant's personal information

Conflict of interest: any real, potential or perceived abuse of the trust placed by research participants or stakeholders in the researcher, generally in the form of bias stemming from financial or personal interests that can affect professional judgment or objectivity

Consent: the free, informed, and ongoing authorization of a medical intervention or participation in research; comprised of disclosure, capacity, and voluntariness, thus ensuring that consent is based on consideration of relevant information about risks and benefits of participation and is provided without coercion

Construct validity: aspect of validity concerning the degree to which a measurement tool (such as a survey) evaluates the intended theoretical background, or construct

Content validity: aspect of validity concerning the degree to which a measurement tool (such as a survey) evaluates all facets or dimensions of a given theoretical construct

Convenience sampling: type of non-probabilty sampling involving the selection of a population for study that is close at hand; method of sampling precludes generalizations to the total population, but is an efficient and simple means of accruing a sample

Correlation coefficient: *see* Pearson's coefficient

Critical appraisal: methodolody used to evaluate research data, highlighting strengths and weaknesses of the study (e.g., sources, methodological rigour, levels of evidence, bias) in order to determine if appropriate conclusions were drawn and to direct evidence-based practice

Critical case sample: the process of selecting a small number of valuable cases, insight on which is most likely to yield the desired objective; can involve a typical case (for general understanding and causal relationships), extreme case (prototypical or paradigmatic to highlight underlying issues), or deviant case (representing extreme ranges of values)

Cronbach's alpha: *see* internal consistency

Cross-sectional study: a descriptive approach, involving observation or investigation of a population at a single specific point in time (e.g., administering a survey to a large and varied group at one time)

Data collection tools: means by which study data is initially recorded, such as templates for inputting observational or extracted numerical data, survey forms, etc.

Data quality: the correctness of the data collected, in that it is complete, valid, consistent, and representative of the truth of what has been measured (e.g., proper units of measurement, lack of transcription or calculation errors, no missing data, etc.)

Data saturation: the point during the data collection process (primarily in qualitative research) where gathering additional data does not lead to new ideas, themes or opinions on the topic being researched, thus suggestive that the data collected is sufficient to answer the research question

Deception: non-disclosure of research intents in order to avoid undesired impact on behaviour or data that can stem from knowingly participating in a research study; contravenes principle of informed consent and is thus rarely justified in ethical research

Degrees of freedom: number of different variables or parameters that are free to vary independently without restriction; relates to the determination of a critical value that will serve as a threshold to reject the null hypothesis (and thus conclude the existence of an effect)

Delphi process: a structured approach to generating consensus to guide practice, based on systematic rounds of questionnaires administered to experts in a given area, to encourage convergence on the most "correct" outcome; a formal and structured approach to pooling expertise will lead to a more accurate or effective decision (such as a set of standards or practice guidelines); generally applied in modified approach that begins with a pre-established subset of a broader scope of elements and/or involves some face-to-face consensus-building or discussion

Deming cycle (PDSA cycle): approach to continuous quality improvement, involving cyclic progression through four phases of implementation and evaluation of a program—plan, do, study (or check), act—to refine and optimize an initiative or program

Dependent variable: represents the attribute that is to be measured in an investigation, to determine if it constitutes any output or effect; observed in the context of independent variables, which are manipulated by the researcher as the input or cause

Descriptive statistics: communicates what data trends looks like and involves the organization, summary, and display of data, allowing the researcher to understand and identify trends; includes percentages as well as the determination of the mean, median, mode, standard deviation, and range of data; cannot be used to generate statements about cause and effect relationships

Diagnostic trials: type of clinical trial that investigates means of detecting disease

Direct costs: budgetary items considered necessary to conduct a given research investigation, beyond the regular operation of the environment in which the research is conducted, such as salaries for dedicated research staff (research assistant, biostatistician), services, equipment, business supplies, etc.)

Disruptive innovation: revolutionary or radical invention or improvement in practice that fundamentally changes a system through necessitating a change in roles or practices to accommodate the innovation, thus marginalizing the previous system

Direct observation studies: qualitative research methodology involving first-hand witnessing and studying of a social phenomenon; the researcher can either remain removed from the environment (non-participation) or engaged in it (participation)

Document review: qualitative research methodology involving extraction of information from paperwork or records, including patient charts, practice guidelines or policies, committee terms of reference or meeting minutes, etc.

Double-blind: study in which bias is minimized by not revealing to either the subject or the researcher whether the subject is receiving the intervention (likely as opposed to a placebo) in a randomized trial

Editorial board: a group of people who provide direction and guidance and set the tone for a publication (such as a journal); usually consists of experts in the field or subject area of the publication

Effect size: a measure of the strength of a phenomenon or relationship, or the difference between two groups; identification of a minimum desired effect size is a consideration in determing the necessary sample size

Ethnography: qualitative research methodology involving immersion in a social situation to investigate the culture or interactions of a population in a natural setting

Evidence-informed policymaking: an approach to making decisions relating to public programs, guidelines, and practices that is based in rigourous objective research; an extension of evidence-based practice as it applies to health services

Exclusion criteria: conditions that would make someone or something ineligible for consideration, even if inclusion criteria are met

Expectation effect: *see* Rosenthal Effect

Expedited review: process of ethical review conducted for a submitted research protocol representing a study expected to involve minimal risk; commonly conducted by a subcommittee of the Research Ethics Board (REB) in a shortened timeline

Experimental study design: a research study involving a controlled investigation, in that effects of variables other than the independent variable are minimized; tends to include an experimental group, where the intervention is performed, and a control group, without intervention

External validity: psychometric measure of the degree to which a finding can be generalized to a broader population, and thus outside of the unique environment in which the research is conducted

Face validity: psychometric measure of the degree to which a survey is believed to address the concept or phenomenon it was designed to measure; transparency or relevance of the tool to the assessment of what participants expect it to assess

Focus group: qualitative research methodology involving facilitated and moderated group discussion designed to obtain perceptions, opinions, beliefs, and attitudes relating to a given topic

Full Board Review: process of ethical review conducted for a submitted research protocol representing a study expected to involve greater than minimal risk; conducted by the entire Research Ethics Board (REB) to assess risk and determine ethical appropriateness of conducting the proposed research

Good Clinical Practice (GCP): a standard for the design, conduct, performance, monitoring, auditing, recording, analyses, and reporting of research (especially clinical trials) that provides assurance that the data and reported results are credible and accurate, and that the rights, integrity, and confidentiality of trial subjects are protected

Grey literature: informally published written material, such as reports, that is not available in conventional commercially-published means such as peer-reviewed journals; literature that is produced on all levels of government, academics, business, and industry in print and electronic formats

Grounded theory: the generation of theory through qualitative study and data collection; hypothesis-generating rather than hypothesis-testing, as concepts are framed inductively based on thematic analysis of data

Hand-searching: an approach to searching the literature whereby a complete volume of a journal thought relevant to a particular topic is searched; this type of search can overcome the possibility of missing key articles through other means, but can be increasingly challenging as journals are less often published in print; also known as "powerbrowsing"

Hawthorne effect: phenomenon where research subjects modify behaviour in response to the knowledge that they are being observed, thus potentially biasing results and compromising external validity of the research; also known as the "observer effect"

Health services research: study of factors impacting access to and quality of healthcare, including social, financial, organizational, technological, and personal factors; consideration of the provision of health care from the perspective of social science and economics

Impact factor: a value assigned to a journal that serves as a measure of the degree to which a publication is valued and recognized by others; a function of the number of times an article in that journal was cited in another article as compared to the number of articles published by that journal in the two preceding years

Implementation research: the study of methods and change strategies to facilitate the uptake of research findings, especially in the area of health services innovations

Inclusion criteria: conditions that must be met in order to participate in a given research study, or, in the case of a literature review, the conditions that would lead to the consideration of a given article

Independent variable: represents the attribute that can be manipulated in an investigation, to evaluate a presumed influence (effect) on the dependent variable

Indexing: process of making a journal or other publication available through specialized searchable databases such as PubMed, to improve visibility and accessibility of the publication's content; based on criteria relating to scope, relevance, representation, and quality of content; indexing may influence the impact factor of a journal

Indirect costs: budgetary items considered inherent to the environment in which the research is conducted, but nonetheless necessary overhead to support and facilitate research (library services, salaries of clinical staff, clinical equipment, research administration services, etc.)

Inference: logical conclusion drawn from analysis of data, or the process of drawing such conclusions; must be appropriate to the scope, scale, and nature of the findings

Inferential statistics: communicates whether there is a relationship between variables, serving to test a hypothesis and determine causation to allow rejection or acceptance of a null hypothesis; involves use of parametric or nonparametric tests (t-tests, confidence intervals, etc.)

Informed consent: *see* Consent

Innovation: a significant improvement to a service, product, or process that allows it to better meet new requirements or existing needs

Innovation Adoption Lifecycle: model that defines the various and sequential approaches to implementing a novel practice, product, or process through suggesting the levels of support and resistance by entities (e.g., individuals, institutions) in a position to adopt the innovation

Instrumentation effect: potential impact on research outcomes of a change or difference in the measurement device, observer, or scorer used to assess the dependent variable; can represent a threat to internal validity

Intellectual property: a legal concept referring to recognized ownership of intangible inventions, such as musical and artistic works, discoveries, and designs; protected by patents, copyright, and trademarks as they define exclusive rights

Internal consistency: a quality of survey instruments representing a measure of the correlation between different items within the instrument, suggesting whether items intended to measure the same construct will generate similar scores from participants; represented by a statistic known as Cronbach's Alpha

Internal validity: psychometric measure of the degree to which a measure is assessing what is intended to be measured, and suggests the minimization of bias and other systematic error; represents whether there is sufficient evidence to support or reject hypotheses

Inter-rater reliability: psychometric measure of the degree of agreement between two or more raters in their implementation of a tool (such as a provider-administered scale assessing severity of side effects) (e.g., whether each of the raters give the same result)

Interval scale: data that have order (can be ranked) and have a consistent degree of difference between items, but for which a measure of zero is arbitrary, thus not permitting ratios between items (such as temperature, where each degree represents the same incremental increase in temperature, but where 20°C is not twice as hot as 10°C)

Interventional trials: controlled experiment testing the impact of a novel treatment, technique, drug, or other intervention, administered according to a defined protocol, on a population, usually as compared to the current standard of care; more commonly referred to as a "clinical trial"

Interview: qualitative research methodology involving conversation between two or more people, to elicit information from the interviewee to contribute to an understanding of a topic; *see also* "structured interview," "semi-structured interview," and "unstructured interview"

Invention: the creation or introductoin of a unique novel product or process, which has not previously existed

Investigator: formal collaborator on a research grant or investigation, engaged in the conduct of the research and responsibility for the ethical, methodological, analytical, and financial aspects of the investigation; *see also* "co-investigator," and "principal investigator"

Item: individual questions in a research survey

Journal club: a group of individuals who meet regularly to review and critique identified journal artcles, in efforts to foster research awareness and inform evidence-based practice

Knowledge gap: the difference between what is known or understood through investigation and published literature, and what is practiced; a function of the degree to which newly-generated knowledge is disseminated and implemented

Knowledge tranlsation: the term for the process of transferring the results of research investigations from the research setting to the practice setting, and the application of that information to inform improvements in healthcare

Kotter's Change Process Theory: an eight step model created to facilitate change within an organization, ultimately leading to future success; involves creating a sense of urgency, creating a guiding coalition, creating a vision for change, communicating the vision, removing obstacles, creating short-term wins, building on the change, and anchoring the change in the institutional culture

Lean strategy: the concept, introduced in the world of manufacturing, of reducing wasteful steps and processes in the creation of a valuable product; step-by-step continuous improvement strategy to generate quality and safety, efficiency, and engagement to reduce the costs of healthcare

Likert scale: ordinal respondent rating scale used in survey research, originating with a 5-option scale of "strongly Approve," "Approve," "Undecided," "Disapprove," and "strongly Disapprove," but with many modifications of wording for option scales

Literature review: navigation of available information on a topic, and the critical evaluation of the relative value of that information; can serve to assess any knowledge gaps to justify a research question, guide the development of a research question, or constitute research in itself

Longitudinal cohort survey: *see* "longitudinal survey"

Longitudinal survey: a survey approach whereby a given suvey instrument is applied to study a particular issue over time, either by surveying the same population multiple times (longitudinal cohort survey), or by administering the same survey more than once over a defined period of time, to different individuals (longitudinal trend survey)

Longitudinal trend survey: *see* "longitudinal survey"

Mean: average of the total of a set of data

Median: the middle value in a set of data

Mentorship: the provision of guidance and direction by an experienced researcher to a novice researcher in the conduct of research, through sharing of knowledge, skills, and advice, facilitating navigation of research processes and conventions, and overseeing of ethical and effective research practices

Meta-analysis: a type of systematic literature review, more specifically a statistical tool used to compile and report results of quantitative studies that address the same research question, to more powerfully estimate an effect size; constitutes the highest level of evidence

Methodology: the study of the methods used to conduct research, including the theoretical models, phases, and techniques to collect and analyze data

Minimal risk research: research in which the probability and magnitude of possible harms implied by participation in the research is no greater than those encountered by participants in those aspects of their everyday life that related to the research

Mode: the most frequently-occuring value in a set of data

Modified Delphi process: *see* "Delphi process"

Multistage random sampling: *see* "cluster random sampling"

Narrative synthesis: a type of systematic literature review that applies a qualitative approach to reporting the categorization of studies into thematic categories according to design, context, or outcome; the qualitative counterpart to a quantitative meta-analysis

Natural Sciences and Engineering Research Council of Canada (NSERC): Canada's federal funding agency for university-based research; one of three federal agencies represented by Canada's Tri-Council Policy Statement

Negative brainstorm: the creative process of considering potential poor solutions to a problem or failures to achieve a goal in order to mitigate the risk of having those become a reality, through actively engaging in solutions that would avoid those eventualities

Networking: the interaction and development of working relationships with others with a common interest or within the same professional sphere, for the benefit of all through the sharing of knowledge, expertise, resources, and professional opportunities

Nominal scale: data that can be categorized according to mutually exclusive groups, but that do not have a ranking order or defined degree of difference between categories (such as hair colour, gender, cancer diagnosis)

Non-parametric test: statistics employed when data or populations do not have an inherent structure or expected distribution, such as ranking or order statistics

Non-participant observation: a type of direct observation study whereby the researcher remains removed from the social environment under study

Non-random sampling: the process of generating a sample of a broader population through means that do not necessarily provide a representative sample, and can thus introduce a degree of bias; includes convenience, quota, snowball, and purposeful sampling

Non-experimental study: a type of prospective study where no intervention is given (such as a qualitative ethnographical study) or where the intervention is not within the realm of control of the investigator, and subjects are thus not randomly assigned to intervention or control groups

Non-probability sampling: *see* "non-random sampling"

Null hypothesis (H_0): the default position, not stated explicitly by the researcher, that assumes there is no difference between groups; results demonstrating a difference can serve to reject the null hypothesis

Nuremberg Military Tribunals: trials held in the 1940s that served in part to hold accountable those who conducted unethical medical research by the Nazis on prisoners of war during World War II; led to the Nuremberg Code

Nuremberg code: standards for judging physicians and scientists who had conducted experiments on concentration camp prisoners and become the prototype of later Codes intended to assure that research involving human subjects would be carried out in an ethical manner

Objective: describes the aim or goal of the research, and guides how the research is going to answer the question being investigated; *see also* "primary objective" and 'secondary objective"

Objective measure: used to determine physical quantities and qualities using an unbiased measure, not impacted by human judgement or perspective

Observational study: *see* "non-experimental study"

Observer effect: *see* "Hawthorne Effect"

One-sided test: statistical measure used to assess a directional hypothesis, or an intervention that is expected to generate a difference in only one direction (positive or negative)

Open-access database: repository of peer-reviewed journals that is available free-of-charge, often generating revenue through charging researchers to publish there, rather than through charging end-users for access

Open-ended questions: qualitative type of survey item that provides an unrestricted field for response, rather than a fixed list of options, thus generating rich data but often requiring a more involved approach to analysis

Ordinal scale: data that can be categorized according to mutually exclusive groups and arranged in a ranking order, such that A>B or A<B, but for which there is no defined degree of difference between categories (such as cancer staging)

***p*-value:** statistical measure of the probability of obtaining an observed result by chance, when there is no real effect, or the probability of H_0 being true when results of an investigation would suggest that it should be rejected; commonly reported as a fraction or percent chance, and often required to be <0.05 or 5% in order to reject H_0 and deem a result to be statistically significant

Paired test: statistic employed to test two measurements obtained from the same subject, usually at different time points (such as before and after an intervention), assuming each subject to be its own control and thus limiting the impact of individual differences

Parametric test: statistics employed when data or populations are expected to have an inherent structure or distribution, such as descriptive statistics that can determine a mean and standard deviation; consideration of the values themselves, rather than just the order or rank of values

Participant observation: a type of direct observation study whereby the researcher becomes immersed or engaged in the social environment under study; a form of ethnographic qualitative research

Patent: legal protection of intellectual property, defining the exclusive rights to an invention or innovation

Pearson's coefficient (*r*): a value assigned to determine the strength of a relationship between two variables, in that a positive *r* suggests a positive linear relationship, and a negative *r* suggests a negative relationship; degree to which one variable tends to change when the other changes

Peer review: the independent and often blinded evaluation of work by qualified members of a profession or experts in a field, prior to publication or presentation of that work; represents the self-regulation of the knowledge dissemination within a field, to provide credibility to published work

Phase I clinical trial: first stage of clinical trial, conducted with healthy volunteers to determine the pharmacological actions of the drug, as well as its safety and side effects; inlcudes pharmacokinetic and drug interaction studies; *see also* "clinical trial"

Phase II clinical trial: second stage of clinical trial, conducted on patients in multiple centres to determine the safety and efficacy of an intervention or drug, including side effects and short-term adverse events; *see also* "clinical trial"

Phase III clinical trial: third stage of clinical trial, conducted on patients in multiple centres to confirm the clinical safety and efficacy of an intervention or drug in the capacity and conditions in which it is expected to be implemented; *see also* "clinical trial"

Phase IV clinical trial: final, confirmatory, stage of clinical trial, conducted after a drug has been approved for market, to further optimize the drug's use; *see also* "clinical trial"

Phenomenology: the objective qualitative study of subjective experience, intended to establish commonalities in how individuals perceive or attribute meaning to a given situation or experience, based on their perceptions, judgements, or emotions

PICO principles: acronym for the considerations in generating a research question—population, intervention, comparison, and outcome

Piloting: preliminary implementation of a survey instrument or other intervention on a limited number of people who are representative of the study population, to test the measurement tool and guide revisions from the generated information; can include questions on flow, clarity and understandibility of the tool itself

Placebo: a sham treatment, made to look and be administerd in the same way as the real intervention, to reduce the potential for bias in having the subjects (or researcher) know whether or not they are receiving the intervention in a randomized trial

Placebo effect: the manifestation of the perception that one is receiving the intervention, when really only recieving a placebo, often attributable to attention or expectation on the part of the healthcare provider (in a single-blind study); can involve either a perceived or actual improvement in the medical condition under consideration

Power: the chance of correctly rejecting the null hypothesis when it is false, generally desired to be on the order of 70–90%; a consideration in the determination of a necessary sample size, statistically represented by $1-\beta$, where β is the rate of type II error

Power analysis: determination of the desired power of a study; *see also* "power"

Powerbrowsing: *see* "hand-searching"

Practice effect: potential impact on research outcomes of a change in behaviour or performance of participants as a result of practice or repeated exposure to the measure; can represent a threat to internal validity

Precision: degree to which the measurement of the same value varies after repeated measurements; increases as random error decreases

Primary endpoint: the measured outcome of interest for two or more groups, constituting the main goal of the investigation (e.g., five year disease free survival rate)

Primary objective: describes the principal aim or goal of the research, and guides how the research is going to answer the question being investigated

Principal investigator (PI): leading collaborator on a research grant or investigation, engaged in the conduct of the research and responsibility for the ethical, methodological, analytical, and financial aspects of the investigation, and managing the contributions of co- investigators

Probability sampling: *see* "random sampling"

Process innovation: novel enhancement of the steps or approach in delivery of goods, devices, or services, to improve access, quality, or efficiency; *see also* "innovation"

Product innovation: development or improvement of physical goods, devices, or services for market; *see also* "innovation"

Profession: a calling requiring specialized knowledge and often long and intensive academic preparation; often considered to include research as a fundamental activity which contributes to the body of specialized knowledge

Professionalization: social process of transitioning from a trade or occupation to a profession; involves the building of a body of knowledge through research, the formalization of educational preparation, and often the establishment of a professional assocation and entry-to-practice requirement

Program evaluation: systematic approach to collection, analysis, and utilization of data relating to the effectiveness and efficiency of a program within the public or private sector, guiding future planning to optimize the meeting of needs of all relevant stakeholders

Prospective study: a study designed to evaluate the change in a population over time, from the current time to a point in the future, focusing on the outcome

Psychometrics: qualities of a test (often a survey instrument) that pertain to how well it measures what it is designed to measure, including validity, reliability, and consistency

Purposeful sample: type of non-probabilty sampling involving the selection of subjects for study that will likely provide the most valuable insight to the investigation, often identified by way of a stratification of necessary variables such as age, gender, experience, professional group, etc.

Qualitative research: broad categorization of research methodology to encompass approaches that are interpretative of behaviours, perspectives, and opinions, relying on subjective experience to assign meaning to social phenomena

Quality Improvement (QI) study: studies that are carried out to directly improve, assess or evaluate the performance of a process, service, practice or outcome of a department, program or organization; will often use the PDSA cycle to guide the methodology

Quality of Life (QOL) trials: type of clinical trial that considers Quality of Life (perceived emotional, social, and physical status of an the individual's life) as an endpoint, particularly in diseases with a poor prognosis, such as palliative treatment for metastatic cancer

Quantitative research: broad categorizatiom of research methodology to encompass approaches that make use of numerical data to obtain information during observation; commonly used for testing hypotheses

Quasi-experimental design: a research study involving a controlled investigation, in that effects of variables other than the independent variable are minimized, but where participants are not randomly assigned to control and experimental groups

Quota sampling: type of non-probabilty sampling involving the hand-picking of subjects by the interviewer based on some key characteristic

Random sampling: the process of generating a sample of a broader population through means that provide all individuals within the population equal probability of being selected for inclusion; makes use of using random number tables, or computer generated random assignment; most likely to provide an unbiased and representative sample

Randomized Control Trial (RCT): the gold standard clinical trial that involves the blinded, non-biased, random assignment of subjects before an intervention to groups that receive different interventions (usually an experimental treatment versus the standard of care)

Range: the minimal and maximal values in a set of data

Ratio scale: data that have order (can be ranked) and have a consistent degree of difference between items, and where a value for zero is fixed and meaningful (such as age, time, etc.)

Rationale: as used in a research proposal, it is the justification for the need to address the proposed question, and the potential contribution to practice of seeking the answer to the question; framed by the literature review which highlights the gap in knowledge

Recruitment: the process of attracting, screening, selecting, and consenting an individual within a sample population to participate in a research study

Reflexivity: the consideration of the impact of the qualitative researcher's personal background, values, and contruction of meanings on the carrying out of research and the interpretation of data; presentation of factors relating to the researcher which might introduce bias to the results of a qualitative research study

Reliability: psychometric measure of the degree to which a tool (such as a survey instrument) consistently produces similar results under consistent conditions; represented by a statistic known as Cohen's Kappa; *see also* "inter-rater reliability" and "test-retest reliability"

Repeated measures test: *see* "paired test"

Response rate: the number of people who completed a survey as compared to the number of people who were eligible and had access to do so (the sample); usually expressed as a percentage

Research Ethics Board (REB): independent arm's length committee of medical professionals and lay people who determine the ethical acceptability of proposed research under the auspices of a given institution, and who act as gatekeepers to the conduct of research investigations within that institution

Research portfolio: a personal collection of evidence of one's body of work, including publications, presentations, speaker scores, either physical, electronic, or theoretical, that can serve to guide future work and reflect one's experience to others, such as employers

Research utilization: process of reviewing, critiquing, and implementing research findings into practice; foundation of evidence-based practice

Research proposal: detailed statement of intent to identify the rationale and feasibility of conducting a research project, to provide justification to stakeholders of the value in supporting the proposed work; analogous to the business case for the need for funding, such as with a grant proposal, ethics approval (such as with a component of a Research Ethics Board [REB] application) or justification of clinical impact of the project

Retrospective study: a study that is conducted through investigation data that has already beencollected, through review of records, often serving to investigate the contributing factors to a given outcome

Rigour: state or quality of a systematic, formal, and thorough approach to research, through striving for validity, reliability, credibility, etc.

Rosenthal effect: phenomenon that can occur when the researcher expects certain effects and biases subjects to perform better towards the desired effect, either in actuality or in the perception of the researcher, compromising external validity of the research; also known as the "expectation effect"

Sample size: the number of participants in a given research investigation, determined through sample size calculations to be powered to identify an effect of an intervention, should one exist

Sampling: refers to the process of selecting study subjects from a defined population

Sampling bias: preferentially selecting certain groups for inclusion in a study population, while excluding others, based on sampling approach

Scale: survey tool, instrument, or individual item with associated response options

Scholarship: engagement in the formal process of generating, evaluating, and communicating new knowledge; considered to involve discovery, integration, application, and teaching, and often contributes to the definition of a profession

Scoping review: exploratory or preliminary literature review, often conducted as a precursor to a full systematic review, serving to determine the amount and quality of information available on a topic, highlighting key findings and gaps

Screening trials: type of clinical trial that investigates and compares approaches to detecting disease

Secondary objective: "by-product" of the primary objective and could be findings that occur as a result of other measures that are being collected

Semantic differential scale: type of survey ordinal scale that provides options for gradations between two antonyms, such as "happy" versus 'sad," allowing for numerical grading and analysis between the two extreme response options

Semi-structured interview: a version of qualitative interview methodology that makes use of an interview script (discussion guide) to provide guidance to the investigator, allowing for deviation from the script to prompt elaboration on emergent themes

Simple random sampling: a rudimentary approach to random sampling, in that a formal method of true sampling is not used to generate a representative sample, but nonetheless intending to provide a sample of a broader population through means that provide all individuals within the population equal probability of being selected for inclusion

Single-blind: study in which bias is minimized by not revealing to the subjects whether they are receiving the intervention (likely as opposed to a placebo) in a randomized trial, while this information is available to the researcher

Snowball sampling: type of non-probabilty sampling involving the consideration of the opinions of non-randomly chosen qualified participants to identify others who may also qualify as respondents

Snowballing: the process in conducting a literature review of scouring the reference list in a article that proved relevant, in efforts to identify other key references cited in that publication

Sponsor: in clinical trials, the person who assumes responsibility for filing an application to the government body (e.g., Health Canada) prior to initiation of the trial; often a private company or industry responsible for the manufacturing a drug, but can also be an individual investigator

Standard deviation: statistical measure of the degree of variation or dispersion around an average measurement; represented by the Greek sigma (σ)

Statistical power: *see* "power"

Statistical significance: the extent to which an observed effect is likely to represent an actual effect, as opposed to having occurred by chance in the investigated situation, often represented by a lower p-value and a low Type I error rate

Stratified random sampling: approach to random sampling, whereby the researcher identifies the need for a sample to contain proportions of participants with a given characteristic; the broader sample population is sorted into predetermined groups and samples are pulled randomly from within each group or strata to generate a final sample

Structured interview: a version of qualitative interview methodology that makes use of a strictly-followed interview script (discussion guide), without permitting the investigator to delve deeper into an emergent theme; akin to a verbally-administered survey

Study protocol: the defined and formalized approach to conducting a given research investigation, including the purpose and hypothesis, study design, study populations, interventions or procedures, as well as data analysis and dissemination of the information learned during the course of a research study; often prepared as a document to be submitted with a research proposal or Research Ethics Board (REB) application prior to the initiation of research

Subjective measures: used to determine physical quantities and qualities by way of human judgement or perspective, acknowledging and even prioritizing the inherent bias

Sustaining innovation: inventions or improvements in practice that support advancement of that practice but that do not disrupt it or require a new model or set of roles; tends to be incremental as opposed to radical

Systematic random sampling: approach to random sampling whereby potential subjects are listed by some order that is unrelated to what is being measured (e.g., alphabetically), and then every *n*th subject is included in the sample

Systematic measurement bias: repeated error or deviation from a "true" value that can occur if a particular measurement tool is not well calibrated, applied incorrectly, or not appropriately chosen to measure the construct in question

Systematic review: a formal, rigourous, and comprehensive review of available literature to compile all published work on a given topic and summarize the state of knowledge and subsequent gaps in that area

***T*-test:** inferential statistic or parametric test used to compare the mean difference of continuous (interval or ratio scale) data between two groups, assuming the data is normally distributed; considers the mean, variance, and sample size of a dataset

Test-retest reliability: psychometric measure of the degree to which scores attained using a given tool are consistent from one administration to the next, under the same testing conditions and assuming no change in the construct being assessed

Theoretical sampling: iterative approach to sampling in qualitative research, whereby samples are sought based on an emerging need for insight in a particular area, as determined by data collected earlier in the investigation; the key approach to grounded theory methodologies, as the researcher works to build a theory out of collected data

Thesis: an in-depth research study or exploration of a given topic, often performed in the course of completing a graduate degree

Transcription: the process of transferring audio- or video-recorded data to verbatim text, for the purposes of qualitative data analysis; often performed using transcription services or software

Triangulation: a process used to validate data by using two or research methods to collect data and check (cross-verify) that the results support the same conclusion

Trustworthiness: representation of the credibility, transferability, confirmability, and dependability of data collected through qualitative research, suggesting the degree to which data is representative of the context and realities in question

Two-sided test: statistical measure used to assess a non-directional hypothesis, where the intervention has the potential to generate a difference in either direction (positive or negative); the default test if directionality is unknown

Type I error: statistical phenomenon that results in the incorrect rejection of the null hypothesis when it is actually true, representing a false positive result; can occur with the use of too small a sample

Type II error: statistical phenomenon that results in the failure to reject the null hypothesis when it is actually false, representing a false negative result; represented by β, and decreases as power increases ($1-\beta$)

Unpaired test: statistic employed to test two measurements obtained from different subjects or cohorts (often with one set having received an intervention, and the other not having received it), not necessarily at different time points

Unstructured interview: a version of qualitative interview methodology that involves a free-flowing discussion between the interviewer and interviewee, without the adherence to an interview script (discussion guide), to allow for in-depth exploration of a subject that could take a different direction for each interviewee

Validity: psychometric measure of the degree to which a tool measures what is intended; *see* "construct validity," "content validity," "face validity," "internal validity," or "external validity"

Variable: term used to describe an attribute to be manipulated, observed, or assessed in a study; *see* "dependent variable," and "independent variable"

White papers: authoritative reports or guidelines on a given topic, often compiled by government agencies, experts in a field, or by a task force on behalf of professional groups or associations

APPENDIX

Examples of Peer-Reviewed Journals Relevant to Radiation Therapy Practice

Journal	NLM Title Abbreviation	Publisher	Country	Affiliation	Impact Factor	Focus
Acta Oncologica	Acta Oncol	Informa Healthcare	England/ Sweden	European Organization for Research on Treatment of Cancer Education Branch	2.867	– clinical cancer research, from applied basic research to nursing and psychology – clinical aim and interest
Clinical Oncology	Clin Oncol	Academic Press	England	British Association of Surgical Oncology	2.858	– all aspects of the clinical management of cancer patients – pathology, diagnosis and therapy (radiation and systemic therapy)
International Journal of Radiation Oncology, Biology, Physics ("Red Journal")	Int J Radiat Oncol Biol Phys	Elsevier	United States	American Society of Therapeutic Radiation Oncology (ASTRO)	4.524	– clinical trials – outcomes research – laboratory studies – innovation

Journal	NLM Title Abbreviation	Publisher	Country	Affiliation	Impact Factor	Focus
Journal of Allied Health	J Allied Health	Association of Schools of Allied Health Professions	United States	Association of Schools of Allied Health Professions / American Society of Allied Health Professions	not yet acquired/assigned	– research and development in interdisciplinary work: education, practice, policy
Journal of Cancer Education	J Cancer Educ	Springer	England	American Association for Cancer Education	0.880	– patient, public and provider education – dissemination of information about improving cancer education worldwide
Journal of Interprofessional Care	J Interprof Care	Informa Healthcare	England	N/A	1.483	– interprofessional education and practice
Journal of Medical Imaging and Radiation Science (JMIRS)		Elsevier	Canada	Canadian Association of Medical Radiation Technologists (CAMRT)	not yet acquired/assigned	– radiation therapy, radiological technology, magnetic resonance imaging, nuclear medicine – advancement of quality and innovation in patient care

Journal	NLM Title Abbreviation	Publisher	Country	Affiliation	Impact Factor	Focus
Journal of Medical Radiation Sciences		Wiley Online LIbrary	Australia	Australian Institute of Radiography (AIR) and the New Zealand Institute of Medical Radiation Technology (NZIMRT)	Not yet acquired/assigned	– radiation therapy and medical imaging disciplines, as well as allied health, physics, oncology, and radiology – timely research to foster evidence-based clinical, scientific, and educational practices
Journal of Pain and Symptom Management	J Pain Symptom Manage	Elsevier	United States	University of Wisconsin—Madison Department of Anesthesiology	2.601	– best practices related to the relief of illness burden – clinical trials of pain or symptom control therapies – development and evaluation of instruments to assess pain
Journal of Radiotherapy in Practice	J Radiother Pract	Cambridge University Press	England	N/A	not yet acquired/assigned	– radiotherapy professional practice – technical evaluation and case studies

Journal	NLM Title Abbreviation	Publisher	Country	Affiliation	Impact Factor	Focus
Radiotherapy and Oncology ("Green Journal")	Radiother Oncol	Elsevier	Ireland	European Society for Therapeutic Radiology and Oncology (ESTRO)	4.520	– clinical radiotherapy – combined modality treatment – imaging, dosimetry, and radiation therapy planning – radiobiology
Medical Dosimetry	Med Dosim	Elsevier	United States	American Association of Medical Dosimetrists	1.009	– developments for the medical Dosimetrist – clinical applications and techniques
Medical Teacher	Med Teach	Informa Healthcare	England	Association for Medical Education in Europe (AMEE)	1.824	– new teaching methods – curriculum, assessment – innovation and research in medical education
Medical Physics	Med Phys	American Institute of Physics	United States	American Association of Physicists in Medicine	2.911	– medical physics of imaging, dosimetry, technology
Nature Reviews: Clinical Oncology	Nat Rev Clin Oncol	Nature Publishing Group	England	N/A	15.031	– diagnosis, therapy modalities, screening and prevention, epidemiology – in-depth reviews, research highlights, case studies

Journal	NLM Title Abbreviation	Publisher	Country	Affiliation	Impact Factor	Focus
Practical Radiation Oncology (PRO)	Pract Radiat Oncol	Elsevier	United States	American Society of Therapeutic Radiation Oncology (ASTRO)	not yet acquired/assigned	– dosimetry – practice guidelines – quality and safety
Radiation Oncology	Radiat Oncol	BioMed Central	England	N/A	2.107	– treatment of cancer using radiation
Radiography	Radiography	College of Radiographers	England	College of Radiographers/ Society of Radiographers (SoR)	not yet acquired/assigned	– radiographic imaging (diagnostic, computed tomography, nuclear medicine, sonography) and radiation therapy (patient care, dosimetry, treatment delivery, oncology)

INDEX

D

S

T

U

V

W